AF182283

MENTAL ILLNESSES AND TREATMENTS

SELF-FRAGMENTATION AND SELF-INTEGRATION IN PEOPLE WITH SCHIZOPHRENIA

VOLUME 1

A MULTI-DIMENSIONAL INTERPRETATION AND RECOVERY

MENTAL ILLNESSES AND TREATMENTS

Additional books in this series can be found on Nova's website
under the Series tab.

Additional e-books in this series can be found on Nova's website
under the e-book tab.

MENTAL ILLNESSES AND TREATMENTS

SELF-FRAGMENTATION AND SELF-INTEGRATION IN PEOPLE WITH SCHIZOPHRENIA

VOLUME 1

A MULTI-DIMENSIONAL INTERPRETATION AND RECOVERY

KAM-SHING YIP

New York

Copyright © 2015 by Nova Science Publishers, Inc.

All rights reserved. No part of this book may be reproduced, stored in a retrieval system or transmitted in any form or by any means: electronic, electrostatic, magnetic, tape, mechanical photocopying, recording or otherwise without the written permission of the Publisher.

We have partnered with Copyright Clearance Center to make it easy for you to obtain permissions to reuse content from this publication. Simply navigate to this publication's page on Nova's website and locate the "Get Permission" button below the title description. This button is linked directly to the title's permission page on copyright.com. Alternatively, you can visit copyright.com and search by title, ISBN, or ISSN.

For further questions about using the service on copyright.com, please contact:
Copyright Clearance Center
Phone: +1-(978) 750-8400 Fax: +1-(978) 750-4470 E-mail: info@copyright.com.

NOTICE TO THE READER

The Publisher has taken reasonable care in the preparation of this book, but makes no expressed or implied warranty of any kind and assumes no responsibility for any errors or omissions. No liability is assumed for incidental or consequential damages in connection with or arising out of information contained in this book. The Publisher shall not be liable for any special, consequential, or exemplary damages resulting, in whole or in part, from the readers' use of, or reliance upon, this material. Any parts of this book based on government reports are so indicated and copyright is claimed for those parts to the extent applicable to compilations of such works.

Independent verification should be sought for any data, advice or recommendations contained in this book. In addition, no responsibility is assumed by the publisher for any injury and/or damage to persons or property arising from any methods, products, instructions, ideas or otherwise contained in this publication.

This publication is designed to provide accurate and authoritative information with regard to the subject matter covered herein. It is sold with the clear understanding that the Publisher is not engaged in rendering legal or any other professional services. If legal or any other expert assistance is required, the services of a competent person should be sought. FROM A DECLARATION OF PARTICIPANTS JOINTLY ADOPTED BY A COMMITTEE OF THE AMERICAN BAR ASSOCIATION AND A COMMITTEE OF PUBLISHERS.

Additional color graphics may be available in the e-book version of this book.

Library of Congress Cataloging-in-Publication Data

ISBN: 978-1-63463-977-4

Library of Congress Control Number: 2015931179

Published by Nova Science Publishers, Inc. † New York

Contents

Preface

Theoretical Underpinnings of Schizophrenia

Schizophrenia has long been regarded as one of the most important mental problems since the twentieth century. There are numerous theoretical underpinnings in explaining and describing the formation, cause, process, and treatment of schizophrenia. Apart from the biochemical model of dopamine (Healy, 1993) as well as the genetic models, there are in fact many psychosocial theories explaining the cause of schizophrenia. These include psychodynamic, cognitive behavioral, phenomenological, existential, biochemical, as well as social construction perspectives. Psychodynamic concepts stress the conflicts of the id and superego to a stage that the individual distorts the sense of reality in order to settle this. It is also a diffusion of ego boundary with the external environment (Freud, 1924/1983; Blatt & Wild, 1976). Cognitive perspective emphasizes the cognitive impairment in hallucinations and delusions in which external stimuli are wrongly perceived, interpreted, and responded to (Costella, 1993). In negative symptoms, individuals even lack the abilities to have emotional responses (blunt affect), to foresake pleasure (anhedonia), to express his/her idea clearly (alogia), and to have clear purpose and behaviors (avolition) (American Psychiatric Association, 1994). Phenomenological and existential perspectives affirmed that persons with schizophrenia face intensive ontological emptiness and insecurity to an extent that the self of the individual is fragmented and split. Individuals with schizophrenia also strive for their own meaningfulness as well as attitude in life (Jaspers, 1946/1963; Laing, 1960). Related studies and literature affirmed that individuals' mental illness, including psychosis, are generated by highly oppressive social environments such as prolonged bullying, previous life trauma, and related cultural context (Al-ssa, 1995; Laing, 1960; Walker, 2005). Within all these perspectives, schizophrenia is interpreted as the manifestation of problems occurring in various layers of a full human being, including the ontological insecurity and meaninglessness of life in existential phenomenological perspective, diffusion of self boundaries, conflict in self-system in psychodynamic schools of thought, cognitive impairment in cognitive perspectives, and interpersonal oppression in social construction and interpersonal perspectives. All of these have strong implications to the recovery of persons with schizophrenia. It implies that for a full recovery of schizophrenia, individuals need to deal with difficulties and problems that occur in their meaning of life, self-system, mind, and social environments.

Mental Health Recovery Movement

Recovery is an upfront trend within this decade, regarded as the most important ideologies and practice orientations in providing service and intervention for persons with mental illness, including those with schizophrenia. In 2004, December, the National Consensus Conference on Mental Health Recovery and Mental Health Systems Transformation was launched in the U.S.A. Related parties in this conference had successfully formulated the National Consensus Statement of Mental Health Recovery (U. S. Department of Health and Health Services, 2004). This statement became the over-riding guidelines in mental health services in the U.S.A. Following this statement were various technical papers, reports, studies of recovery processes for different types of clients, in different life spans as well as in different social sectors such as family, community, organizations and society (Yip, 2012). Mental health recovery, defined by the Consensus statement, is as follows:

> Mental health recovery is a journey of healing and transformation enabling a person with a mental health problem to live a meaningful life in a community of his or her choice while striving to achieve his or her full potential. (U.S. Department of Health and Human Services, 2004)

In this definition, several personal components include

1. Personal Journey
2. Healing and Transformation
3. Living a Meaningful Life
4. In a community
5. Individual's Choice
6. Achieve the full potential

The Consensus statement consists of ten principles in recovery. These ten principles can be regarded as ten fundamental principles for mental health recovery. They are self-direction, individual and person centered, empowerment, holistic, non-linear, strength based, peer support, respect, responsibility and hope.

The recovery movement, which happened in this decade, can be described in terms of three main types of recovery, personal and subjective recovery, functional recovery, and social recovery. It started with personal experiences and narration of clients with various mental illnesses, in particular those with chronic schizophrenia. All these personal experience narrations affirmed that recovery is a highly subjective and personal journey in which hope and will to recover occurs for patients who are determined to get well. Since it is highly subjective and personal, every person may have his/her own pace and process, as well as one's own interpretation of recovery. It seems that subjective and personal recovery is very good in asserting one's own will responsibly, and experiences in getting well from mental problems. However, it creates difficulties for policy makers and practitioners in measuring their input and outcomes in a recovery based mental health service.

To input objective measurement in related services, related scholars tried to develop various types of scales in ensuring the effectiveness of services and programs in implementing principles of recovery for clients with mental illness. All these objective scales assume that people with mental problems undergo similar stages, processes, and outcomes in recovery in which measurement can be imposed. It enables service providers and policy makers to ensure proper implementation of services. The outcome of these services is measured by the social functioning of clients with mental problems as well as their drug compliance. All this literature implies a focus on functional recovery of clients with mental problems. However, an objective articulation of recovery, in many ways, is contradictory to subjective paradigm in interpreting recovery of persons with mental illness. The assumption of a unified path for every client with a mental problem is a highly reductive and simplified articulation about the complex natures of human beings and mental illness. It violates the uniqueness of clients in terms of individuality, and self-directedness.

Apart from subjective personal recovery and the objective functional recovery in the development of the recovery movement, related pressure groups organized by mental health consumers attempted to advocate an accepting social environment as well as related policies and services, which are accessible and adequate in ensuring a holistic recovery for clients with mental illness. They disclose the conspiracy of pharmacological companies and psychiatry in advocating psychiatric drugs as well as electric shock therapy. They criticize related stigmatization and discrimination of people with mental illness in accommodation, employment, and other aspects of life. They also advocate for sufficient social support, respect, and acceptance for persons with mental problems. Coupled with this mental health consumer movement is the continuation of the self-help movement, flourishing since the 1970s. Within the 12-steps self-help wisdom, self-help groups have been developed for different sorts of people with mental problems. Together with this is also the spontaneous development of relatives and friends support groups. Within these self-help groups are individuals' own wisdom, insight, and experiences in helping members to recover from various types of mental problems. The mental health consumer movement can be described as a development of social recovery in which consumers advocate for a better and more acceptable social environment for recovery of mental problems. Whereas the self help wisdoms can be considered a social environment formed by the clients and patients to combat their own mental problems.

Within the recovery movement in this decade, there seems to be unresolved theoretical dilemmas and controversies within the development of subjective personal recovery, objective functional recovery, as well as social recovery. The subjective personal recovery considers that every one's recovery process is unique, subjective, and individual based. The functional recovery stresses objective measurement and scales assuming the recovery process and outcomes can be commonly observed and measured by related scales and measurement. The social recovery presumes that individuals with mental problems have to fight for their own rights in counteracting adverse social labeling, stigmatization, inadequate mental health services, and social control oriented mental health legislation and policy. They should create their own social environment and self-help group for their own recovery. While subjective recovery is contradictory to the objective oriented 'functional recovery', social recovery provides no answer in which this dilemma can be resolved. In many cases, even if there is a good and accepting social environment, without appropriate clinical help or support, clients with mental problems with traumatic and experiences and memories may feel reluctant to come from their pathological subjective experiences of mental symptoms. The whole recovery movement tends to neglect the importance of clinical recovery for persons with mental symptoms, in particular those with schizophrenia.

Clinical Recovery for Persons with Mental Problems

All these developments have a vital impact on clinical practice and psychosocial intervention for clients with mental problems. Within the influence of post-modernist thinking, studies of resilience, as well as the recovery movement, intervention models such as the empowerment model, strengths based orientation, positive psychology, narrative therapy, solution-focused therapy, or brief therapy are evolving. In all these intervention models, therapists presume that related approaches and theoretical frames could be applied to people with different types of mental problems. In comparison with traditional models of psychotherapies, such as psychodynamic approaches, cognitive behavioral approaches, as well as existential approaches, these post-modernist and recovery based models are good if assuming that people with different mental problems can embrace their own strengths, abilities, and resilience to recover from their mental problems. However, they have the problems of neglecting the rich traditions and profound conceptual underpinning in every type of mental illness.

The situation is particular problematic in persons with schizophrenia. The traditional psychotherapeutic interventions for people with schizophrenia are still well known for their richness and depth in describing and analyzing clients with schizophrenia. However, they presume deficits, deterioration, and even impairment in the process of intervention. Some may even deny the subjective and personal recovery of clients with schizophrenia. They presume that over-whelming professional authority and power is the only magic in helping clients to treat their mental problems.

Unreachable Theoretical Gap in Recovery from Schizophrenia

That means, up to now, a huge theoretical gap exists between concepts research in schizophrenia and mental health recovery. This theoretical gap makes related intervention and services for recovery of patients with schizophrenia become shallow and superficial in theoretical underpinnings. They may follow the recovery orientation closely but they cannot connect with the rich and solid foundation of related theories in schizophrenia in past centuries. It also makes traditional in-depth clinical practice, for people with schizophrenia, fail to meet the challenge from the upfront trend of mental health recovery.

Self-Fragmentation and Self-Integration Dilemma in Recovery from Schizophrenia

This book serves to bridge this theoretical gap by a profound revisit of different perspectives and concepts in self-fragmentation of persons with schizophrenia. Within a phenomenological and existential orientation, the writer re-articulates clients' intense urge for an integrated self-system and ontological existence behind their fragmented psychotic experiences. The writer revisits psychodynamic theories to search the urge of ego in attaining its integrity and harmony within intensive conflict of superego and id in psychotic manifestation. The inclination for consolidated ego boundaries behind the diffused ego boundary is also articulated. The inherent search for meaningfulness within ontological meaninglessness, and the emptiness of psychotic experiences are described. The prevailing urges and needs for an accepting, empathic, and genuine social environment for people with schizophrenia, in facing their highly oppressive reality, are clearly expressed. The inherent urge and potentials of self-integration behind various symptoms of self-fragmentation, once fully recognized and developed, assist in mental health recovery of clients to become clinically valid and effective. It also facilitates related professionals, clients, and their significant others to participate in a multi-dimensional recovery within supportive and caring social and service contexts. The self-fragmentation and self-integration dilemma can be further elaborated into three dynamic forces, self-splitting versus self-cohesion, self-preservation versus self-destruction, as well as self-visibility versus self-concealment. These three dynamic forces have a crucial influence on positive, negative, and first rank symptoms of clients with schizophrenia. In this book, the writer describes the details and process of self-fragmentation in terms of self-concealment, self-destruction, and self-splitting on one hand. On the other hand, he points out how every client with schizophrenia contains an intense urge for self-preservation, self-visibility, and self-cohesion. However, within a highly oppressive environment, self-preservation, self-visibility, and self-cohesion can only be attained within a self-constructed delusive reality. If related professionals can nurture and provide a supportive, caring, and developmental social environment, the client with schizophrenia can actualize his/her self-preservation, self-visibility, and self-cohesion within an actual reality. Then, related psychotic symptoms in self-fragmentation are gradually alleviated and the client is on the road to mental health recovery.

The Layout of This Book

Since the self-fragmentation and self-integration dilemmas in schizophrenia are highly complicated, they can hardly be covered in one volume. This book is divided into three volumes.

Volume one is a multi-dimensional interpretation of self-fragmentation and self-integration dilemmas in people with schizophrenia. Its implication to mental health recovery is also fully discussed. It consists of three chapters.

In Chapter One, with reference to related stories and clients' self narration, the writer describes how people with schizophrenia experience related symptoms and how their subjectivity is being fractured and disturbed by psychotic self-fragmentation.

In Chapter Two, external and internal causes of fragmentation in schizophrenia are fully described. Related literature shows that, psychosocially, schizophrenia is nurtured by a highly depowering and oppressive environment. Prolonged engulfment, implosion, and depersonalization by significant others in particular parents may develop psychotic self-fragmentation. Traumas and victimization experiences also play a crucial role in psychotic self-fragmentation. Related implication to mental health recovery is also suggested.

In Chapter Three, the process of and dynamics of self-fragmentation and self-integration dilemmas in people with schizophrenia are fully described. The three dynamic forces in terms of self-splitting versus self-cohesion, self-visibility versus self-concealment, as well as self-preservation and self-destruction, are elaborated. In that way, related professionals can resolve these three forces and channel them towards mental health recovery when clients with schizophrenia are discussed.

Volume Two consists of eight chapters (Chapter 4 to 11). It is a full and comprehensive interpretation of positive and negative symptoms including diagnosis, etiology, psychosocial causes, and how they contribute to, as well as are influenced by, the three dynamic forces in psychotic self-fragmentation.

Chapter 4 is a description about the diagnosis and a multi-dimensional articulation of positive symptoms in people with schizophrenia. In fact, for every client with schizophrenia, his/her delusions and hallucinations represent an endless struggle to their unavoidable but highly oppressive or even abusive social environment.

In Chapter 5, the writer begins with a full articulation of related psychosocial concepts and theories of paranoid delusions and hallucinations. The self-fragmentation and self-integration dilemma in paranoid delusions and hallucinations is fully mentioned. Its implication to mental health recovery is also suggested.

In Chapter 6, the writer reviews various psychosocial theories in grandiose delusions and hallucinations. Their relationship with paranoid delusions and hallucinations are also discussed. In what ways they are influenced by the three dynamic forces, self-preservation versus self-destruction, self-visibility versus self-concealment, as well as self-splitting versus self-cohesion are fully described. Related implication to mental health recovery for clients with schizophrenia is also suggested.

Chapter 7 is a comprehensive account of catatonic stupor and fixation in people with schizophrenia. Related literature shows that catatonia in clients with schizophrenia is not a stagnant and inert state of mind. Instead, clients are trapped with a dilemma of existence and non-existence from external threats within a highly oppressive environment.

In Chapter 8, the writer gives a comprehensive description of how people with schizophrenia shift and interchange among paranoid, grandiose, and catatonic delusions and hallucinations. Related interventions for mental health recovery are also discussed.

Chapter 9 is a description about the diagnosis and etiology of negative symptoms in schizophrenia. The related literature is dominated by concepts of cognitive difficulties and impairment. However, in 2006, the NIMH had induced a project on the measurement and treatment research to improve cognition in schizophrenia (MATRICS). The findings illustrated that negative symptoms are not correlated to cognitive impairment and difficulties.

Thus, in Chapter 10, the writer provides a multi-dimensional articulation of negative symptoms including existential, phenomenological, and psychodynamic concepts. The writer formulates a comprehensive mechanism in negative symptoms in terms of dissociation, detachment, fixation, regression, and fixation. The self-fragmentation and self-integration dilemma in negative symptoms is then fully articulated in Chapter 11. Related implication to mental health recovery is fully mentioned in this chapter.

Volume Three is comprehensive articulation of self-fragmentation and self-integration dilemma in first rank symptoms. It consists of 6 chapters (Chapter 12 – 18).

It begins with an articulation of diagnosis and subjective experiences of first rank symptoms in people with schizophrenia in Chapter 12. In fact, in recent literature and diagnosis, particularly in DSM V, related scholars and practitioners have neglected first rank symptoms, partly because of their complexity and ambivalence. The writer tries to clarify and reassure the importance of first rank symptoms in schizophrenia.

In Chapter 13, a comprehensive conceptual review of first rank symptoms in terms of ego boundary diffusion is described. Its implication to mental health recovery is also mentioned. It shows that within the first rank symptoms, one's self-boundary is diffused. S/he has poor senses of individuality, self, and agency. In addition, his/her self-structure is loose and confused.

In Chapter 14, disturbances of self-consciousness, senses of reality, being in first rank symptoms in people with schizophrenia are fully mentioned. It is clear that people with schizophrenia may have a diffused self-consciousness, as well as dual consciousness, in reality and their delusive inner world.

In Chapter 15, the writer gives a refined account of Jaspers' phenomenological interpretation of first rank symptoms. According to Carl Jaspers, the individual's awareness in every daily life consists of awareness of object, experiences of space and time, awareness of body, feeling and affective states, urge, drive and will, as well as awareness of self. Within psychotic first rank symptoms, all these are being disturbed, confused, and split.

In Chapter 16, hyper-reflectivity and first rank symptoms in people with schizophrenia are fully interpreted and its implication with mental health recovery is discussed. For clients with schizophrenia, because of their self-fragmentation and diffused consciousness, they are over-self-reflexive on others' perception and self-evaluation with a spontaneous struggle about whether or not they are good or not, or others are good or not. It is a kind of exaggerated self-consciousness with self-alienation as well diminishing self-affection. All of these have a close relationship with first rank symptoms in people with schizophrenia. Its implication to mental health recovery is also discussed.

In Chapter 17, based on related conceptual review, the writer formulates a multi-dimensional perspective on self-fragmentation and self-integration of first rank symptoms. Its implications to mental health recovery are also described.

Related clinical practice reveals that psychotic symptoms in people with schizophrenia are not in a stable and stagnant state. Instead, there is continuous shifting and interchange among positive, negative, and first rank symptoms according internal and external conditions. In Chapter 18, the writer describes this fully.

References

Al-ssa. I. (1995). 'The illusion of reality or the reality of illusion, hallucination and culture' *British Journal of Psychiatry,* 166: 368-373.

Blatt S.J. & Wild C.M. (1976). *Schizophrenia: a Developmental Analysis,* New York: Academic Press.

Costella, C. G. (1993). (Edited) *Symptoms of Schizophrenia*, New York: John Wiley

Freud. S. (1924/1983). `Neurosis and Psychosis' in *Sigmund Freud: on Psychopathology,* London: Penguin Books.

Healy D. (1993) *Psychiatric Drugs Explained*, London: Mosby

Jaspers K. (1946/1963). (7th edition) *General Psychopathology*, (J. Hoenig, & M.W., Hamilton trans.) Manchester: Manchester University Press (Original work published 1923)

Laing R.D., (1960) *The Divided Self*, London: Tavistock Publication.

Walker, M. T. (2005) `The social construction of mental illness and its implications for recovery model', *The International Journal of Psychosocial Rehabilitation*, 10(1): 35-64.

United States Department of Health and Health Sciences (2004) *National Consensus Statement on Mental Health Recovery,* Washington, DC: United States Department of Health and Health Sciences.

Yip, K.S. (2011) `Resilience and recovery: Implications to clients with mental problems' in K. S. YIP (Ed.) *Recovery and Resilience of Persons with Mental Problems: Interpretation, Interaction and Intervention* pp. 15-210. New York: Nova Science.

Chapter 1

Experiencing the Psychotic Process: From Subjective Experiences to Subjectivity

Experiences in Being a Person with Schizophrenia

While normal persons enjoy daily experiences of a well-functioning and integrated self-system, in forms of negative and positive as well as first rank symptoms, individuals with schizophrenia suffer from painful experiences of self-fragmentation. Facing these painful experiences of self-fragmentation, every individual with schizophrenia has a prolonged daily struggle. What below is the self-narration of a person with schizophrenia in his daily struggle with his related symptoms in self-fragmentation.

> `More than by any other one thing, my life has been changed by schizophrenia. For the past 20 years, I have lived with it and in spite of it – struggling to come to terms with it without giving in to it. Although I have fought a daily battle, it is only now that I have some sense of confidence that I will survive my ordeal.....I attempt to keep in touch with my feelings and to attend immediately to difficulties, including symptoms of paranoia. For example, instead of worrying about the police surprising me, I always choose a seat where I can face the door, preferably with my back to a wall, not to other people. In general, instead of working myself up emotionally over some threatening possibility, I will check out reality by asking the people I am with questions like who they are calling, where they are going, or whatever. It clears the air immediately, and usually I am satisfied with their answers and can go on about my business. In other words, I cope by recognizing and confronting my paranoid fears immediately and then moving on with my life, freeing my mind for other things. Also, I have learned to suppress paranoid response and I make an effort not to talk to myself or to my voice when others are near. It can be done through self discipline and practice.' (Leete, 1989: 198)

Leete's self-narration clearly showed that he was in a state of self-fragmentation with prevailing paranoia and that he had to talk to himself. He kept on hearing voices commenting on him, and he was spontaneously wary of others in the nearby environment possibly planning to arrest or pick on him. Indeed, all these paranoid experiences were painful and unbearable. Thus, he used various means to conquer and adapt his fear and ignore his paranoia by asking others for validation. Leete was actually aware of both his delusive world as well as the reality. On the one hand, he was self-fragmented as he constantly heard voices commenting on him. On the other hand, he embraced a strong urge to integrate himself by constantly validating the reality and ignoring all these paranoia.

He also learned to suppress all these paranoid ideas and self-talk by engaging his mind in other things in the actual reality. Similar feelings of self-fragmentation in thinking also occurred in Leete's situation.

> `Sometimes I still find it difficult to keep my thoughts together. I therefore request communication to be simple, clear and unambiguous. It helps me if the information is specific, as vague or diffuse responses only confuse me. When speaking to someone, I may need more time to think, and understand before responding and I take this lime. Likewise, I have learned when working on a task to be careful, perhaps taking more time than others and to concentrate fiercely on what I am doing. And I must be persistent.' (Leete, 1989: 198)

Leete (1989) described his difficulties in putting his thoughts together. He seemed to be in a state of dual consciousness (Yip, 2007). He was both conscious about his delusions or hallucinations as well as the realistic outer world. To free himself from the delusive inner world, he forced himself to concentrate on the outer world.

Together with a struggle with self-fragmentation is a prolonged sense of loneliness and ontological emptiness.

> `In addition, I suffer from feelings of isolation, alienation, and loneliness. This is difficult to deal with because on one hand, I need to be with people, but on the other hand I am frightened of it. I have come to realize my own diminished capacity for really close relationships, but also my need for many acquaintances… .' (Leete, 1989: 198)

Leete's description also showed that he was being kept within an approach and avoidance complex in being together with other. On the one hand, he wanted to be with others to deal with his sense of loneliness. On the other hand, he was afraid of being diminished by close relationships. This complex, in fact, represents a dilemma of self-visibility and self-concealment. When he felt lonely, he wanted to be visible to others hoping that he could be accepted and get along with others. However, the closer he got to others, he kept himself concealed among others to protect his risk of being diminished

The life of having schizophrenia is indeed painful, ambivalent, and confused, especially with the intensive labeling and stigmatization from the public.

> `Life is hard with a diagnosis of schizophrenia. I can talk, but I may not be heard. I can make suggestions, but they may not be taken seriously. I can report my thoughts, but they may be seen as delusions. I can recite experiences, but they may be interpreted as fantasies. To a patient, and even an ex-patient, is to be discounted. Your label is a reality that leaves you with it. It gradually shapes your identity that is hard to shed. (Leete, 1989: 198).

From Symptoms to Person Disorder Interaction

Symptomatic Diagnosis`

Related professionals, especially psychiatrists, are merely concerned in making a diagnosis of schizophrenia for related clients. Once the diagnosis is being made, they may not be interested in listening to the clients' subjective experiences in living with schizophrenia. Even in the process of diagnosis, they try to categorize clients' experiences to fit into common features described by the criteria of diagnosis. That means, they care only about the common form of clients' experience, but they ignore the details and unique features and content of the individual client experience in living with schizophrenia.

In DSM IV, schizophrenia is diagnosed with the following criteria:

A. Characteristic symptoms: Two (or more) of the following, each present for a significant portion of time during a one month period (or less if successfully treated)
   1. Delusion
   2. Hallucination
   3. Disorganized Speech
   4. Grossly disorganized or catatonic behavior
   5. Negative symptoms i.e., affecting flattening, alogia, or avolition

   Note: Only one criterion. A symptom is required if delusions are bizarre or hallucination consists of a voice keeping up a running commentary on the persons' behavior or thoughts, or two or more voices conversing with each other

B. Social/ occupational dysfunction

   For a significant portion of the time since the onset of the disturbance, one or more major areas of functioning such as work, interpersonal relations, or self-care are markedly below the level achieved prior to the onset (or when the onset is in childhood or adolescence, failure to achieve expected level of interpersonal, academic or occupational achievement)

C. Duration

   Continuous signs of the disturbance persist for at least 6 months. This 6 month period must include in at least 1 month of symptoms (or less if successfully treated) that meet criterion A (i.e., Active phase symptoms) and may include periods of prodromal or residual symptoms. During these prodromal or residual periods, the signs of the disturbance may be manifested by only negative symptoms or two or more symptoms listed in criterion A present in attenuated form (e.g., Odd beliefs, unusual perceptual experiences)

D. Schizoaffective and Mood Disorder Exclusion
E. Substance/general medical examination exclusion
F. Relationship to a pervasive developmental disorder

Classification of longitudinal course (can be applied only after at least one year has elapsed since the initial onset of active phase symptoms)

(American Psychiatric Association, 1994: 275)

From the symptoms listed in DSMIV, there are three main groups of symptoms. They are positive symptoms, negative symptoms, and the first rank symptoms. Positive symptoms include delusion, hallucination, catatonia, and disorganized speech. According to DSM IV, delusions are erroneous beliefs or misinterpretation of perceptions:

> 'Delusions are erroneous beliefs that usually involve a misinterpretation of perceptions or experiences. Their content may include a variety of theme (e.g., Persecutory, referential, somatic, religious, or grandiose).... The distinction between a delusion and a strongly held idea is sometimes difficult to make and depends on the degree of conviction with which the belief is held despite clear contradictory evidence...`Delusions are deemed bizarre if they are clearly implausible and not understandable and do not derive from ordinary life experience... Delusion that expresses a loss of control over mind or body (those included among Schneider's first rank symptoms) are generally considered to be bizarre... thought withdrawal (taken by others)... thought insertion (thought input by others) ... delusion of control (mind or body control by outside force).' (DSM IV, 1994: 275)

Hallucination is defined by DSM IV as follows:

> `Hallucination may occur in any sensory modality (e.g., auditory, visual, olfactory, gustatory, and tactile, auditory hallucination is by far the most common and characteristic of schizophrenia. Auditory hallucinations are usually experienced as voices, whether familiar or unfamiliar, which are perceived as distinct from the person's own thoughts. The content may be quite variable, although pejorative or threatening voices are especially common. Certain types of auditory hallucinations (i.e., two or more voices conversing with one another or voices maintaining a running commentary on the person's thought or behavior) have been considered to be particularly characteristic of schizophrenia and were included among Schneider's list of first rank symptoms. If these types of hallucinations are present, then only this single symptom is needed to satisfy Criterion A. (American Psychiatric Association, 1994: 275)

Disorganized thinking, according to DSM IV is interpreted as follows:

> `Disorganized thinking (formal thought disorder, "loosening of association" has been argued by some (Bleuler, in particular) to be the single most important features of Schizophrenia because of the difficulty inherent in developing and objective definition of "thought disorder" and because in a clinical setting inference about thoughts are based primarily on individual's speech, and the concept of disorganized speech... . Because mildly disorganized speech is common and nonspecific, the symptom must be severe enough to substantially impair effective communication.' (American Psychiatric Association, 1994: 276)

Negative symptoms include alogia, avolition, and blunt affect. They are defined as follows:

> 'Affective flattening is especially common and is characterized by the person's face appearing immobile and unresponsive, with poor eye contact and reduced body language. Although a person with affective flattening may smile and warm up occasionally, his or her range of emotional expressiveness is clearly diminished most of the time.' (American Psychiatric Association, 1994: 276)

`Alogia (poverty of speech) is manifested by brief, laconic, empty replies. The individual with alogia appears to have a diminution of thought that is reflected in decreased fluency and productivity of speech. This must be differentiated from an unwillingness to speak, a clinical judgment that may require observation over time and in a variety of situations.' (American Psychiatric Association, 1994: 277)

'Avolition is characterized by an ability to initiate and persist in goal-directed activities. The person may sit for long periods of time and show little interest in participating in work or social activities.' (American Psychiatric Association, 1994:277)

First rank symptom, according to Schneider (1959), represents a loss of self-identity and boundary.

`We are far from being able to presume a common structure for all these symptoms of first rank importance. Some can certainly be regarded as a group, which represents the `lowering' of the `barrier' between the self and the surrounding world, the loss of the very contours of the self. That is the group of symptoms, which constitute "loss of identity" (ego disturbance): thought withdrawal, passivity thinking, diffusion of thought, and all passivity experiences, whether feeling, drive or volition, may be involved. The characteristic hallucinations (by no means all hallucinations are symptoms of first rank importance) and delusional perception, however, cannot be brought into this group formally without resorting to speculative construction.' (Schneider, 1959: 134)

According to Schneider (1959), first rank symptoms included the following:

- Voices heard arguing
- Voices heard commenting on one's actions
- Experience of influences playing on the body (somatic hallucination)
- Thought withdrawal
- Thought insertion - Thoughts are ascribed to other people who intrude their thoughts upon the patient
- Thought diffusion (or called thought broadcast)
  (Schneider, 1959, 154)

In DSM IV, both delusions and hallucinations can be classified as first rank symptoms if they represent a diffusion of ego boundary and identity.

'Delusions are deemed bizarre if they are clearly implausible and not understandable and do not derive from ordinary life experience....Delusion that expresses a loss of control over mind or body (those included among Schneider's first rank symptoms) are generally considered to be bizarre... thought withdrawal (taken by others)... thought insertion (thought input by others)...delusion of control (mind or body control by outside force)... . Certain types of auditory hallucinations (i.e., two or more voices conversing with one another or voices maintaining a running commentary on the person's thought or behavior) have been considered particularly characteristic of schizophrenia and were included among Schneider's list of first rank symptoms. If these types of hallucination are present, then only this single symptom is needed to satisfy. (American Psychiatric Association, 1994: 277)

Person-Disorder Interactions

Within the process of diagnosis, individuals with schizophrenia are being put into groups of symptoms. Their individual needs and feelings behind experiences of symptoms are suppressed. Also, once the diagnosis of schizophrenia is made, the individual professional is no longer interested in listening or understanding clients' experiences of psychosis.

Instead of separating patients themselves from their symptoms or labeling clients by their categorization of disorder, Strass (1989) proclaimed that based on his studies in subjective psychotic experience, person-disorder interactions are crucial. These person disorder interactions involve the person with schizophrenia as a goal directed being, the personal feeling, interpretation, and the existence of regulatory mechanism. That means, individuals are active agents in interacting with their own mental illness. Their subjective experiences coupled with their responses towards such experience intermingle with their manifestations of symptoms and their process of treatment and recovery.

Goal Directedness

Strauss (1989) asserted that persons with schizophrenia are the same as other normal persons, their behaviors, and cognitions, including their symptoms such as delusions and hallucinations, are goal directed, meaningful and with an effort to satisfy one's needs.

> `First, we must attend to goal-directed aspects of the person. This involves attention to what Aristotle called "final cause" in contrast to the "efficient" cause, immediate precursor, Attending to goal-directedness in spite of the problems such teleology entails making it possible to consider other important concepts as well, the existence of alternative pathways to the same end, and the possible existence of regulatory mechanisms - mechanisms that adjust processes to attain a particular goal. Considering goal-directedness provides a basis for identifying a range of functions that a particular phenomenon might have instead of assuming, for example, that a particular type of experience merely and always reflects pathology. For instance, participants in a conference held by Romme and Escher (1989) described several possible functions that hearing voices may have, including companionship or advice-giving as well as more frightening or undermining effects.... It is valuable to refrain from forging definitive "explanations" about how such negotiations may reflect different parts of the self, incorporation of others, etc. Holding back from such interpretation allows further collection of data before jumping to a premature "answer". We continue to try to understand various possibilities about what these voices indicate for this subject. At the very least, however, the evolution of interaction appears to reflect a way in which a goal-directed person relates to the disorder and some possible effects of the person's effort.' (Strauss, 1989:182)

Feeling About Disorder and Its Course Affects Its Evolution

Based on his studies on subjective psychotic experience, Strauss (1989) stressed that persons with schizophrenia actually have their own feeling about their own disorder. Their understanding and feeling strongly affect the evolution and process of the disorder. Thus, the process of illness, treatment, and recovery is unique and individual for every person with psychoses.

> `We have suggested that the evolution of schizophrenia and of the person-disorder interaction is neither linear nor homogenous. Rather, distinctive phases and processes can be identified and occur at different times in the course of disorder and improvement.' (Strauss, 1989:183)

The treatment and recovery process is actually intermingled with a person's feeling and interpretation in many ways. Individual subjective responses to their relapse, process of treatment, have an immense impact on the patients' own recovery and treatment. They can either be stimulated to get better or rid one's determination to get well.

> `Also the possibility that a person's feelings and understanding of his current situation might influence that situation and its evolution is described in many fields and seems likely to operate in severe mental disorders as well.... Such responses are certainly not surprising, but their implications can be all too readily overlooked. What the person has experienced has an impact on the feeling state. That feeling state probably has immense impact on active role and subsequent experience, and on the further evolution of disorder and improvement. And this chain continues. Improvement for such a patient can acquire a meaning "look out; you are just going to get your hopes up and then fall apart again." The course itself becomes loaded with feeling and meaning, which influence subsequent actions and course' (Strauss, 1989:183)

Regulatory Mechanism

Strauss (1989) further articulated that facing the manifestation of symptoms of schizophrenia; the individual actually has his/her own unique regulatory mechanism. Within this mechanism, the individual interacts with his own symptoms, as a sane response to the highly oppressive world, and s/he is able to preserve his/her self-esteem. Strauss stressed that a person with psychoses has his or her own regulatory mechanism in facing their symptoms

> `But attempts at adjusting oneself to mental disorders appear to go far beyond how the person deals with auditory hallucinations. As suggested by Bleuler, Freud, and others, symptoms themselves may reflect an unconscious and conscious effort at adjustment to provide the person with what is needed to survive - even at a low level.' (Strauss, 1989: 183)

Strauss' research on subjective experience showed that clients are interacting with their hallucinations and even with negative symptoms.

> `It is common to hear people with hallucinations talk about their interaction with their voices, where one rejects the other, accept what they say, or even negotiates. These kinds of interactions are also discussed in other reports in this issue, reports based on a wide range of methodologies. Thus, people who hear voices often try consciously to achieve their goals through various ways of dealing with the voices. The negotiations often suggest a kind of adjustment between two or more conflicting forces or processes.... Even many of the so called "negative symptoms" including apathy, withdrawal, and muteness, may reflect a self protective mechanism that the person with severe mental disorder uses to avoid the numerous discouragements and psychological assaults inflicted by the disorder, by society, and even by oneself.' (Strauss, 1989:184)

Strauss even found out that such negative symptoms might be a sane response in facing the dynamics and conflicts in the process of illness.

> `Withdrawal, apathy, and even muteness seem not an unreasonable way of protecting oneself from combined problems with stigma, the loss of social security benefits with improvement, the doing to the family, the experience of repeatedly making some progress only to be undermined by recurrent psychoses, and the many other experiences of that kind that patients describe.' (Strauss, 1989:184)

Strauss (1989) stressed that by means of all types of regulatory mechanisms, persons with psychoses are able to maintain a certain level of self-esteem, structure, involvement with the world, social contact, or analogous goals.

> `The person, consciously or unconsciously, often appears to adjust perception, interpretations and action to maintain a certain level of self esteem, structure, involvement with the world, social contact or analogous goals.' (Strauss, 1989:184)

Subjective Experience in Schizophrenia

As mentioned above, in the diagnosis of schizophrenia, positive symptoms, negative symptoms, as well as first rank symptoms, are strictly considered by related psychiatrists. They are inclined to use objective scales in making an accurate diagnosis. At first, they would listen to the experiences, problems, difficulties described by the clients and their relatives or related parties. In the process of diagnosis, they tried to put all these descriptions in related categories within diagnosis. Only the common forms in terms of prescribed symptoms rather than content, context, details, and process of occurrence of symptoms are noted. Once the diagnosis is clear, related professionals may not have the patience to listen to any subjective account of the client. Instead, they incline to a simple solution by rendering anti-psychotic medication to the client and reminding him/her to follow medication regularly. If the client is reluctant to do so, coercive treatments will be given accordingly. However, with a person-symptoms interaction perspective, subjective experiences of schizophrenia are meaningful, unique, and crucial for clients themselves. Recovery and treatment are incomplete or even apathetic without a clear understanding, recognition, and encounter with all these subjective experiences of symptoms.

Subjective Experiences of Positive Symptoms

In diagnosis, only the form and commonality of positive symptoms are considered, however, in subjective experiences, individuals' feelings, and needs are represented in refined details of related symptoms. This is particularly true for positive symptoms, in which paranoia, grandiosity and catatonia, mentioned by Strauss as meaningful, feeling embedded and need oriented.

Meaningful Subjective Experience of Hearing Voices

In facing paranoia, individuals with schizophrenia are always threatened by its contents. They feel fearful and helpless in the occurrence of paranoia especially when it first occurs.

Below are some narrations from persons with schizophrenia recorded by Romme and Escher (1989) in their study of hearing voices.

> Narration 1:
> `On a Sunday morning at 10 o'clock, it suddenly was as if I received a totally unexpected enormous blow on my head. I was alone and there was a message - a message at which even the dog would turn up their noses....I instantly panicked and could not prevent terrible events from happening... .' (Romme & Escher, 1989: 210)

> Narration 2:
> `Perhaps it sounds funny but I had two egos. A normal child-ego, fitting with my age, and an adult ego. The voice adapted itself to the ego. It spoke a child language of the child and an adult language to the other ego.' (Romme & Escher, 1989: 210)

> Narration 3:
> `Painting is like bringing something from your head into your hands. I start to paint a dark forest on the wall with a reptile on the foreground. I have always been able to hear colors. They transmit vibrations. I can hear black, red, and deep brown. During the painting, it was deathly quiet in the room. The radio was not on. In this silence, something frightening was slowly growing. Something threatening was coming up. I had the feeling I was not alone in the room any more. Then I heard a monotonous sound in my ears, that did not come from me and which I could not explain. It was a bit like the squeaking you hear when your ears are closed. Only this sound was lower and monotonous. It was like an emotion, but deeper. I had the feeling something was looking at me.' (Romme & Escher, 1989: 209)

In all these three narrations, it was clear that individuals with paranoid schizophrenia were threatened and frightened by all these external voices. Although they were all similarly diagnosed by their psychiatrists as suffering from paranoid schizophrenia, their content, context and meaning of these voices were different and unique. The individual in narration 1 was `afraid of dogs turning their nose'. The individual in narration 2 was involved in `a highly divided ego system talking with one another'. The individual in narration 3 was deeply threatened by deep voices that possibly came from the colors of his paintings.

Meaningful Subjective Experiences of Grandiose Identity

Apart from paranoid delusions and hallucinations, individuals with schizophrenia also experience grandiose delusions and hallucinations. In many ways, grandiose delusions may represent a change of an individual's identity from his/her own normal ones to someone with supernatural power. Below was a self-narration from a client with grandiose delusive identity. His consensus in using his story for academic purpose is sought. For the sake of confidentiality, his/her personal identity and related information was properly disguised.

> A said: `I have been suffering from schizophrenia for more than twenty years. During the days of my first onset, I had a strong feeling that I was the Chief Disciple of the Buddha. In fact, up to now this sort of feeling and self-identity was still there. But, comparing with the days of first and second onset, this sort of feeling is much less and remote now. In fact, when I was very small, my parents were dedicated followers of the Buddha. I learnt to follow rituals and lessons from Buddhism. I lost my mum in a car accident when I was only twelve years old. I lost my father when I found my first job. Life was full of misfortunes and suffering for me. I had to struggle for my own survival.

In my job, colleagues around me, including my boss, was highly oppressive and insulting. They tried to humiliate me in all aspects. They gossiped about me. They trapped me to be responsible for all the problems that they had done to the company. One day, my deceased parents kindly introduced me to a kind Buddhist voice. This voice continuously told me that I was the Chief Disciple of the Buddha in my previous life. Because I had done some misdeeds and showed no respect to the Buddha, my status was temporarily taken away. I had to overcome various suffering, hardship and trauma in this life before I could resume my status as the Chief Disciple in this life or the next life (In Buddhism, people usually have three lives, the previous life, the present life and the next life. What one has done in one's life properly may be the cause and effect of the previous and next life.) To attain this, I must show deep respect to the words of Buddha. I must dress like a faithful follower of the Buddha. I must change my name to the Chief Disciple of the Buddha. By doing so, all my sufferings, hardship, and torture in this life were all meaningful. They served as pre-requisites for me to transcend myself back to the Buddha.'

From A's self-narration, it was clear that A harbored a grandiose delusion that he was in fact, the Chief Disciple of the Buddha. This was a grandiose self-identity in which he could be empowered in facing the adversity in his life. It gave him meaningfulness in encountering various suffering and hardship in life including the death of his parents, being oppressed by his colleagues. It also helped him to develop hope in the future - to be transcended back to the Disciple of the Buddha. The formation of this grandiose self-identity was rooted from his family involvement in Buddhism. In many individuals with schizophrenia, grandiosity works together with paranoia. In facing the over-whelming paranoid delusion and hallucination, many clients say that they possess supernatural powers to beware of any external threat, or they are actually people with power, such as descendants of royal family or political leaders, great bankers, gods or goddesses. All these help them to boost their own delusive power to face the over-whelming threatening environment.

Stagnancy by Autonomous Subjective Experience on Catatonia

Catatonia is also regarded as one of the positive symptom. What below is a self-narration of an individual with schizophrenia in describing her experience in catatonia.

`To me, two things happen when I become catatonic. One is that I enter a state of profound indifference so extreme that I, ordinarily an extremely modest person preferring never be seen naked, refusing even to have the usual female medical exams/tests, can be stripped of all clothing and have all sorts of catheters inserted and even be toileted by strangers without the slightest reaction, either internally felt or externally apparent. I no longer care what happens to that body. Everyone is fussing over, and I feel an almost Buddhist-like detachment from it, from all the concerns and bother going on about me.

The other thing is that along with this indifference comes the more obvious slowing down, even to the point of immobility. While I may seem immobile and non-responsive to those trying to elicit a reaction, in fact my experience is one of reacting quite appropriately, just in glacial time, which to me feels perfectly normal. In fact, other people seem to be moving way too fast and only the clock tells me that I am the slow one rather than the reverse.

My indifference allows me to perceive all of this without distress, merely a detached curiosity, like a scientist observing natural phenomena, while my psychomotor retardation doesn't feel particularly slow except in comparison to others. It does prevent

> me from communicating quickly enough to be heard though, and no one notices that I am answering a question, or performing an action, because they are in such a hurry!
>
> Meanwhile, whether my actions truly make sense or not, that is, whether they are motivated by psychotic thoughts, they are purposeful. I am, for example, reaching out to wipe my nose, even when my arm seems "stuck" or "posturing" in mid-air apparently nowhere near my nose. It just hasn't gotten there yet, and it's extremely frustrating when others, trying to be helpful, replace my arm "more comfortably" down on the bed, because then I have to start all over again. Though they can't see it or hear it, I am moving, I am answering, only in a time frame they do not perceive or won't wait for.
>
> Does this sound familiar to any of you? Supposedly, it's a rare state, yet I've heard many people say that they've been catatonic. (Pamwagg, 2004)

From Pamwagg's (2004) description, it is clear that subjective experiences of catatonic schizophrenia are contained the following component.

A distant feeling of self-dissociation from one's own body

1. A detachment from related persons and things happening in immediate social environment
2. Immobility of body allows one to observe the mobility in the reality more clearly and more independently
3. The individual can choose his/her right time, the right way, and the right pace to respond to the immediate environment. That means, one can be free from any influence in the immediate environment. The individual can be truly autonomous and independent from the oppressive environment

It was clear that Pamwagg (2004) had some unbearable experiences with the oppressive psychosocial environment. In facing this highly oppressive social environment, she felt shameful and humiliated as well as being controlled. That means she had a strong urge to regain her own integrity, uniqueness as well as autonomy. Thus, the state of catatonia served as a means to be distancing from both herself (her body), as well as the oppressive environment. The sense of distancing was attained by keeping herself in a form of immobility (mutism), as well as closely and defensively watching oneself and others in the environment (excitement). Within this form of immobility and watchfulness, she felt that she could regain her sense of autonomy, as she was no longer controlled by her social environment. Instead, she could choose the right time, right place, and right pace to react and respond. She could also preserve her own integrity, as the humiliating body in the body check up process in the admission to psychiatric ward was not so humiliating if the body did not belong to her. At the same time, she felt she was unique and special among the people around her. Within the catatonia, she could comment, criticize, and undermine the aimless mobility of people in her immediate environment. Interestingly, she attributed special meaning to her own catatonic gestures that were unknown to others. With that sort of special meaning, she embraced a sense of owning special power, and the ability to overcome and dominate others.

Nevertheless, all these special meanings, needs and interpretations in subjective experiences of catatonia, were in fact, unknown and uncared by others, in particular the nursing staff. They interrupted all these by the input of psychiatric medication.

`Nurses caring for me sometimes believed I had to somehow have been faking the catatonic state, (though how that could be done I don't know) because they could not understand how I could go from immobility to agitation without any switching of gears. Understandably, they wanted something, anything indicating that the changeover was coming. Instead, I woke up, so to speak, and immediately went bananas.

All this remains a curiosity to me, but even now, I cannot feel distressful in remembering it, only the same detachment from my body, as well as a pervasive perplexity why any of it mattered. The only time I felt upset was after being given four Ativan, which according to the doctor often relieves catatonia, though no one is sure why. Then I knew something was supposed to happen, and suddenly, before I could physically move, I finally cared. I wanted the bolt of electricity to hit and arouse me, whereas before then I could not have cared less. It suddenly mattered that I could not, or at least did not, move properly...and it felt for the first time like the eternity as it was, for me to begin to react.

It wasn't that I wanted to please the doc, though I admit I felt like he was showing off in front of his students and residents, by coming back the way one might in a TV movie, but it was certainly what I expected. (By the way, for those of you who don't know this, in such a state, the brain, the mind is nonetheless aware of everything; one just doesn't react or respond to the world. But one hears and sees just fine, a warning to those who talk in front of people in catatonia as if they were zombies.) Soon after he injected the Ativan into my body, I felt the slowness of my actions and understood how awful it must have seemed that I lay there completely motionless for so long.

Finally, the drug began to take effect on my body, several minutes after my brain felt it; that is, I wanted to move before I actually could. Anyhow, eventually I could feel my muscles returning to me, could feel the impulses at the neuromuscular junction connecting normally, and soon I found myself able to blink on command, or give a feeble squeeze of the doctor's fingers. Then slowly, over a couple of days, I became able to talk and walk on my own again.

Mind you, all this is what happens under the effect of four Ativan; if however I wake on my own, and then it is to frenzy with no agonizing or gradual coming to. Even with the help of Ativan by IV, I usually flip into a super-reactive state, but at least then there is some warning before it happens, however slight.

As I said, all these still fail to disturb me. I've often wondered how other people felt when catatonic, or whether they too have no emotional recall of the state, not caring about it now, just as perhaps they did not when in the midst. Paranoia and such often seem an extreme exaggeration of feelings everyone can relate to, but catatonia seems to me to be a state with which there is no ordinary analogy. Anyhow, that's -- briefly -- my story. Anyone with comments about their own experience is welcome to add them here.' (Pamwagg, 2004)

Related professionals tended to neglect the unique meaning, needs and purpose behind Pamwagg's catatonia, they instructed her to take Ativan. They affirmed that it was the only way to relieve her state of catatonia. She rejected it at first, as it might alter her stay of catatonia. That means, taking away her uniqueness, detachment, as well as autonomy in the state of catatonia. However, she was also bewildered that the state of catatonia hindered her freedom and will to move her body. Thus, she also regarded the taking of Ativan as a kind of electricity that sparked and aroused her own natural tendency to move again. That means, there is a dilemma facing the individual with catatonia. On one hand, the individual enjoys autonomy, uniqueness as well as detachment from the highly oppressive environment. On the other hand, the individual also feels the actual restriction, dissociation, as well as the paralysis of his/her feeling, needs, movement and body.

Subjective Experience of Negative Symptoms

Bouriclus (1989) did a study on the subjective experience of negative symptoms of a 32-year-old man, who had suffered from schizophrenia for 12 years. He was rated by five professionals, using the Scale for the Assessment of Negative Symptoms. These rating were compared with samples of the client's own writing that reflected his own emotions. The results suggested that a client exhibiting moderate negative symptoms might be experiencing feelings that s/he did not display through either verbal or facial expressions (Bouriclus, 1989: 201).

Objective Items of Negative Symptoms

Within negative symptoms, there are four major components, blunt affect, alogia, anhedonia, and avolition. Blunt affect refers to impoverishment of emotional expression, reactivity, and feeling. Alogia refers to impoverished thinking and cognition. Thought processing is described as seeming empty, turgid, and slow. Avolition is a lack of energy, drive, and interest, but not due to sadness or depression. Ahendonia is an inability to experience pleasure in recreational activities, sex, or intimacy (Bouriclus, 1989:201). According to Scale for the Assessment of Negative symptoms (Andreason, 1982: 201), it consists of the following items:

Blunt Affect:
1. Unchanging facial expression
2. Decreased spontaneous movements
3. Faculty of expressive gestures
4. Poor eye contact
5. Affective non-responsivity
6. Inappropriate affect
7. Lack of vocal inflections

Alogia
1. Poverty of speech
2. Poverty of content of speech
3. Blocking
4. Increased latency of response

Avolition-apathy in:
1. Grooming and hygiene
2. Impersistence at work or school
3. Physical anergia

Anhedonia-Asociality
1. Recreational interests and activities
2. Sexual interest and activity
3. Ability to feel intimacy
4. Relationship with friends and peers

(Andreasen, 1982)

Subjective Feelings behind Negative Symptoms

From all these items, it clearly shows related professionals in diagnosis only focus on objective and external observable behaviors and response for individuals with schizophrenia. They tend to neglect their inner feelings and subjective experiences behind negative symptoms. Bouriclus' (1989) record of her son's subjective experiences in negative symptoms in schizophrenia clearly showed that he was not emotionally or cognitively inert. Instead, he experienced intensive senses of loneliness, unbearable pain in his mind and body, feeling of being trapped or confined in hospital, and anger and stagnancy due to prolonged institutionalization. Despite the fact that he had been rated high in the Scale for the Assessment of Negative Symptoms (SANS) by five psychiatrists, he was not emotionally dull. Actually, his emotions rapidly and intensively occurred inside his mind. However, because of various reasons, he was unable to express his emotional dullness.

Below is the client's subjective writing account of these feelings

1. Intensive sense of loneliness

> `Who is this deluded fighter? His mane is torn and soiled; His thoughts are tired and frail. Who is this lonely dreamer?
> Who was thrown down and cast out of this own dream?
> His soul is cracked and crying at the seams.
> His desires are still there.
> More faithful than eternity
> And stronger than death and Hell
> Holding Never as All goes by
> Holding on to himself, tears inside....
> I am a lonely nothing, a being but pass me by. Forever pass me by. Strangers, I don't see you. My afflictions till the place that was meant for sharing love. I am crying by despair.' (Bouriclus, 1989: 204)

From the client's writings, it was clear that he was in a state of extremely loneliness. No one around him understood him. His chronic and prolonged loneliness implied an inner vacuum, an inner cry for help, and an inner emptiness. In fact, negative symptoms in terms of blunt affect, anhedonia, alogia, as well as avolition, are only external behavioral articulations of clients' symptoms but they neglect their intensive inner pain and feelings.

2. Intensive anger towards hospitalization and coerced treatment as well as an intensive urge to escape

Apart from loneliness, the client also described his intensive anger towards apathetic treatment and institutionalization induced by mental health professionals in mental health services.

> `Hot blood keeps me up nights;
> Tranquillizers keep me down days.
> Doctors with kaleidoscopic eyes peer into me;
> `Are you healthy now?'
> No Doctor, and I don't want to be.
> I want to burn and shatter.......I want to lose sleep.....I want to blow up in your face,
> I want to destroy your important papers. I want to eat little and talk loudly...
> I want to develop cracks in my brain and escape out into the sunshine...
> I want to isolate myself. I want to be free and never see another psychiatrist or pill or asylum again.
> I want to listen, I want to touch, taste and smell.
> I want to shatter myself and die. Then I will be happy.' (Bouriclus, 1989:205)

The writing of client described by Bouriclus (1989) clearly demonstrated that he was very angry with the apathetic treatment imposed by his psychiatrist who merely imposed medication, labeled his symptoms without a clear and empathetic understanding of his inner conditions and pains in his body as well as prolonged suffering in life. He deeply felt that his autonomy and freedom was deeply constrained by the psychiatrist as well as by the institutionalized mental hospital.

3. Difficulties in expressing his intensive feeling as well as thinking

Clients with schizophrenia suffer intensive confusion in their mind. They are not having impairment in cognitions, emotions, and interaction with others. Instead, their minds are too confused and too painful to express their highly complicated and boiling feelings and emotions. The client described by Bouriclus had this sort of difficulty.

> `Why can I laugh and cry with others?
> O Beloved, I mean not to kill my soul!
> I was embarrassed to sing in harmony and to be emotional and enthusiastic.
> Why am I filled with hate and sorrow?....
> How many times have I lost? What will the cost?
> Will I go on losing? Who will be a worm in a hole in the ground?
> Please let me be that much at least...
> Stuck in my thinking, brain paralyzed between fear and love. Stuck on you.
> Stuck between that last word and the next.
> Stuck by confusion, the inability to proceed and further in understanding or speech.
> Oh well, I'm just stuck again... (Bouriclus, 1989: 204)

From the above description, it was clear the client was stuck between his strong emotion of love and hate, pain and sorrow to a degree that he was unable to express them. He was stuck within his confusion of thinking, fear, and love. No words could actually express his pain and predicament. In fact, within a highly institutionalized service hospital setting, even if the client tries every means to express his/her pain and complicated feelings, apathetic medical professionals may only regard severe symptoms that require further coerced treatments, restraints, and longer hospitalization.

4. Unbearable pains all over his body

Bouriclus (1989) suffered from unbearable pains all over his body. It was a kind of suffering that the mind was observing the sufferings of the body without being able to heal or cure it.

> `My affliction: hard upper inside head, mucus, and rough throat, prickly feeling, head fragmented, stemness, lack of simplicity. Too much thought of body, body can heal if I stop thinking. For months, I have had pain, which has not been healed. Perhaps the mind is too sharp and it cuts the body. I must rest alone with myself. Pain is in my chest. Sorrow is in my head and neck. Anguish is in my shoulder. All suffering is truly in me.' (Bouriclus, 1989: 204)

5. A spontaneous and endless struggle between sanity and insanity

Facing all these unbearable pains all over the body, endless sufferings from coercive treatments and institutionalization as well as difficulties in expressing one's highly complicated emotions; the client still kept on his struggle and endeavor. He still harbored hopes and dreams with the beauty of his desires.

> `The pain of my body keeps my company. I have been fooling myself, but now I see selfish me, dependent me, ugly me. I have no life but I have pain. I have despair. I want to be no more at all, for life goes on without me, and sometimes without me...I am sick with an unknown disease and no cure in sight. I have the immensity and beauty of dreams and desires, and the conflict that make it all impossible... (Bouriclus, 1989: 205)

Subjective Experiences of First Rank Symptoms

First rank symptoms, according to Schneider (1959), represent a loss of self-identity and boundary. It consists of several 'symptoms' that become the crucial ingredients in diagnosis of schizophrenia:

- Voices heard arguing
- Voices heard commenting on one's actions
- Experience of influences playing on the body (somatic hallucination)
- Thought withdrawal
- Thought insertion - Thoughts are ascribed to other people who intrude their thoughts upon the patient
- Thought diffusion (or called thought broadcast)
  (Schneider, 1959, 154)

That means, both delusion and hallucination can be classified as first rank symptoms if they represent a diffusion of ego boundary in which the individual no longer feels s/he is an integrated and cohesive person. S/he continuously is aware that his/her thinking and perception can be diffused outside. At the same time, objects, persons, and events in the outside reality can diffuse into his/her mind and body without any boundaries or burden. Within an observer's objective view, first rank symptoms appear to be odd and bizarre, irrational and not understandable. However, within a subjective view, first rank symptoms represent the individual's intensive urge to escape from the oppressive reality that s/he has nowhere to hide. The individual's self identity, self competence, self image and self boundary is gradually dissolved and diffused with a result of unbearable but spontaneous painful sense of self confusion with a dual consciousness of his/her massive inner world and detached reality (Yip, 2007). Perhaps, the following citation from the case of Peter described by Laing (1960) can describe that sort of massive feeling of confusion and dissociation in the painful experiences of first rank symptoms.

> 'This was expressed by a dream he had at that time. He was in a fast moving car. He jumped off; hurting himself but not seriously, while the car went on to crash.... He finally opted out as completely as he knew how; he dissociated himself both from himself and from other people.... His sense of pointlessness, of lack of direction, of futility was enhanced, as was his conviction that he was nobody `really', he felt that it was pointless to pretend any more. He formulated this to himself in these words: "I am nobody, so I'll

do nothing." He tended to be detached and away from everything including himself…' (Laing, 1960: 125)

From Laing's description, Peter embraced an intensive sense of diffusion and dissociation in which he thought that he was nothing and at the same time, nothing was 'him'. He was away from himself as well as from others. He did not have substantial consciousness and sense of being. His self-image was confusing and diffusing as well as non-existential. By means of doing this, he was able to regain his own autonomy over another. He was not controlled by anything or anybody by being nothing or not being anything. For Peter, all these were effective measures to keep him consciously away from a highly oppressive social environment.

Subjective Experiences of First Rank Delusions

According to Schneider's description, delusions are first rank if an individual's thought can be inserted or withdrawn by others. In some cases, the individual feels his/her thought can be diffused or broadcasted to others. For the former, it represents the individuals are being controlled by others. For the latter one, it represents the individual consists of power to control others. Both of them are peculiar, strange and even threatening experiences for the individuals.

Below is the self-narration of a client who experiences thought insertion and thought withdrawal. Her consensus to use her story for academic purpose was sought. For the sake of confidentiality, her personal identity and information were properly disguised.

> Miss L was a well-educated woman. Before the onset of her schizophrenia, she was a successful scholar in a well-known university in China. She came from a rural family in which her father was a poor farmer struggling for a hand to mouth life within poverty. Fortunately, L was sponsored by a charitable organization to have a good education in the urban city. She was diligent, clever, and enduring in study. Later, she was sent to one of the famous universities in the United States where she graduated as a bachelor of computer engineering. She continued her post-graduate studies there by earning a good scholarship. However, at that time, she encountered a highly oppressive supervisor, and she had to follow his highly unreasonable, and even humiliating, advice and criticisms in study or else she would fail in her study. Apart from that, she was spontaneously isolated and bullied by her schoolmates saying that she had committed adultery with her supervisor and that was why she could get the most well known scholarship in the post-graduate school. L was deeply puzzled by all these humiliating experiences. She began to harbor intrusive delusions that her thoughts and mind were in fact, being controlled by her supervisor and her classmates.
>
> L affirmed that her supervisor was highly manipulating and powerful. He conspired with her dentist when she had a normal dental check up; the dentist implemented a micro computer chip somewhere in her gums or teeth so that she was unable to remove it. Thus, no matter where she went, they could still control and manipulate her. They could insert some painful thought that she was useless and her life was complete nonsense. Very often, when she went to some place she would get a feeling that she should not go there. She studied hard for hours, however, after a very short while; all she had remembered and understood would suddenly be forgotten. She strongly felt that her supervisor and her classmates managed to steal her thoughts away.
>
> To counteract her supervisors' control and intrusive delusion, she gradually harbored delusive thought by means of using the computer; she could broadcast her ideas to others

and sought help from other colleagues and classmates. Once their thoughts were collected together, they could fight back and eliminate her bad supervisor's influence. However, her supervisor managed to disturb all these electronic broadcasts by sending strong electronic waves from his extremely powerful computer in his office. She affirmed that once the dominant computer in his supervisor's office was damaged, she could collect all these thoughts together and get rid of her supervisor's control and be free again.

Thus, she went into her supervisor's office, destroyed the things, including the computer, there. Finally, she was caught by the police, and sent to a nearby mental hospital, and was diagnosed as having paranoid schizophrenia. In the mental hospital, she committed self harm act by using a knife to cut her teeth and gums saying that this was the only way to remove the implemented electronic chip and free herself from the control of her supervisor and classmates. Six months later, her mental condition became stable and she returned China and got a job as a research assistant in a famous university in China. She managed to finish her PhD study in computer engineering and became a scholar there. Though she managed to have a decent job, she still harbored delusions that someone was chasing and controlling her. Below was her self-narration.

L said: 'though my psychiatrist always said, I should be diagnosed as paranoid schizophrenia as I harbored symptoms of thought insertion and thought broadcasting. They did not recognize the vividness and fear of being controlled and manipulated in every aspect of life by a superior authority. My supervisor was very powerful in the academic field in the States. He was so powerful that he managed to manipulate every PhD student to serve his own purpose and build up his own kingdom. He was also so skillful in computer systems. That was why I fully believed that he could control my thoughts once the computer chip was implemented in my body. It was so small that could even be absorbed within our capillaries. That was why I could not find it. Though, I am of no more use to him, he can still control me. Because I am so smart in computer engineering, he tries to steal my inventions and my thoughts away. There is no way I can hide from his overwhelming control, the only way I can survive now was to declare his plan openly, letting everybody know that he is controlling, manipulating and oppressive. In fact, he extends his control over many unknown bodies around the world. He is in conspiracy with the President as well as the Intelligence Department of the United State of America. Only by doing so, can I collect and unite with those people who are oppressed or going to be oppressed by the American government. We can work together by uniting our thoughts together to counteract the overwhelming control by electronic waves.

From L's self-narration and her life experiences, it was clear that she harbored thought insertion as well as thought broadcasting. All these were originated from L's highly oppressive experiences with her overwhelmingly controlling and manipulating supervisor and classmates. His supervisor's oppression and manipulation were so powerful and overwhelming that she had nowhere to hide or to escape. Gradually, she harbored delusions that her supervisors could insert thought to control her everywhere through the computer chip implemented in her body. Her first rank persecutory delusive thoughts were thus understandable as a delusive symbolization for unavoidable oppression and humiliation from her supervisor and her classmates. To defend herself from this persecutory, she had to develop thought broadcasting to everyone around her so to declare her supervisor's control as well as to collect and crystalize collective brainpower to counteract the control of her supervisor. For her, it was certainly a kind of self defense mechanism to protect her from unavoidable control and manipulation.

Subjective Experiences of First Rank Hallucination

According to Schneider's description, hallucinations are of first rank of importance in diagnosing schizophrenia if they are voices commenting or criticizing the individual or they are arguing with one another. In many ways, persecutory hallucinations are founded on persecutory delusions in which the individual's ego boundary is highly diffused. Individuals not only feel that others control their thoughts; they may also hear voices commenting on him/her continuously. These voices are highly threatening, annoying, and disturbing to the individuals. The following client's narration recorded in Jasper (1923/1946) can clearly demonstrate that sort of pain and suffering in facing endless commenting hallucinations in one's life.

> `It is amazing, horrible, and for me, humiliating, to think what acoustic exercises and experiments – musical ones too – have been conducted with my ears and body for nearly 20 years. Sometimes, I could hear one and the world repeated without interruption for two to three hours. I had to listen to long continuous speeches about me; frequently the content was insulting and there was often an imitation of well-known persons. Thus, lectures, however, have little truth about them, usually they were infamous lies and slanders about my person, sometimes also others often proclaimed that `I' said all these things...the scoundrels wanted to pass the time with onomatopoeia, paronomasia, and other figures of speech, and kept up a perpertual mobile of speech. (Jaspers, 1923/1946: 73)

From the above description, it was clear that the commenting hallucination was horrible, dreadful, and humiliating for the client. It had been long lasting and continuous for twenty years. These hallucinations were continuously criticizing him by well-known but nasty and immoral persons. Although the client knew all these criticisms were faulty, unreal, fragmented, and repetitious, however, he was deeply disturbed by them. He had nowhere to hide but tolerated them day-by-day, week-by-week, and year-by-year.

> `Sometimes one could only just hear these incessant, uninterrupted sounds but sometimes one could hear them a half or full miles away. They were being catapulted out of my body and the most varied sounds and noises going about, especially when I entered some house or village or town. This is the reason I have been living like a hermit for the last few years. All the time my ears keep ringing, and sometimes so loudly that it can be heard far and wide. When I am among woods or brush and the weather is stormy, some horrible, demoniacal poltergeist is aroused; when it is quiet, each tree starts rustling and uttering words and phrases when I approach, also with water – all elements are being used to torture me.' (Jaspers, 1923/1946: 73)

These commenting voices might occur close or alienated to the client. They might also come out from one's body or happen suddenly entirely out the prediction of the client. To avoid these voices, the client lived everywhere and changed from one place to another. Nevertheless, such commenting hallucinations still followed. When he was in forests and woods, they might occur in the form of horrible large voices, and every object in the related environment, including tress and sounds, seemed to torture him continuously.

Subjective Experiences of Other First Rank Symptoms

Apart from hallucinations and delusions, there are other forms of first rank symptoms including the experience of influences playing on the body (Schneider, 1959).

Similar situation occurs in the catatonic state. As mentioned above, Pamwagg's (2004) state of catatonia manifested features of first rank symptoms such as diffusion of ego boundaries.

> `To me, two things happen when I become catatonic. One is that I enter a state of profound indifference so extreme that I, ordinarily an extremely modest person preferring never to be seen naked, refusing even to have the usual female medical exams/tests, can be stripped of all clothing and have all sorts of catheters inserted and even be toileted by strangers without the slightest reaction, either internally felt or externally apparent. I no longer care what happens to that body. Everyone is fussing over me, and I feel an almost Buddhist-like detachment from it, from all the concern and bother going on about me.
>
> The other thing is that along with this indifference comes the more obvious slowing down, even to the point of immobility. While I may seem immobile and non-responsive to those trying to elicit a reaction, in fact my experience is one of reacting quite appropriately, just in glacial time, which to me feels perfectly normal. In fact, other people seem to be moving way too fast and only the clock tells me that I am the slow one rather than the reverse. (Pamwagg, 2004)

From Pamwagg's (2004) description, it was clear that her state of catatonia consisted of an ambiguous ego boundary, in which she detached her sense of being from her own body. By doing so, she could avoid facing the humiliating feeling of being naked in front of the related medical staff. She also detached herself from the surrounding environment. By being stagnant in front of others, she was able to regain her sense of being without being swallowed by the fast changing external environment. The clear ego boundary with a clear ego identity as well as a constant and meaningful exchange between the ego and the surrounding environment, in individuals with catatonic schizophrenia, the ego boundary became blurred and ambiguous. In Pamwagg's situation, the ambiguous and blurred ego boundaries allowed her to detach herself from the oppressive environment. It also facilitated her to detach her sense of body from a sense of being and separated her sense of being from the sense of being humiliated. All these senses of detachment from body, from one's own feeling, and from the external environment, imply a painful process of self-fragmentation.

From Objective Diagnosis to Inter-subjective Understaning: Implications to Mental Health Recovery

From Objectivity to Subjective Experiences

Subjective experiences in people with schizophrenia are always neglected by related professionals in mental health services. The current trend of treatment and rehabilitation merely focuses on the diagnosis of symptoms in schizophrenia and is then followed up by medical treatment as well as evidence-based psychiatric programs and training. All these are founded on objective empirical and evaluative studies with a tight control on resources input and outcome measurements. Objectivity is stressed by related professionals in formulating and justifying the effectiveness and efficiency of related interventions, programs, and training. Behind the objectivity is an assumption that subjective experiences of schizophrenia can be undermined or neglected in the process of treatment and rehabilitation. However, in actual practice, subjective experiences and subjectivity of people with schizophrenia should be regarded as the most fundamental requirement in the process of recovery.

Deegan's Articulation of Lived Experience in Recovery

Patricia E. Deegan was a crucial figure in originating the concepts of recovery. Deegan (1988) experienced mental illness in her young age and was hospitalized in a mental hospital for a long periods of time. As time passed by, she lost his initial hope of recovery and was kept in a stage of stagnancy. She painfully narrated the following:

> `We experienced time as a betrayer. Time did not heal us. Our pasts deserted us and we could not return to who we had been. Our futures appeared to us to be barren, lifeless places in which no dream could be planned and grew into a reality. As for our present, it was a numbing succession of meaningless days and nights in a world in which we had no place, no use, and no reason to be. Boredom and wishfulness becomes our only refugee (Deegan, 1988: 5)

She also experienced despair and anguish. She did not have any hope for recovery.

> `Our denial gave way to despair and anguish. We both give up. Giving up was a solution for us. It numbed the pain, our despair, because we stopped asking "why and how will I go on" ... When one lives without hope (when one has given up) the willingness to do is paralyzed as well.... `It is living in darkness without hope, without a past or a future. It is self-pity. It is hatred of everything that is good and life giving. It is rage turned inward. It is a wound with no mouth, a wound that is so deep that no cry can emanate from it. Anguish is death from which there appears to be no resurrection. It is an inertia from which there is no hope. It is being truly disabled, not by a disease or injury, but by despair. This part of the recovery process is a dark night in which even God was felt to have abandoned us.' (Deegan, 1988: 13)

Deegan's aspiration to recover was sparked by some who loved her and supported her. It re-vitalized Deegan's will to recover.

> `We do remember that even when we had given up, *there were those who loved us and did not give up. They did not abandon us. ... Their love for us was like a constant invitation*, calling us forth to be something more than all of this self pity and despair.... I began to hear and respond to this loving invitation.... But one day, something changed in us. A tiny, fragile spark of hope appeared and promised that there could be something more than all of this darkness. This is the third phase of recovery. This is the mystery. This is the grace. This is the birth of hope called forth by the possibility of being loved. All of the polemic and technology of psychiatry, psychology, social work, and science cannot account for this phenomenon of hope. But those of us who have recovered knew that this grace is real. We lived it. It is our shared secret. (Deegan, 1988: 15)'

Deegan later became a well-trained psychologist and tried her best to advocate, and to develop the concept of recovery, and challenged the rehabilitation concept and practice of behavioral oriented skill training with a set of baseline measurements, procedural manuals, and outcome orientation. They simply regard people with mental illness as passive and inadequate in their lives. To rehabilitate, they have abandoned their own life experiences or wisdom and learn the sets of skills imposed by related professionals.

> `Rehabilitation refers to the services and technologies that are made available to people with disabilities so that they might learn to adapt to their world. Recovery refers to the lived and real experiences of people as they accept and overcome the challenge of disability… 'The recovery process cannot be completely described with traditional scientific, psychiatric, or psychological language. Although the phenomenon will not fit neatly into natural scientific paradigms, those of us who have been disabled know that recovery is real because we have lived it.' (Deegan, 1988: 12)

In terms of sea rose, Deegan (1996a) stressed the importance of enduring hope in the process of recovery. It grows quietly within darkness. It bends towards light.

> 'It did not grow straight toward the light at first. No. First, its growth sought a downward course, reaching, stretching, and blindly groping through shifting sands to find a solid place. A place to be rooted…and then, having rooted itself in this way, the sea rose began its journey toward the light. Poking through the darkness, that sea flower emerged tiny, lovely, insistent, and courageous. On frail and trembling limbs, this small thing rose to a new life…' (Deegan, 1996a:3)

People with mental illness should not be reduced to objects for medication and oppression, treatment, and dependence on hospitals and institutions. Similar to sea rose, the conspiracy of hope becomes will power, a strong driving force for the recovery. No matter how humiliated and helpless their current situation is, their environment should be changed so that they can grow to their full potential as a full human being (Deegan, 1996a). In the article 'Recovery as a Journey of the Heart', Deegan asserted that recovery should be an affirmation that people with a diagnosis of mental illness should live as a full human being. This includes the following features:

1. A full human being can act to change the situation.
2. A full human being can have a voice and speak for himself/herself. S/he has a right that his/her voice should be heard and be listened to.
3. A full human being should have his/her self-determination.
4. A full human being should have a stand in facing his/her distress without being passively victimized by this distress.
5. A full human being should be the expert of his/her own experiences, in particular, resilience from difficulties and hardship and recovery from illness and trauma.
6. A full human being should have his own uniqueness and individuality without being hindered by mainstream society.
7. A full human being can search for his/her own meaning of life without being labeled, hindered or shattered by mainstream society. (Yip, 2012)

Apart from these seven features in humanization, Deegan (1988 & 1996a) added three more features of a full human being.

1. A full human being should embrace long lasting hope for their current and future life.
2. A full human being should have the opportunities and rights in exercising his/her aspiration to live, work and love in a community in which s/he makes a significant contribution.
3. A full human being should establish a new and valued sense of integrity and purpose within and beyond the limits of disability.

The trip of the mind or the conspiracy of hope is never completed in the road of recovery. Deegan (2007 and 2008) affirmed that persons with mental illness should not be a passive receiver of medication. It is also highly unrealistic to presume that simply taking medication prescribed by medical professional is the only way to recover from mental illness. Apart from taking appropriate medication, they should develop their own useful strategies in counteracting hallucinations, delusions, depressive moods, and elated moods as well as prevailing anxiety. An active stance regarding psychiatric medication and medical treatment implies that individuals with mental illness should be accessible to learn related information about medication; create an accurate journal in recording their own physical and psychological response in taking different types of medication; and have their own agenda in psychiatric consultation.

Subjective Experiences and Subjectivity in Recovery

Deegan's self-narration shows that recovery should be a restoration of the full human nature of people with mental illness. In fact, recovery should be a full manifestation with respect of clients' subjective experiences, and their subjectivity in everyday life.

Strauss (1996) preferred an open attitude of respecting regarding the subjectivity of the person with schizophrenia.

He thought that subjectivity should include six major areas of concern. They are:

1. mental integration and dissolution amidst the onslaught of life;
2. specificity - the life is in the details;
3. E Pluribus Unum - The Overall Picture of the Parts
4. the nature of change;
5. competence and dysfunction in mental disorder - what's from outside, what's from inside;
6. what is the basic phenomena of disorder
   (Strauss, 1996)

1. Mental integration and dissolution amidst the onslaught of life

Strauss (1996) advocated that individuals with schizophrenia are similar to others in extreme stress and adversity, which leads to dissatisfaction of life. In facing this issue, one will try his or her best to have mental integration. This kind of struggle is the subjective concern of every person with schizophrenia in facing the torture of illness (Yip, 2012).

> 'That's what schizophrenia may be about. That's where subjectivity comes in, the massive effort to coordinate, integrate, understand, command, adapt and readapt. Subjectivity is all that coming together - figuring out "Will I be well? Will I be sick?" It is the equivalent of managing an air force, army, and navy, troops from different countries, the weather, surprise, success, failure, judgment, feelings, intuitions, hopes and fears, the whole damn things' (Strauss, 1996:209)

2. Specificity - "The Life Is in the Details"

Strauss (1996) stressed that to respect one's subjective experience is to respect his or her specific details about life. To figure one's subjectivity, we have to go into the details of this person, including his or her family life and every particular bit of his or her daily life pattern. For persons in schizophrenia, schizophrenia is only part of their life. They also experience every detail and particular in his or her daily life. Subjectivity is actually the experience of every detail in one's life. (Strauss, 1996)

3. E-Pluribus Unum - The Overall Picture of the Parts

Strauss (1996) was concerned about the overall picture of parts and details. The experience in facing every detail and particular is unique and special for every individual. Every individual may have different interpretations or feelings in facing every similar experience.

> 'And the strange thing about these specifics is that, perhaps many of them together can build a meaningful picture or construct. Our writing group presented a grand round at the Yale Department. Six of us read short pieces from our creative writings about clinical experiences. Each of the writings was very different, very much reflecting the personality of the particular writer' (Strauss, 1996: 209)

4. The Nature of Change

By change, Strauss (1996) actually means the subjectivity of change, improvement, and deterioration in mental disorders. It also implies the momentum required to initiate change and getting well. We may just assume someone who cares can provide the change, but in real life, it is another struggle.

> 'Someone who cares is the right stimulus, but the process? That is the process, fear and taming.... Someone we say the right things to, like: caring about, but often assumes that is all that needs to be known. If we say them with brief terms like that, abstractly enough, they sound important and we have saved ourselves, and the scientific world, the pain of having to feel. But "the life is in the details". A human science, without the details, without the feeling, has no life, is not human.' (Strauss, 1996:210)

5. Competence and Dysfunction in Mental Disorder - What's from Outside and What's from Inside

Strauss (1996) proclaimed that competence or dysfunction in mental disorders, to a certain extent, is what other people perceive. It is entirely subjected to individual explanation. Sometimes, what is observed from the outside may be entirely different from the inside (Yip, 2012).

6. What Are the Basic Phenomena of Disorder?

Strauss (1996) critically reflected that the basic phenomena of disorder are what the person subjectively felt about the experience of the disorder. The person with hallucinations may have his or her own way of dealing with that kind of voice. That sort of mechanism or feeling, in fact, is quite normal in reacting to such disorders (Yip, 2012).

Reconstruction of a Holistic Person

In terms of the specificity, wholeness, and subjectivity of individual regulatory mechanisms, Strauss (1992) tried to formulate a constructive perspective in interpreting the subjective experience of people with schizophrenia. Similar to other normal persons in society, it is a trip for a human mind:

1. to search for meaning from experience;
2. to induce interaction between the individual and his/her related environment;
3. to have vigorous integration among normal and abnormal functioning regulatory mechanisms;
4. to have one's unique and distinctive constructive entity;
5. to put meaning into delusional beliefs;
6. and to facilitate interaction among different systems.

(Strauss, 1992)

1. Human mind searches for meaning from experience

Based on the work of Piaget and rationalistic philosophy, Strauss (1992) stressed that every human mind searches for and builds concepts and meaning from experience and from internal and external stimuli. S/he constructs his/her world of mentality. It is a sense of world and self with interaction to one another.

> 'Thus, the mind is seen as constructing from experiences a sense of the world, of self and of how the world and self interact. Construction is essentially a psychological process, but at the same time it is influenced by the person's biology, by the environment, and by the past experience.' (Strauss, 1992: 22)

2. Interaction between the person and the environment

Strauss (1992) suggested a person with schizophrenia is interacting with as well as constructed by his or her social environment. The social situation and environmental contexts tend to construct the psychological mechanism of the patients. They interact with the normal aspects as well as symptoms of clients with mental illness (Strauss, 1992).

> 'A wide range of normal constructive activities appear to occur in different processes. On one occasion, these processes may be at the very heart of psychopathology and improvement. At other times though, they may be part of psychological functioning in situations not related to mental illness. Yet in all contexts in which they occur, these processes may have definable underlying psychological mechanisms; a study of these can help us further our understanding of human coping styles and their abbreviations, and of how we construct and deal with our world.' (Strauss, 1992: 24)

In other words, the person constructs their environment as well as the environmental context influences the person.

> 'The postulate of constructivist processes suggests rather that there are many psychological mechanisms, varying from normal to pathological in their functioning and outcome, that these processes may reflect a range of coping, developmental, and regulatory mechanisms (perhaps following a Piagetian person-environment-interaction model), and that they are triggered, guided and modified by a range of specific environmental and personal factors' (Strauss, 1992: 24)

3. Interaction among the normal and abnormal mechanism

The construction process integrates both normal and abnormal mechanisms.

Strauss (1992) suggested that within the constructive perspective, both the normal and abnormal mechanisms are actually interacting with one another.

> 'Thus with the constructive view, as exemplified in Klemperer's hypothesis about hallucination and delusions, we can be begin to have a model for thinking about normal and abnormal processes as potentially interacting as dimensions on continua, and as continua across different kinds of abnormality. We also have a way of integrating such important factors as self-esteem and functioning across a range of areas, all this feeding into the construction process.' (Strauss, 1992: 22)

4. Schizophrenia as a distortion of the construction process

From a constructive perspective, schizophrenia is a distortion of the constructive process instead of a continuum of abnormal functioning (Strauss, 1992: 25)

> 'From the constructive perspective, it may be best to view schizophrenia as a range of distortion of these constructing processes, or as a segment, the borders of which are more or less arbitrarily defined, in a matrix of dimensions of functioning. Thus, the conceptualization of schizophrenia carves out a segment of several of these intersecting dimensions, and we have often come to believe that this segment is an isolated, discrete entity, rather than part of a continuum in these various functions. The notion of schizophrenia as a discrete entity has probably been useful up to a point' (Strauss, 1992: 25)

5. A Constructive perspective on delusional perceptions

Strauss (1992) formulated that delusional perception is constructed by the individuals themselves. The construction process is correlated with a person's belief and their own meaning of life. The result of this construction process may be both destructive and constructive for persons with schizophrenia.

> `Delusional perception is an experience in which the person perceives something and then makes a delusional interpretation.... This seems, in many ways, a normal analogue (although in a person with mental illness) to the notion of delusional perception: a particular experience leads to a whole change in belief, and the change becomes a new and central structure in a person's life. The same form of mental construction appears to be going on in both instances. In many delusional perceptions, this underlying process can generate a result that may be destructive. However, in other instances, as with Mr. M,

this process reflects something that occurs for many people in their lives and may actually be quite normal and even helpful.' (Strauss, 1992: 23)

Strauss even used a case, Mr. M, to illustrate the constructive power of this underlying process.

'The man I interviewed, Mr. M., had, before he developed a mental illness, been involved with business. One evening, a colleague said to him "You have a very strong faith in God, but I probably never will." Mr. M. said he thereupon decided to quit business and become a preacher. Although not strictly speaking a perceptual one, the experience with colleague, generated in him an entire change in how he saw the meaning of his life. He did, in fact, become a preacher, but was never very successful, went through many years of mental illness, and then, still in and out of periods of disorder, began preaching again. He became more and more successful and this mental illness began to fade. Mr. M. developed a societal network of other preachers, who were helpful in guiding him, and shortly before our follow-up interview, he received official recognition of his success in this field. He said that in the last year, his life had changed entirely: he had finally been able to follow the calling that he had received many years previously' (Strauss, 1992: 23)

6. Complication Interaction among various systems in the process of treatment

Within the constructive perspective, treatment can be viewed as the interaction among various human processes rather than relying on medication or any single clinical approaches.

'Treatment can be viewed as the interaction of numerous psychological, biological or social impacts on these basic human processes. Even drugs for which our hopes may be have been highest, such as clozapine; usually do not result in the total qualitative change that one might anticipate from a simple diagnostic category or treatment model. Rather, results are best from the combination of intensive and sophisticated psychological treatment programs with the medications' (Strauss, 1992: 25)

Conclusion

As a conclusion, this chapter describes the importance of subjective experiences in persons with schizophrenia. Despite clients with schizophrenia having the same psychotic symptoms and diagnosis, each one of them has their own subjective experiences in symptoms, treatment, and daily life, and in coping with their life stress and frustration. Related professionals should respect clients' subjective experiences. The whole chapter describes clients' subjective experiences in positive symptoms such as paranoia, grandiose and catatonic delusions, and hallucinations; negative symptoms and first rank symptoms. Both Deegan and Strauss affirmed that empathic understanding of clients' subjective experiences is the first step to understand, to restore, and to reconstruct the clients' sense of subjectivity, individuality, and self-cohesion. In fact, clients' subjective experiences are the pre-requisites of recovery. Onken (et al., 2007) and U.S. Department of Health and Human Services (2004) definitions clearly demonstrate this in detail.

> `When recovery from psychiatric disability is identified as the primary challenge, recovery is defined as a process of gaining mastery over the illness - this is largely accomplished by the individual and results in the elimination or alleviation of symptoms. The deviance status, however, and the accompanying stigma of mental illness imposed by society carries with it a host of barriers to successful recovery, including poverty and social marginalization. In this sense, the recovery process emphasizes social inclusion and meaningful roles the person with psychiatric disability is able to inhabit, along with the need to build inclusive communities' (Onken et al. 2007: 10)

In 2004, the U.S. Government regarded the concept of recovery as the sole concern in mental health policy and services. It defines mental health recovery as follows:

> 'Mental health recovery is a journey of healing and transformation enabling a person with a mental health problem to live a meaningful life in a community of his or her choice while striving to achieve his or her full potential.' (U.S. Department of Health and Human Services, 2004)

Within all these mentioned definitions, recovery should have the following elements:

1. A process
2. With ups and downs
3. Personal journey
4. Healing and alleviation of symptoms
5. Living a meaningful life
6. Personal choice
7. Manifestation of individual fullest potential
8. Social inclusion and community life
9. Dealing with exclusion, marginalization and stigma (Yip, 2012)

This means that the concept of recovery should not only focus on medication, alleviation of symptoms, and social functioning of clients with schizophrenia (functional recovery). Instead, it should start with clients' restoration of their senses of subjectivity and individuality as well as their sense of agency (subjective personal recovery) so that they can live a meaningful life within their own personal choice. All these should be done within a supportive, non-discriminatory and inclusive social environment (social recovery) so that clients' full potentials can be fully manifested and developed. In the following chapters, the writer is going to describe the dilemma of self-fragmentation and self-integration in people with schizophrenia. In fact, clients with schizophrenia, under the prolonged influence of an oppressive environment, try to undergo a process of self-fragmentation so that they can be detached from the oppressive environment. That means, the underlying force of self-fragmentation is to preserve a self-integration within clients' delusive inner world. Along this line of thinking, recovery should start from a full recognition and respect of clients' subjective experiences in self-fragmentation manifested within their positive, negative, and first rank symptoms. Then, related professionals should provide or nurture a supportive and inclusive social environment so that clients' inherent urge in self-integration can be restored in reality. By doing so, his/her sense of agency, subjectivity, and individuality can be rebuilt within their own social contexts.

References

American Psychiatric Association (1994). *Diagnostic Systematic Manual* (4th Edition), Washington, D.C. American Psychiatric Association.

Andreason, N. C. (1982). `Negative symptoms in schizophrenia: Definition and reliability, *Archives of General Psychiatry*, 39: 784-788.

Bouriclus, J. K. (1989). `Negative symptoms and emotions in schizophrenia', Schizophrenia *Bulletin*, 15(2): 201-208.

Deegan, P.E. (1988). `Recovery: The lived experience of rehabilitation', *Psychosocial Rehabilitation Journal*, 11(4): 11-19.

Deegan, P.E. (1996a). `Recovery and the conspiracy of hope', paper presented at the *The Sixth Annual Mental Health Services Conference of Australia and New Zealand.* Brisbane: Australia.

Deegan, P. E. (1996b). 'Recovery as a journey of the heart', *Psychiatric Rehabilitation Journal*, 19(3): 91-97.

Deegan, P. (2004). 'Rethinking rehabilitation: Freedom', Symposium conducted at the 20th World Congress of Rehabilitation International, Norway: Oslo.

Deegan, P.E. (2007). 'The lived experience of using psychiatric medication in the recovery process and a shared decision making in mental health care,' *Psychiatric Rehabilitation Journal*, 31(1): 52-70.

Deegan, P. (2008). *Reclaiming Your Power During Medication Appointments with Your Psychiatrist*, National Empower Centre, www.power2u.org/articles

Laing, R.D., (1960). *The Divided Self*, London: Tavistock Publication.

Leete, E., (1989). 'How I perceive and manage my illness' *Schizophrenia Bulletin*, 15(2): 197-200.

Onken, S. J., Dumont, J.M., Ridway, P., Dorman, D. H., & Ralph, R. O. (2002). *Mental Heath Recovery: What Helps and What Hinders? A National Research Project for the Development of Recovery Facilitating System Performance Indicator Phase One Research Report: A National Study of Consumer Perspective on What Helps and Hinders Recovery*, Alexandria, V.A: National Technical Assistance Center for State Mental Health Planning.

Panwagg, J. (2004). *On Catatonia - A Description of My Personal Experience with Catatonia*, http://www.schizophrenia.com/pam/archives/000916.html

Romme, M. A. J., & Escher, A.D. (1989). `Hearing voices' *Schizophrenia Bulletin*, 22: 209-210.

Schneider, K. (1959). *Clinical Psychopathology* (translated by Hamilton M.W., & Anderson E.W.) New York: Grune and Straton

Strauss, J. S. (1989) `Subjective experience of schizophrenia: toward a new dynamic psychiatry II', *Schizophrenia Bulletin*, 15, 179-187.

Strauss, J. S. (1991). `The person with delusions', *British Journal of Psychiatry,* 159: 57-61.

Strauss, J. S. (1992). `The person-key to understand mental illness: towards a new dynamic psychiatry III', *British Journal of Psychiatry*, 162: 19-26.

Strauss, J. S. (1994). `The person with schizophrenia as a person II: approaches to the subjective and complex', *British Journal of Psychiatry*, 164: 103-107.

Strauss, J. S. (1996). `Subjectivity', *Journal of Nervous and Mental Diseases*.184: 205-212.

Strauss, J. S. & Estroff, D. (1989). `Forward to subjective psychotic experience issues' *Schizophrenia Bulletin*, 15: 177-178.

Yip, K. S. (2007). *Clinical Practice of Persons with Schizophrenia: A Humanistic and Empathetic Encounter*, New York: Nova Science Publishers.

Yip, K.S. & Yip, T.W. (2012) (Edited) *Resilience and Recovery of Persons with Mental Illness: Conceptualization and Interpretation*, New York: Nova Science Publishers.

United States Department of Health and Health Sciences (2004). *National Consensus Statement on Mental Health Recovery,* Washington, DC: United States Department of Health and Health Sciences.

Chapter 2

External and Internal Causes of Self-Fragmentation in Schizophrenia and Its Implication to Mental Health Recovery

Introduction

There are various perspectives in explaining self-fragmentation in schizophrenia. Apart from biochemical causes, there are also existential and phenomenological, psychodynamic, sociological explanations. In this chapter, the writer tries to describe various types of conceptual underpinnings in describing the internal and external factors leading to self-splitting and self-fragmentation in schizophrenia. Its implication to social recovery for clients with schizophrenia is also discussed.

Social Construction of Mental Illness Including Schizophrenia

Language, Discourse, Social Exclusion and Labeling

Within a postmodern perspective, mental illness including schizophrenia is socially constructed. Postmodernism asserts that there are no absolute truths, and instead, there are only different interpretations formed in language. Postmodernism acknowledges how human relationships and communications create vocabularies that interpret our experiences. In other words, our realities are socially constructed by our language and linguistic articulation (Walker, 2005: 2). That means mental health professionals construct vocabularies, such as mental illness 'and schizophrenia'. These vocabularies describe disease and deficit. They view the human being as something that can be assessed, diagnosed, and treated like a machine. Under such pathological terms, people are classified into different categories like `normal' and `pathological' with different 'symptoms', 'disorder' and 'disease' of which 'schizophrenia' is regarded as one of the serious mental illness. Along this line of thinking, 'schizophrenia' is not a reality but rather a term, a perspective constructed by mental health professionals to describe a group of behaviors, thoughts, and feelings. Underlying the term `schizophrenia', there is a set of the following vocabularies and ideologies:

1. a set of diagnostic symptoms in terms of positive symptoms, negative symptoms and first rank symptoms
2. a set of deficits, disabilities, disorders, and impairment in social functioning
3. a set of prescribed treatments, dependencies, and restrictions imposed on the individual with schizophrenia
4. a label, a stigma and a disabled identity that is imposed on the individual
5. a tool or a set of language to communicate among related parties, including clients, their relatives, members in the society, as well as related professionals and service providers
6. a means to moralize, legalize and conceptualize the term `schizophrenia' (neurocognitive science in terms of `chemical imbalance', prescribed anti-psychotic medication, institutionalized mental hospital, coerced and involuntary detention and treatment.)

People with schizophrenia are described as having problems of chemical imbalance of dopamine. Thus, anti-psychotic medication is imposed on them. Their ways of thinking, behaviors, and feelings, are labeled as hallucinations and delusions in terms of `psychotic' symptoms. People with psychotic symptoms should be controlled, labeled, excluded, institutionalized, and even detained. With reference to Szazs's (1961) labeling of madness and social construction of pathological discourse, people with mental illness, including schizophrenia, are socially excluded and controlled by powerful actors (professionals, mental health service providers, as well as other normal people) in the society. Within continued social exclusion, social labeling, and social control as well as manipulation by others, people with schizophrenia suffer constant devaluation, humiliation, and defeating experiences by others. All these tend to create the following insurmountable destructive effects for the individual:

1. The individual is involuntarily isolated and excluded by others. Prolonged social isolation and social exclusion may lead to self-isolation and self-exclusion from others that is highly defeating to the social functioning of the individual. Social isolation and self-isolation as well as self-exclusion and self-exclusion may also result in detachment from the social environment and actual reality, which can be a powerful breeding ground for psychotic delusion and hallucination. That means, the individual has to construct his own reality and social environment.
2. The individual is spontaneously stigmatized, humiliated, and labeled by the others. Prolonged stigmatization, humiliation, and labeling by others will result in self-stigmatization, humiliation, and labeling. Prolonged self-stigmatization, self-labeling and self-humiliation may result in self defeating and self-torture, which may result in weakening or even fracturing one's self image and identity as well as ego functioning and self-structure. All these are a breeding ground for developing psychotic symptoms, such as paranoid and persecutory delusion, severe regression in negative symptoms in terms of anhedonia, blunt affect, avolition, and alogia.

Implications for Recovery of People with Schizophrenia

All these have strong implications for recovery of people with schizophrenia. There may be various degrees of social constructionism in formulation of schizophrenia. *In the first level, there is no such thing such as mental illness and/or schizophrenia.* The term 'schizophrenia' is socially constructed by related human professionals. In other words, if everyone is being treated normally and equally, schizophrenia will not be formulated as well as constructed. In other words, the recovery of people with schizophrenia should mean that despite their diagnosis and labels such as schizophrenia, they should be treated normally and equally. Related mental illness labels should thus be diminished. *In a second level, the individual's mental problems are actually constructed by related social exclusion, humiliation, institutionalization, restriction, and medicalization.* In other words, normal respect and community integration should be the only way for a holistic recovery in which the individual can re-experience the sense of a full human being in his/her meaningful life within his/her normal community. In the final level, people with schizophrenia, being labeled, excluded, institutionalized, and humiliated by society for a very long period of time, have already lost their trust and confidence in normal social interaction and social functioning in daily life. *They are not only socially constructed but also self constructed to have schizophrenia, in particular.* In that occasion, they need extra and long-term caring, respect and support to regain the trust and confidence in their actual reality so that they can develop their own confidence in designing their own meaningful and constructive reality.

Power, Truth and Reality vs. Delusive Empowerment

Foucault's Civilization of Madness, and History of Madness

In the book, 'Civilization of Madness, and History of Madness' (Foucault, 2006) Foucault examined related ideas, practices, institutions, art, and literature relating to mental illness in western history. This book was Foucault's first major book. It was written while he was the Director of the Maison de France in Sweden. In this book, Foucault had a full description of history from the Middle Ages in which lepers were totally excluded from the main society. Gradually, during the Renaissance, madness was regarded as unacceptable to the Reason of God. Insanity represented a full manifestation of human desires and dissimulation that should be rejected, labeled, and excluded. Following this was a large confinement of people with madness starting from the 17th century, and in full swing in the 19th century. The house of confinement was only limited to the mentally ill, but also to the poor and the sick including the vagrants, the unemployed, impoverished and orphaned. It was not only a phenomena happening in French but also in other regions in Europe.

Foucault affirmed that confinement of madness not only demonstrated a sort of social control and order, but also a manifestation of power and disciplinary actions, including punishment to those deviants to the norms of the society. Despite the rising of a comparatively humanistic scientific way in the related treatment of mental illness, the abuse of power, confinement, and different degrees of confinement, such as involuntary detention, use of straitjackets, and coerced medication were still imposed on persons with mental illness in the 19th and 20th centuries. People with mental illness were forced to internalize that all these punishments. Confinements were necessary and doing some good for them. In addition, all these punishments and confinements, as well as social exclusion are moralized, legalized, and even humanized by those powerful in the society.

Foucault's Power, Truth and Knowledge

Foucault's *Civilization of Madness* and *History of Madness* was his first book. In fact, he did not contest the reality of madness or mental illness. Instead, as what he addressed in his later publication, he explored how madness was being constituted by knowledge and power. Asylum and institution is a disciplinary power imposed on patients with mental illness.

Foucault (1976; 1980) based on his remarkable articulation of truth, knowledge, and power, asserted power is not something one has, but what one exercises. Foucault (1982; 2002) brought along a change from structural view to a genealogy of power by stressing the circular, capillary, and exercise of power implementation. Foucault's views of power, truth, and knowledge can be summarized as follows:

1. The truth and right is constructed by power
2. Those in power can construct the reality, the truth for the powerless
3. Those in a powerless position have to speak the truth, and act upon the truth being constructed by the powerful figure
4. Those who do not follow the truth should be punished, condemned and labeled as deviant by those in power
5. Power exercise in its capillary form with a full set of network
6. Power concern about the intention and consciousness of those in power
7. Power exists in a circular form
8. Power can be constructed and exercised through mechanisms of knowledge and control
9. The mechanism of knowledge and control exercised by those in power to those who are powerless can pass through related professionals and their professionalization process. (Foucault, 1976; 1980; 1982; 2002).

Loss and Distortion Power, Truth and Knowledge in Powerless Persons

Foucault's view of power, truth, and knowledge is a good postmodernism explanation of those in the position of power. However, Foucault did not mention those in powerless positions. Along Foucault's line of thinking, it can be formulated in Table 1.

Table 1. Distortion of Power, Truth, Right, and Knowledge of the Powerless

Foucault' Orientation	The Dominance of Those Powerful (Power, Truth, Right and Knowledge)	The Submissiveness and Loss of the Powerless (Distortion of Power, Truth, Right and Knowledge)
Power, Truth and Right (Construction)	The truth and right is constructed by power	The truth and right is alienated from the powerless
Power, Truth and Right (Construction)	Those in power can construct the reality, the truth for the powerless	The reality and the truth does not belong to the powerless
Power, Truth and Right	Those in powerless positions have to speak the truth, act the truth being	For the powerless, the powerful figure is the truth, the reality that they have to

Foucault' Orientation	The Dominance of Those Powerful (Power, Truth, Right and Knowledge)	The Submissiveness and Loss of the Powerless (Distortion of Power, Truth, Right and Knowledge)
(Dominance)	constructed by the powerful figure	follow, submit and obey involuntarily
Power, Truth and Right (Dominance)	Those who do not follow the truth should be punished, condemned and labeled as deviants by those in power	For the powerless, the reality and truth is oppressive, humiliating, frustrating and intolerable
Genealogy of Power (network)	Power exercise in its capillary form with a full set of network	The powerless is depowered by a capillary with a full set of networks of oppressive and humiliating others
Genealogy of Power (right)	Within the capillary, the power is exercised in regional and local institutions where individual rights are being controlled or even coerced.	The right and integrity of the powerless is denied, ignored and rejected
Genealogy of Power (intention)	Power concern about the intention and consciousness of those in power	The consciousness and the intention of the powerless is totally ignored, rejected, denied and excluded by others
Genealogy of Power (circularity)	Power exists in a circular form	The depowering process exists in a circular form. The more they are oppressed and depowered by others, the more vulnerable they become, and the easier they can be oppressed
Genealogy of Power (Knowledge of control)	Power can be constructed and exercised through mechanism of knowledge and control	The depowering process and related oppression on the powerless are moralized, legalized and sanctioned by mechanisms of knowledge and control
Genealogy of Power (Knowledge and Professionals)	The mechanism of knowledge and control exercise by those in power to those powerless can pass through related professionals and their professionalization process	Related professionals in the exercise of disciplinary knowledge and/or serve as control agents in oppressing, depowering and humiliating the powerless

Delusive Empowerment and Psychotic Reality

Along Foucault's line language and power, the process of becoming a schizophrenic patient is actually a depowering process with which the dominant parties, including related professionals, members in the society use 'medicalized' and `pathological' language to get rid of individuals' ability and integrity including their social status, social functioning, social identity and social position. The more one becomes schizophrenic, the more intensive the depowering process is. In terms of Foucault's genealogy of power, individuals with schizophrenia are spontaneously oppressed, humiliated, isolated, and depowered by powerful groups in the society. As their reality, truth and right are constructed by the oppressive and humiliating others, they cannot construct a pleasant and accepting reality. Instead, their truth and reality are painful and intolerable. All they can do is to be submissive and depowered by the highly oppressive and humiliating environment, which is highly intolerable and unbearable for the individual. Consequently, all people with schizophrenia can do is to construct their own delusive reality. That is, individuals' may construct an acceptable paradigm of truth, justice, and right. That means, individuals with schizophrenia delusively are empowered by self-constructed reality, within which they can make their own meaning, and detach from the intolerable and unbearable as well as oppressive and humiliating reality. This can be shown in the following Table 2.

Table 2. Delusive Reality of Truth, Right, and Power by Persons with Schizophrenia

Foucault' Orientation	**The Dominance of Those Powerful (Power, Truth, Right and Knowledge)**	**The Submissiveness and Loss of the Powerless (Distortion of Power, Truth, Right and Knowledge)**	**Delusive Reality of Truth, Right and Power in Persons with Schizophrenia**
Power, Truth and Right (Construction)	The truth and right are constructed by power	The truth and right are alienated from the powerless	The powerless have to construct their own truth and rights. However, all these are only delusive and unacceptable by the powerful
Power, Truth and Right (Construction)	Those in power can construct the reality, the truth for the powerless	The reality and the truth does not belong to the powerless	The self-constructed delusive truth and right are the delusive reality for the powerless
Power, Truth and Right (Dominance)	Those in powerless positions have to speak the truth, and act the truth being constructed by the powerful figure	For the powerless, the powerful figure is the truth, the reality that they have to follow, submit to, and obey involuntarily	The actual reality is highly oppressive and humiliating that is intolerable for the powerless. The powerless must involve the delusive reality so that they can detach from the oppressive reality constructed by the powerful
Power, Truth and Right (Dominance)	Those who do not follow the truth should be punished, condemned and labeled as deviant by those in power	For the powerless, the reality and truth is oppressive, humiliating, frustrating and intolerable	The powerful try to oppress the powerless through the oppressive and humiliating reality in terms of truth, rights, and knowledge. The powerless try to isolate themselves from this oppressive reality by their own constructed delusive reality. The powerful try to label all these delusive realities as pathological, abnormal, insane, and even risky to the dominant society, and should be institutionalized, isolated, and detained.
Genealogy of Power (network)	Power exercise in its capillary form with a full set of networks	The powerless are depowered by a capillary form with a full set of networks of oppressive, and humiliating others	The dominance, oppression, and humiliation of actual reality are overwhelming and inescapable for the powerless. Thus, in constructing the delusive reality, the powerless have to develop paranoid delusions and hallucination in assuming the dominance and the oppression is overwhelming and everywhere. In doing so, in paranoia, the powerless also assume that they have a special ability to detect all these known or unknown, predictable and unpredictable oppression, and humiliation from the powerful. All these are labeled by professionals as positive symptoms

Foucault' Orientation	**The Dominance of Those Powerful (Power, Truth, Right and Knowledge)**	**The Submissiveness and Loss of the Powerless (Distortion of Power, Truth, Right and Knowledge)**	**Delusive Reality of Truth, Right and Power in Persons with Schizophrenia**
Genealogy of Power (right)	Within the capillary, the power is exercised in regional and local institutions where individual rights are being controlled or even coerced.	The right and integrity of the powerless is denied, ignored and rejected	Within the delusive reality, individuals build up their own power and right to dominate others. That means, within the delusive reality, they are the powerful. This form of delusive right, truth, and power may be labeled by professional knowledge as grandiose delusions and hallucinations. To increase the capillary of the power of the delusive reality, individuals' grandiose delusions and hallucinations may be connected with supernatural forces.
Genealogy of Power (intention)	Power concern about the intention and consciousness of those in power	The consciousness and the intention of the powerless is totally ignored, rejected, denied and excluded by others	In the delusive reality, individuals engage in a constant dilemma between their own consciousness and intention and the consciousness and intention of the powerful others. At one time, individuals' consciousness and intention can diffuse into others and can control others' thinking in terms of thought insertion and through broadcasting. At the other time, oppressive others' consciousness and intention can diffuse into the individuals' mind and control the individual in terms of thought insertion by others. All these are labeled by professionals as first rank symptoms
Genealogy of Power (circularity)	Power exists in a circular form	The depowering process exists in a circular form. The more they are oppressed and depowered by others, the more vulnerable they become, and the easier they can be oppressed	The more flourishing the delusive reality is constructed, the more individuals are detached from the actual but oppressive reality and the more they are labeled by the oppressive but powerful others as pathological, deviant and mad that should be further excluded, detained and excluded by institutionalized mental health services. As a consequence, individuals' actual social function, and self image are all doubly oppressed in the actual reality and in the delusive reality to a degree that they have intensive emotional detachment (blunt affect), loss of their interest in any actual meaningful and pleasurable activities (avolition and anhedonia) as well as loss of interest in expressing their needs, idea or feeling (alogia). All these are labeled by professionals as negative symptoms.

Table 2. (Continued)

Foucault' Orientation	**The Dominance of Those Powerful (Power, Truth, Right and Knowledge)**	**The Submissiveness and Loss of the Powerless (Distortion of Power, Truth, Right and Knowledge)**	**Delusive Reality of Truth, Right and Power in Persons with Schizophrenia**
Genealogy of Power (Knowledge of control)	Power can be constructed and exercised through mechanism of knowledge and control	The depowering process and related oppression on the powerless are moralized, legalized and sanctioned by mechanism of knowledge and control	The self-constructed delusive reality is being labeled by professional knowledge as schizophrenia, in which delusive defense against oppression is regarded as 'paranoid delusion'. Delusive empowerment is diagnosed as grandiose delusion. The loss of interest and engagement in actual oppressive reality is considered as negative symptoms. The confusion of actual and delusive reality is labeled as first rank symptoms. Those in the state of delusive reality for more than six months are diagnosed as schizophrenic and obliged by the powerful to have treatment, exclusion, and even detention in mental institutions Medical knowledge in terms biochemical explanation is imposed to legalize and moralize all these diagnostic labeling, medical treatment, institutionalized detention and social exclusion of the powerless with delusive empowerment and reality.
Genealogy of Power (Knowledge and Professionals)	The mechanism of knowledge and control exercise by those in power to those powerless can pass through related professionals and their professionalization process	Related professionals in the exercise of disciplinary knowledge and or serve as control agents in oppressing, depowering, and humiliating the powerless	Medical professionals are trained to exercise all these diagnostic labeling, medical treatment, institutionalized detention, and social exclusion of the powerless with delusive empowerment and delusive reality. Medical professionals are moralized and legalized by the powerful as sole agent to exercise control, manipulation to the powerless with delusive empowerment and delusive reality

Implications to Recovery

Foucault's orientation of power, truth, and reality in fact has a strong implication to mental health recovery for clients with schizophrenia. As mentioned above, Deegan's orientation asserted that recovery is founded on an experience of being a full human being. It includes the following components:

1. A full human being can act to *change the situation.*
2. A full human being can have a voice and *speak for himself/herself.* S/he has a right that his/her voice should *be heard and be listened to.*

3. A full human being should have his/her *self-determination.*
4. A full human being should have *a stand in facing his/her distress* without being passively victimized by this distress.
5. A full human being should be the *expert of his/her own experiences*, in particular *resilience from difficulties and hardship* and recovery from illness and traumas.
6. A full human being should have their own *uniqueness and individuality* without being hindered by the main stream society.
7. A full human being can search for *his/her own meaning of life* without being labeled, hindered or shattered by the mainstream society. (Yip, 2012)
8. A full human being should embrace *long lasting hope* for their current and future life.
9. A full human being should have the opportunities and rights to *exercise his/her aspiration to live, work and love* in a community in which s/he makes a significant contribution.
10. A full human being should establish a *new and valued sense of integrity and purpose* within and beyond the limits of the disability

Deegan's sense of a full human being, clearly showed that recovery of mental illness, including schizophrenia, should not be founded on a social environment in which the individual can actualize his/her self determination, establish a sense of integration, search of his/her own meaning, embrace his/her sense of uniqueness and individuality, speak for himself/herself, manifest a sense of hope, exercise his/her aspiration of hope, and be an expert in resilience of difficulties and hardship, and can change the situation. All these imply that the individual is free from the negative influence of the powerful group. That means, the individual is not obliged by the truth and reality constructed by the powerful group. Instead, s/he can construct his/her sense of reality and s/he can determine his/her fate, way, and own life. In other words, instead of constructing his/her own reality and truth within psychotic delusions and hallucinations; s/he has substantial influence, sense of autonomy, respect, integrity, determination, uniqueness, and individuality within an actual and healthy reality. All these can be shown in the following case illustration. Related parties' consensus in using their stories for academic purposes was sought. For the sake of confidentiality, their personal information and identities were properly disguised.

Peter: The Oppressed Inspector with Psychosis

Peter was born in a middle class family in which his father was a police officer in China. He was stern, strict, and autocratic. His mother was quiet and diligent, serving the needs of the whole family. Peter had a younger sister who was active, naughty, but clever. During his childhood, Peter was accustomed to be strictly disciplined by his autocratic father. He needed to regard his father's words as a strict command without any argument. In Foucault, his father constructed the truth and reality that Peter needed to follow and oblige. In fact, for his whole life, Peter tried his very best to meet his father's expectation. He studied hard and became one the top students in his primary and secondary school. He entered into a degree program of Business Studies in a famous university and graduated with a good second up honor.

While everything looked good and Peter seemed to have good future in his career life, Peter did not feel happy at all. Instead, he felt that he lived under the strong shadow of his father. Despite this, he was quite successful in his academic performance; his father did not feel happy at all. According to his father's wish, he wanted Peter to be a tough policeman, at least a chief inspector, or even a senior superintendent. Peter's father was only a rank and file for his whole life. He casted his unfulfilled wish on Peter. In fact, Peter had no interest in being a policeman, nor did he want to be a businessman or fund manager. He was interest in making a movie or reading fiction. In no way would his father allow him to do so.

Under his father's strict command, Peter was finally admitted as an inspector trainee in the police force. Under the half-year training period, his colleagues and his seniors continuously bullied Peter since he was too polite and artistic. They called Peter a 'womanish policeman'. Peter tried to react by yelling at them but they pushed him away. When Peter returned home, he told his father about this and refused to enter the police academy again, but his father smashed him and pushed him to tolerate any command, even bullying from seniors. Finally, Peter graduated from the police academy and became a junior inspector.

He was responsible for investigating crime in drug addiction. At first, Peter worked well under his seniors as well as his father's advice. He got along well with his supervisor, a senior inspector who was kind and considerate. He enabled Peter to perform well and taught Peter how to be a good police officer. Unfortunately, he was promoted and transferred to another section in the police force. The new supervisor was completely different. He was apathetic, autocratic, and even abusive to his subordinates. Peter always cursed him as irresponsible, lazy, and even inert in crime investigation. One night, he required Peter to go to his house for case discussion. After he had drunk a bottle of wine with Peter, he raped Peter. In the process, they had a fight, but he was very strong and knocked Peter down. After that, he threatened to Peter that if he wanted to be promoted in the police force; he ought to be his homosexual partner.

Peter was deeply hurt by his issue. He intended to charge his supervisor but quit the police force. However, his father deterred him to do so. His father even said that homosexual rape or harassment was a very common practice in the policy force. Peter had to tolerate this and use it as a threat to his senior for promotion. After he had been promoted, then he could take revenge. Peter really got sick for his father's suggestion. He determined to ignore his father's advice and took action. However, his father kneeled down to him and begged him to fulfill his unfulfilled aspiration in life - to be an outstanding superintendent. He even threatened Peter that if he quit the policy force, he would commit suicide. Peter was deeply disturbed.

Under this father's advice, Peter had to be a junior inspector under the leadership of his oppressive supervisor. He tried every means to keep a distance from this one. However, his supervisor kept on seducing him. The more he refused him, the more his supervisor hated him and assigned him some difficult tasks and duties. Whenever he failed to complete all these duties, his supervisor would curse him and threaten him to oblige his seduction. Gradually, Peter felt high stressed and oppressed. In carrying out his normal police duties, he always assumed that sooner or later, he would fail in this duty, and his father and his supervisor would blame him severely. At night, he always woke up by the nightmare of being raped by his supervisor. In addition to this, he always felt that other colleagues were gossiping around him about his homosexual relationship with his supervisor. He was tense, anxious, and highly oppressed. Apart from normal duties, he isolated himself from interacting with others. He became more and more isolated and self-absorbed. Finally, he developed active hallucinations that there were two voices commenting on his behaviors saying that he was the homosexual partner of his seniors. Other voices said that he was an upright policeman being appreciated by others and his father as well. All these two tracks of voices argued with one another. He felt deeply annoyed.

One day, when he failed to accomplish a duty assigned by his supervisor, he suddenly had a severe outburst of anger. He picked up his gun and tried to shoot at his supervisor saying that he was assigned by God to kill his bastard supervisor. Fortunately, his colleagues came along and deterred him from doing so. He was thus taken by an ambulance to an emergency unit and diagnosed as suffering from schizophrenia.

From the above-mentioned case illustration, it was clear that Peter's psychosis was a result of external oppression. According to Foucault's idea, Peter's mental illness and delusions were actually shaped by the truth and right constructed by the powerful group, including his father and his supervisor. Under his father's oppression, he had to become a policeman. Under his supervisor's oppression, he was homosexually raped. Both his father and his supervisor constructed an oppressive reality that required him to follow and to oblige. As he failed to follow this oppressive truth and reality, he was punished and isolated by powerful figures. His father blamed and cursed him whenever he failed to follow his instruction. His supervisor punished him, assigned him difficult tasks, and coerced him to commit homosexual acts for him. Peter had no way to go. The more Peter was oppressed, the more vulnerable Peter became, and the more he was easily oppressed. Thus, the only way Peter could empower himself was through self-constructed paranoid delusion in which two voices argued with one another. One voice said that he was an upright policeman. One voice told him that he was a homosexual partner of his seniors. These two voices clearly indicated his internal conflicts towards the oppression imposed by the powerful group. They were conflicting to one another. Thus, finally all he could do was to diminish his senior by shooting. This was the only thing he could do to regain his self-constructed reality, truth, and right. It also represents a full onset of Peter's psychosis. However, it did not help much. Instead, he was labeled by society as a schizophrenic, with an authority's diagnosis from a medical practitioner. The label of insanity, along with hospitalization and coerced treatment depowered Peter further. Prolonged institutionalization plus a high dosage of anti-psychotic injections made Peter became inert, passive, and withdrawn. Below is Peter's own narration in reviewing his own experiences and feelings in the process of treatment.

> Peter: `My father wanted me to be an outstanding policeman. My oppressive senior wanted me to be his submissive homosexual partner. They wanted me only to be their own tools in actualizing their egocentric and selfish wish. In front of them, I was nothing but obedient, submitting to their order and manipulation. When I fought back, when I tried to actualize and manifest my anger towards them, I was labeled as insane and crazy. I wanted to shoot my senior to death so that he could not oppress others any more. But I was caught and locked up in the mental hospital. I harbored delusions to kill this bastard but they labeled me as schizophrenic and abnormal and should be locked up in the mental hospital. This was indeed an unfair treatment to me. I was further oppressed by detention, coerced treatment, and involuntary treatment. The only way I could do this was further submission and depowerment. I was nothing but an insane person. I was hopeless in such an insane place…

The Recovery of Peter As a Full Human Being

As mentioned above, the only appropriate way for Peter to recover was to become an integrated and full human being. That means, Peter should be free from the negative influence of the powerful group. He should not be obliged by the truth and reality constructed by the powerful group. Instead, he could construct his/her sense of reality and s/he could determine his/her fate, way, and own life. In other words, instead of constructing his own reality and truth within psychotic delusions and hallucinations, he could exert his substantial influence, sense of autonomy, respect, integrity, determination, uniqueness, and individuality within an actual and healthy reality.

> `Peter was involuntarily hospitalized in a statutory mental hospital for one year. During this period of time, his father deeply regretted what he had done to Peter in his life. He began to realize that he should not oppress Peter to fulfill his own unfulfilled wish in his life. He should not force Peter to suffer homosexual rape and continuous oppression from his supervisor. He knew that Peter's onset of schizophrenia was partly his own fault. He felt deeply sorry for that. To compensate for his sense of guilt, he hired a private detective to search for evidence in proving Peter's supervisor immoral homosexual rape. He visited Peter frequently in the mental hospital.
>
> During this period of time, his supervisor repeated his unlawful act to other colleagues and other people in the community. Peter's father united all these victims secretly together. They searched for further evidence to legally charge Peter's supervisor. As his homosexual rape got worse and worse, he engaged in raping some male children in the community. Some of them were seriously hurt in the raping process. Their parents were furious, and all related victims all legally charged Peter's supervisors. He was thus sentenced for 15 years imprisonment. At the same time, Peter's case was put forward for review in the court. Instead of being sentenced as mentally confused with a lethal act to hurt others, he was re-sentenced as a victim and his mental confusion was actually a result of the oppression. In addition, he complied with medical professionals' order in the mental hospital. They regarded his compliance as a good progress of his mental state. Based on all that, Peter was discharged from the forensic ward of the mental hospital.
>
> His father no longer pushed Peter to be a policeman. Instead, Peter studied a two-year master course of filmmaking. After he graduated, he engaged in a film and advertisement company as an assistant director. As Peter could make his own choice in his own career path, he was happy and autonomous. He was able to exercise his own power, right, and creativity in his film making process. As a film director making his own film, Peter became a full human being with his own integrity, with respect from others.

Power of Delusive Self in Psychosis

Glass (1995) articulated power in delusion in persons with psychosis. He combined a psychoanalytic approach, phenomenological articulation, and a social construction perspective in describing delusive power in psychotic times in persons with psychosis.

Freud affirmed that delusion in schizophrenia is a process of psychotic regression

Glass (1995) started with Freud's orientation of delusion and psychotic regression.

> 'Freud viewed the frightening closed system of belief embodied in delusion as dangerous to the self and a serious threat to the stability of the society and the organization of political life. He was particular disturbed by the power of delusion to attack secondary process functions (the ego separation of reason, moderation, compromise, limitation, and negotiation) and to induce more violent primary process aggressions that assault the ego and, in the case of political life, these institutional artifacts capable of containing it. The Freudian approach to dreams provides a context for understanding the power of delusion, a kind of all encompassing wide attack wide-awake dream that organizes reality and consciousness.' (Glass, 1994: 11)

Freud (1937 & 1939), in fact, affirmed that the power of delusion encourages the regressive mechanism of the individual in a way that resembles the rejected reality, the choice of staying in one's own inner and primary world of aggression and instinct.

> 'Freud considered delusion as a fundamental dimension of the self's infantile past. Delusion owes its convincing power to the element of historical truth, which is inserted in the place of the rejected reality.... (1937: 268)
>
> 'Those who are subject to delusion are suffering their own reminiscences...We have long understood that a portion of forgotten truth lies hidden in delusional ideas, that when this returns it has to put up with distortions and misunderstandings (1939: 85)

In addition to that, Glass (1993) affirms that power is a form of tyranny and domination in which the self of the individual is being fractured by the delusion.

In other words, according to Freud, the power of delusion is as follows:

1. It impairs the secondary functioning of the ego including the ego separation of reason, moderation, compromise, limitation, and negotiation.
2. It induces more violent primary process aggression that assaults the ego and, in the case of political life, these institutional artifacts capable of containing it.
3. It facilitates the individual to create his/her own delusive reality in which his/her sense of reality and consciousness is deeply disturbed.

Delusion Power in Dreams

Freud (1900) affirmed that dreams are a royal road to the unconscious. Similar to delusion, the dream consists of full clues to demonstrate the repressed and denied. *Dreams represent mental antiquities...the reconstitution of the earliest and most obscure periods of the human race* (Freud, 1900: 588; Glass, 1993). In fact, the dream represents the power of the inner mind in terms of the following:

1. the self-constructed reality,
2. the manifestation of inner but repressed drives and instincts,
3. the discharge of unhappiness and frustrated experiences and memories,
4. the representation of one's inner urge and unfulfilled wishes and needs, and
5. the loosening of one's inner inconsistency, conflicts and dilemmas.

Power in Collective Delusion

> 'If we consider mankind as a whole and substitute it for the single human individual, we discover that it too has developed delusions which are inaccessible to logical criticism and which may contradict reality.' (Freud, 1937: 269)

Glass (1993) further elaborated that the collective may be overwhelmed by the distortion of reality in forms of ideology, war, intolerance, fanaticism, and murderous rage because of the collective delusion. Paranoia can be highly institutionalized in public policy, fantasy in searching quick but ineffective solutions. Coupling this is also a regression of collective and rational wisdom in terms of long-term planning and democratic participation in dealing with problems and difficulties. (Glass, 1993: 14).

Regression As a Loss and Suppression of Power in the Psychotic Self

'Regression destroys secondary process structures, pushes the self into a state of boundlessness, releases enormous amounts of aggression and intensifies feelings of psychotic reality anxiety and panic. Living without limits possessed by an epistemology, the self faces a loss of continuity and being...What psychosis releases - intense vulnerabilities, rage and hatred. ' (Glass, 1993: 19)

Within the psychotic self, individuals embed strong destructive urges and instincts to destroy not only the ego functioning and sense of reality, but also others in the external social environment, if they are within a powerful position or with the ability to stir up the connected with collective delusions.

Democracy and Regression in Delusive Power

It also destroys democratic participation within a social circle and science Democracy is, in its politics as well as epistemology, a defense against psychotic modes of being and power. It also leads to a splitting off of self, with a highly violent raging part of self in destroying rationality, participation, and political stability.

'Democracy respects conflicts, works to contain its entropy, the dynamic is dialectical, and the relationship between the container and the contained is reciprocal..... It is a political theory that protects the values of liberty and autonomy, which at the level of individual psychology are parallel to the acceptance of boundary, proportion, and limitation. Democracy opposes the affect or symptom of nonreciprocal power; unrestrained narcissism, unlimited entitlement, perceptions of omnipotence, delusions or images of grandeur and dominance.' (Janet, 1907: 23)

In other words, democracy represents a mechanism to inhibit the manifestation of collective delusive power or individual's delusive power in oppressing others. It regulates affect being stirred up by raging emotions, omnipotence, and grandiosity.

Psychotic Times: Transcendence from External Time to Inner Time

Psychotic time moves the self out of historical or consensual time. It is a time of non-being, full of delusive power in which the individual defines his/her inner time. Within the psychotic time, the individual can transform himself/herself into any form of anything, any person, or any event. They can perceive anything or cause anything to happen within their own consciousness. Glass (1993) illustrated this by various cases with psychosis.

'Jenny believes that she turns into a camel or a monkey every day. She claims that meal trays are made of dangerous plastic.... Chuck comments he has been thrown into shock, that his voice which he called Ed, 'electrocuted me.....I ask him how the voices changes his face. ...but they make me ugly for fifty years... I was young and beautiful ... once ...' (Glass, 1993: 32)

By means of the delusive power, individuals become highly powerful, able to fight back any external oppression. They are able to manifest their own aggression in a prevailing way.

'In the dominion of psychotic time, the helpless become powerful; the lonely discover themselves surrounded by immense populations; the rejected become leaders

> reversed by millions; the weak turn into strong heroes, rescuers of the victimized and tormented....the small grow to great stature and dominate entire nations, world galaxies....Time circulates around these imperatives; distorted forms of power floating without anchor, no historical relationships. (Glass, 1993: 32)

According to Glass (1993), delusion and grandiosity is a way to regain power that has been oppressed and deprived in the process of psychosis. That means, in reality, they are oppressed, deprived, rejected, weak and small. In psychotic time, they are the powerful, the accepted, the strong, the rescued, and the huge.

> `Psychosis attacks the self's sense of its public being; it pulls consciousness away from an awareness of the public world and locates knowledge in an internal, hidden reality accessible only to the subject, its erodes attachments to community, it radically distorts normal duration.... The psychotic self lives with the specificity of whatever events occupies the consciousness, and time is represented in the action of a continuing parade of images related by the logic of the unconsciousness. ... Psychosis provides the psychological space where it self-expresses its nature.... Psychotic time fragments the ego. It refracts destruction in images circulating around the self like a spinning top. It pushes the self into a face-to-face confrontation with the object.... Psychotic time is global, absolute, and total; states of dread, fear, horror, fragmentation, destruction, and imminent annihilation develop within psychological environments in which conventional notions of time have no significance. ' (Janet, 1907: 34)

Despite the power and grandiosity in psychotic time, individuals' ego and sense of reality are continuously fragmented, fractured and destructed. The destructive effects are so strong that they dominate the whole functioning of the individual.

Psychotic Time As a Withdrawal from Consensual Reality

In terms of delusive power, Glass (1995), within psychotic delusion, individually demonstrates an overwhelming state of inner power. That sort of power penetrates into the individual's consciousness as well as sense of reality. Glass (1995) used the term 'psychotic time' to describe the delusive power of the psychotic state of mind.

> `In regression to psychotic states, the self experiences a form of time having absolutely nothing to do with linear historical time understood as part of public or consensual reality.
>
> `Psychotic time, as I call it, exists beyond the self; psychotic consciousness....
>
> ...absorbs linear time, it is the time of the unconsciousness... . It surrounds the self with the narcissistic projection of a total projection of a totally closed system of belief and perception. It is the time of absolute power, tyranny, and freedom. It transforms otherness into torture, domination, and hate.
>
> `To be within psychotic time is to be in the space of torture, a realm of nonbeing where power appears as torture, tyranny, and destruction of individuality. Schizophrenics experience psychotic time as fragmented duration, so that normal temporal sequences have no meaning. Psychotic time can possess an oppressive power....
>
> `In the domination of psychotic time, the helpless becomes powerful, the lonely discover themselves surrounded by immense population; the rejected become leaders revered by millions; the weak turn into strong heroes, rescuers of the victimized and tormented. (Glass, 1995: 28-30)

In other words, in psychotic time, the individual is full of power to control rather than being controlled, energy to exercise their abilities and determination as well as creativity to act upon anything they want, unlimited space and time in actualizing their own needs, drive and determination. All these can be presented in the following table.

From External Oppressive Power to Internal Destructive Power

Delusive but destructive power in psychotic time constructed by Glass (1995), in many ways are similar to Foucault's (1976, 1980 & 1982) orientation of prevailing power and dominance constructed by the powerful and authority figures in the society, within institutions as well as related professionals. Both stressed that psychosis or insanity are constructed and related to power and dominance.

Table 3. Individual State of Mind in Psychotic Time and in Reality for Persons with Schizophrenia (Summarized from Glass, 1995)

Various Dimensions of a persons	**In the reality**	**In the psychotic time**
Power	Being Oppressed by others	Being empowered by the self constructed delusion
Relationship	Being rejected by others as lonely and isolated.	Being respected and appreciated by self construction delusion
Resources	Being deprived by others	Self constructed resources, money, status and position
Self Image	Timid and inferiority	Being superior and determined in self constructed delusion
Meaning of Life	Emptiness and Ontological Insecurity	Substantial and concrete in self constructed delusion.
Body	Feel weak and physically impaired or deteriorated	Feel strong and physically capable in self constructed delusion
Time	Time in reality is condensed, distorted, fixated and neglected	Time in psychotic time is exaggerated, expanded, diffused, transformed and moved according to the hidden needs of the individuals
Consciousness	Consciousness in reality is blurred and diffused	Consciousness in psychotic time is sharp, responsive and delusive
Space	Confined, narrowed and limited with a sense of suffocation and deterioration	Fully extensive, transforming and changing from one space to another one

While Glass described, in full detail, about the inner delusive power of the individual within psychotic time, Foucault described in what ways individuals with madness are depowered by external powerful society, institutions, and professionals in the society.

Within Foucault's orientation of power, for persons with schizophrenia, they cannot construct their own delusive reality of truth, right, and power in the oppressive reality. Others, in forms of civilization, culture, institutions, and power, construct their madness. Following Foucault's line of thinking, all they can do is to construct their delusive reality. This self-constructed delusive reality, in Glass's (1995) terms, is psychotic time in which the individual becomes highly powerful, respectable, grandiose, resourceful and extensive. *There are differences between Glass's and Foucault's orientation.* Glass presumes that delusive power in psychotic times is self-constructed while Foucault's orientation is constructed by oppressive and powerful others in social environment. Another difference is that *Glass stressed all these self constructed delusive but powerful psychotic time for the individual is highly destructive.* It shatters the integrity, and cohesiveness of the individuals. It distorts the sense of reality, time, and space. However, Foucault did not go into the details of the inner psychic of a person with mental illness, including those with schizophrenia. *He affirmed the prevailing oppression of the powerful figures.* In terms of circulatory of power, oppression by the powerful figures is overwhelming and all around. It not only exists in the form of oppressive powerful social structure, but also in forms of network, knowledge, institutions, and intentions. In other words, under the prevailing powerful external environment, individuals are totally depowered. Foucault affirmed that madness is constructed by civilization. He did not go into the inner world of people with madness. He only asserted that madness is socially constructed. That means, he normalized the so-called 'mad' responses of 'mad' people. They are actually constructed by a powerful but 'mad' society, professionals, institutions, and knowledge that label deviants as mad to remain in power and in control for their own benefit and rights. In fact, *the inner orientation of powerful but delusive psychotic times and external destructive external depowering social environment can be complimentary to one another in formulating a full picture of external and internal process of fragmentation for persons with schizophrenia.* Foucault's view is outer violent, oppressive, and destructive forces imposed on individuals. Glass's view is internal destructive and powerful forces constructed by the individuals themselves. There seems to be a theoretical gap regarding how his destructive external reality is being internalized to form the internal destructive reality of the individual. The external destructive force and internal destructive force can be combined in the following ways:

1. The individual has a constant and strong need to have its own power in terms of uniqueness, integrity, and respect in the actual reality in order to sustain his/her sense of existence and ego functioning.
2. Once this need cannot be satisfied in the external environment, the individual can only construct his/her own uniqueness, power, and integrity, within his/her delusive inner world.
3. In constructing this delusive inner world, the oppressive external reality is still there. The individual has two choices, either internalizing the oppressive reality as an ingredient to construct his inner delusive world or being totally isolated and separated from it.
4. In internalizing the oppressive reality, the individual can develop delusion and hallucinations that counteract it (grandiose power to fight again oppressive reality) or exaggerate it (prevailing paranoia that oppression delusively exists everywhere).
5. In isolating of the oppressive reality, the individual can create his/her own inner delusive reality that is totally out touch with reality in terms of superstitions, imaginations, religious beliefs, as well as bizarre thinking.

All these can be shown in Figure 1.

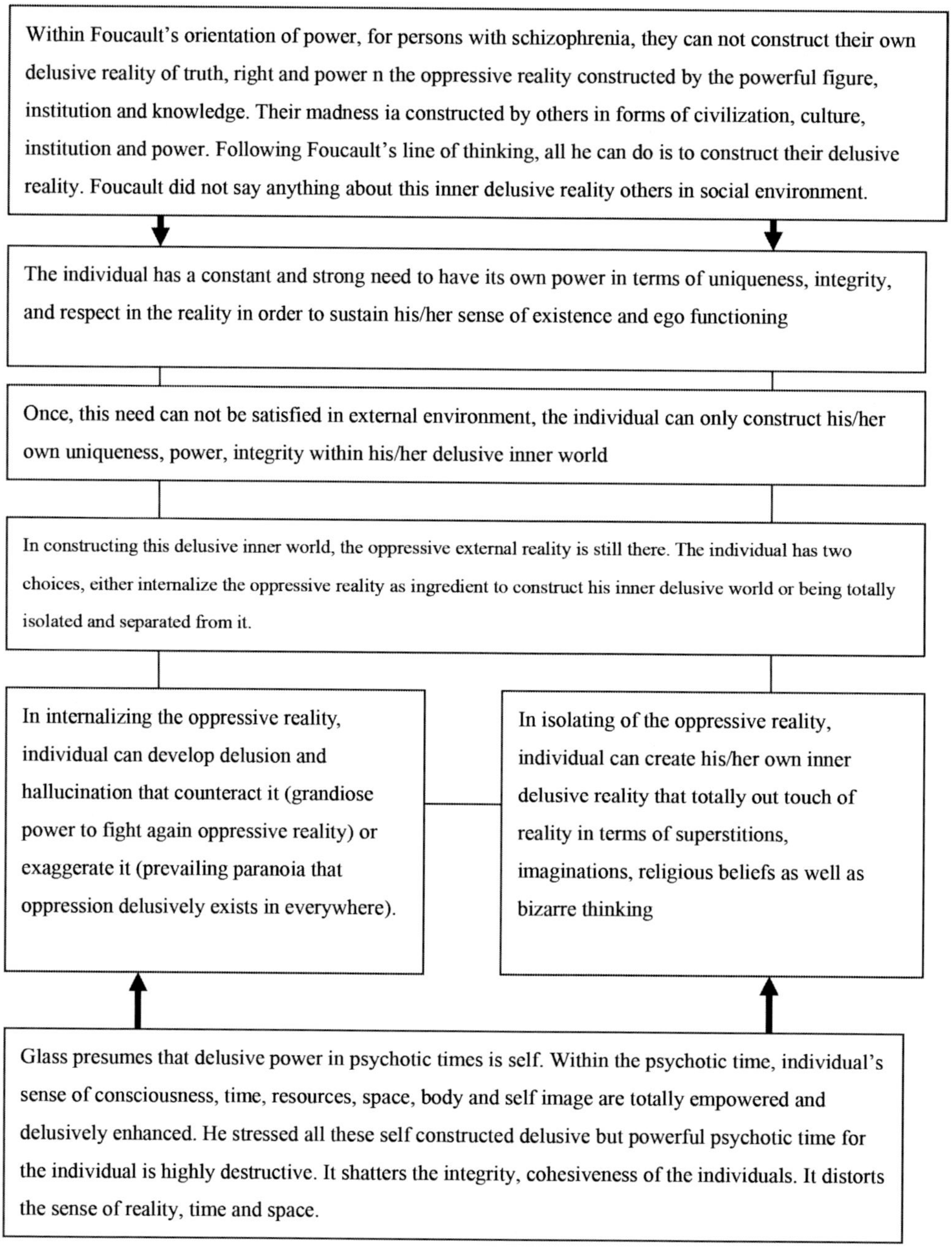

Figure 1. Connection between Foucault and Glass Orientations of Power and Psychotic Time.

Implications to Recovery

The combination of Glass and Foucault's view on onset of mental illness, particularly in schizophrenia, has strong implications to recovery. It is clear that mental health recovery of clients with schizophrenia should be founded on gratifying the individual's needs of having their own power. The individual should have a constant and strong need to have its own power in terms of uniqueness, integrity, and respect in the actual reality in order to sustain his/her sense of existence and ego functioning. In doing so, the following stages should be attained.

1. Remove the oppressive environment that makes clients feel impotent, being oppressed, and loss of uniqueness, integrity, and respect.
2. Cultivate conditions that clients can regain his sense of subjectivity and existence by being a full human being with substantial contribution to his/her family, community, and career.
3. In doing so, there should be a gradual decrease of dependence on medical treatment and social rehabilitation programs. In other words, clients with schizophrenia can regain a normal life within their community.

All these can be demonstrated in the following case illustration. Related parties' consensus in using their stories for academic purpose was sought. To ensure confidentiality, their personal information and identities were properly disguised.

The Chief Disciple of the Buddha Became a Normal Human Being

Paul was an adult male with schizophrenia for ten years. Before his onset, he worked as a manual laborer in a factory. He was born in a single parent family in which his father died when he was only two years old. His mother had to work very hard to sustain a hand to mouth living.

Paul had to take up all the household chores and he was in fact, lacking in discipline and care from his mother. His academic performance was entirely unsatisfactory in primary school life. He was then admitted by a secondary school, which was notorious for delinquent students. Apart from this, he was also bullied by others in his school life. His classmates always teased him as a stupid pig as Paul was a bit fat and inert in his school life. Paul was deeply hurt by that. He looked depressive and boring in his life. Consequently, he joined a delinquent gang and engaged in illegal triad activities. At first, Paul felt highly excited. He was able to threaten those classmates who bullied him. No sooner, the discipline master discovered that and Paul was caught by the police.

As Paul was only 14 years old, the superintendent in the police office only warned him. Because of that, Paul was expelled from his school. Then, Paul became an apprentice in a manufacturing company. He worked very hard day and night but his coach was very demanding and oppressive to him. He cursed Paul every time when Paul did not work up to his standard. He was also isolated and bullied by his colleagues. Paul had to tolerate all that, as it was the only way for him to earn a living. At that time, his mother was severely ill. Paul was under severe stress. On one hand, he had to take good care of this dying mother with a traumatic fear that sooner or later his mother would die and leave him. On the other hand, he had to face the severe stress from being bullied by his colleagues and was oppressed.

Six months later, his beloved mother died of lung cancer. As Paul's mother was a committed Buddhist follower, he firmly believed that she would be in heaven with the Buddha. In order to unite with his mother, Paul began to isolate himself from others and continuously recited the Buddhist bible. He quit his job and lived on his limited savings for three months. Within these three months, he locked himself up and was totally involved in reciting the Buddhist bible. Gradually, he harbored a strong delusion that his mother was next to the Buddha and he became the Chief Disciple of the Buddha with magnificent power to defeat the evil in the society.

From that time onwards, Paul dressed up like a monk with a long garment and bare head, and he continuously recited the Buddhist bible on the street. Whenever he saw someone who appeared like a delinquent, he would approach him and advise him to be good and kind and get rid of their evil acts. In doing so, he would occasionally be cursed or even hit by others. But he did not mind that. He firmly believed that if he could advise one thousand delinquents to be free from delinquency, he could sooner or later became a real Buddha and then he could unite with her deceased mother in the Buddhist heaven. Paul's delusive act was highly disturbing to others.

One day he repeated the same act in a shopping arcade, and had a severe conflict, and fought with several delinquent gangsters. He was then taken into a mental hospital and was diagnosed as having schizophrenia with grandiose delusion. In the mental hospital, Paul was lucky enough to encounter a kind-hearted nurse N who was empathic and tried to understand the unfulfilled wish and needs behind N's grandiose delusion. She listened with an empathic ear to the life stories of Paul. Under this condition, Paul felt deeply understood and respected. He possessed a good recovery in which his grandiose delusion was successfully alleviated. One year later, the medical social worker in the mental hospital referred him to a psychiatric half way house for rehabilitation.

In the half way house, Paul was encouraged to join the therapeutic community program in which every resident in the house was expected to make decisions, to participate and to contribute their view in everyday living in the half way house. Despite that Paul sometimes still elaborated some odd bizarre ideas, such as insisting on vegetarian food for every meal, advising other residents to become Buddhist followers, and telling others that in his previous life, he was the Chief Disciple of the Buddha, he was still respected by other residents and workers in the half way house.

Under this kind of deep respect, Paul's mental health condition was drastically improved. Two months later, he actively required help to search for open employment. Some humorous residents teased Paul that the Chief Disciple of the Buddha did not need to work or search for open employment. All he needed should be purely reciting the Buddhist bible and waiting for the day that he would be transformed into a real Buddha. Facing that sort of challenge, Paul simply laughed happily saying that the Chief Disciple still needed to eat and drink as others. He even said his mother appeared in a dream telling him that having a good employment was also a good means to contact others and spread the good news of Buddhism to others. With the help of the social worker in the half way house, Paul successfully found a job as a manual laborer in a nearby factory. He worked hard and was appreciated by his supervisor.

Six months later, Paul was promoted to a foreman on the manual labor team. Paul was deeply excited by this arrangement and promotion. His sense of integrity and uniqueness were successfully restored. Following this was a drastic decrease in the occurrence of grandiose hallucination and delusion. He no longer named himself as the Chief Disciple of the Buddha. Instead, he required us to call Forman Paul.

The attainment and self-confidence of Paul made him become an attractive young man with admiration from his female colleague as well female residents in the half way house. Finally, Paul fell in love with a female colleague who was a young and beautiful lady. With love and courtship, Paul had a strong determination to live a normal and fruitful live. Finally, he determined to live a normal life with indicators of a good wife, a good job, and a good home. He worked very hard to save a good sum of money to get married and rent a small flat for his sweet home. Two years later, they gave birth to a lovely baby boy. Paul assured that he was completely recovered, and from the time he moved out of the half way house, he was no longer dependent on psychiatric drugs and medication.

From Paul's case, it was clear that his symptom of psychosis, including grandiose identity, delusions, and hallucinations of being the Chief Disciple of the Buddha, was a delusive response to his highly oppressive environment. The delusive identity, Chief Disciple of the Buddha was clearly a symbol of grandiose power to fight his oppressive reality. By means of that, Paul affirmed that he had prevailing power to counteract the evil power in the world. In addition to that, it was also a way to unite with his deceased mother. In other words, in terms of a person with full respect, dignity, uniqueness and rights, the oppressive and frustrating reality, including the loss of his mother, bullying by his classmates, and oppression by his supervisors made him become an incomplete person. To make him complete, the only thing he could do was to construct his/her own delusive omnipotence in the grandiose delusive identity as a Chief Disciple of the Buddha in which he could use magical powers to get rid of his opponent and evil ones in his society, as well as reconnect with his deceased mother. In others words, in oppressive reality, his integrity, dignity, uniqueness and meaningfulness was deeply threatened to the degree his ontological security was evolved. To make him feel ontologically secure, the only way he could do this was to create a delusive reality and a delusive identity in which his integrity, dignity, uniqueness, and meaningfulness was delusively restored. That means, the only way to recover from his delusive identity and completeness was to provide an accretive, caring, and supportive reality in which he could actualize his sense of uniqueness, meaningfulness, integrity, and dignity realistically. The recovery of Paul was based on the following supportive, caring and respecting elements in his psychosocial environment.

1. The therapeutic community in which every resident in the house was respected and expected to make decisions, to participate and contribute their own view in the house
2. Paul was respected by other residents and workers in the half way house
3. Paul successfully found a job as a manual laborer in nearby factories with the help of the social worker in the half way house
4. Paul worked very hard and was deeply appreciated by his supervisors. Six months later, he was promoted to a foreman. He required others to call him Forman Paul.
5. He was attractive to other female colleagues and female residents in the half way house.
6. With love and courtship, he determined to live a normal and fruitful live.
7. He became a good husband and a good father.

All these certainly were crucial ingredients for the individual to rebuild his sense of a full human being with full integrity, dignity, rights, and responsibility in life. In Strauss' (1996) terms, they enabled Paul to regain his sense of subjectivity. They facilitated Paul to have a good mental integration in which he was free from bullying and oppression with a full sense of integrity in determining his choice, and actualizing his responsibility in life. They also helped Paul to dissolve amidst the onslaught of life, such as being bullied, rejected and isolated by others. It also implied that Paul could regain his/her sense of agency through being a full and responsible father, husband, worker, and resident in his life.

Existential and Phenomenological Explanation

In bridging Glass's internal but destructive power in psychotic times, and Foucault's external oppression due to overwhelming and circulatory power, an existential and phenomenological stance, proposed by Laing (1960) in his renowned book, Divided Self, can serve this purpose. He clearly described the ways an individual suffers from ontological insecurity because of external oppression in terms of engulfment, implosion, and depersonalization, which may gradually develop into schizophrenia in forms of self-splitting and self-fragmentation.

Laing's Ontological Security and Insecurity in Self-Splitting

Laing (1960) affirmed that self-splitting and self-fragmentation in people with schizophrenia originates from ontological insecurity from a highly humiliating social environment. His argument started with the emphasis of ontological security in normal human beings. Those who lack ontological security may have a sense of threatening of one's being. The sense of ontological insecurity, according to Laing, is a drive for self-splitting and the formation of embodied and unembodied selves.

Ontological Security in Normal Human Being

Laing (1960) stressed that the sense of ontological security is crucial for a mentally healthy individual.

> `The individual, then, may experience his own being as real, alive, whole; as differentiated from the rest of the world in ordinary circumstances so clearly that his identity and autonomy are never in question; as a continuum in time; as having an inner consistency, substantiality, genuineness, and worth; as spatially coexistent with the body, and usually, as having begun around our birth and liable to extinction with death. He thus has a firm core of ontological security.' (Laing, 1960: 41)

From Laing (1960) description, the sense of ontological security is actually a sense of existence and a sense of substantiality within the reality. It consists of the following component.

a) Experience his own being as real, alive, whole
b) Differentiation from rest of world
c) Clear and unquestionable identity and autonomy
d) Continuum in time (past, present and future)
e) Internal (inner consistency, substantiality, genuineness and worth)
f) Spatial co-existence with body (body and mind fusion)
g) Continue from birth to death, the whole life.

It is also a full sense of existence and being in which the individual can fully beware of his/her own unique self in terms of a clear self-identity, self worth and self-boundary. The sense of existence and being also contains a sense of agency in which the individual can fully exercise his/her own autonomy, perform what s/he needs and wants. It also includes a sense of substantiality with a good integration as well as an interaction among one's body, mind and related environment. It is also a sense of consistency of the individual's past, present and future. It is also a sense of cohesiveness in which the individual experiences his body, his mind and his environment as a highly cohesive whole.

That means, in phenomenological and existential terms, Laing's sense of ontological security is actually a full sense of existence and being. It consists of five elements:

1. A sense of uniqueness in one's self-identity, boundary and worth
2. A sense of agency in which one exercises ones' autonomy
3. A sense of substantiality of having an actual substance of one's body, mind, and related environment
4. A sense of consistency of one's past, present and future.
5. A sense of cohesiveness of the mind, body and externality.
6. A sense of integrity of being respected by oneself and others

Laing's articulation of sense of ontological security exercises within an interpersonal context.

> `That is to say, when two sane persons meet, there appears to be a reciprocal recognition of each other's identity. In this mutual recognition, there are the following basic elements:
>
> 1. I recognize the others to be the person he takes himself to be
> 2. He recognizes me to be the person I take myself to be' (Laing, 1960:35)
>
> `Within two (or more) persons are in relation, the behavior of each towards the other is mediated by the experience by each of the other, and the experience of each is mediated by the behavior of each. There is no contiguity between the behavior of one person and that of the other. Much human behavior can be seen as unilateral or bilateral attempts to eliminate experience. A person may treat another person as though he was not a person, and he may act, himself, as though he was not a person. There is no contiguity between one person's experience and another. My experience of you is always mediated through your behavior. Behavior that is the direct consequence of impact, as of one billiard-ball hitting another, or an experience directly transmitted to another experience, as in the possible cases of extra-sensory perception, is not personal.' (Laing, 1967:22)

Laing (1967, 1960) assumed that ontological security rests on an interpersonal context in which the individual recognizes another's existence by mediating others' behaviors within a spontaneous interpersonal interaction. However, every human being embraces an inherent tendency to eliminate other's behaviors, especially when other's existence creates a threat to one's sense of being. To preserve one's own sense of being, one needs to remove such a threat by eliminating his/her experiences with related threats. That means, within an interpersonal context, ontological security exists in a form of mutual recognition of one others' sense of uniqueness, agency, substantiality, and consistency.

> `Each has his own autonomous sense of identity and his own definition of whom and what he is. You are expected to be able to recognize me. That is, I am accustomed to expect that the person you take me to be, is me. And the identity that I reckon myself to have will coincide by and large.' (Laing, 1960: 36)

This sort of mutual recognition should also be found and spread to other related actors within individuals' social environment. All these can be briefly summarized in Figure 2.

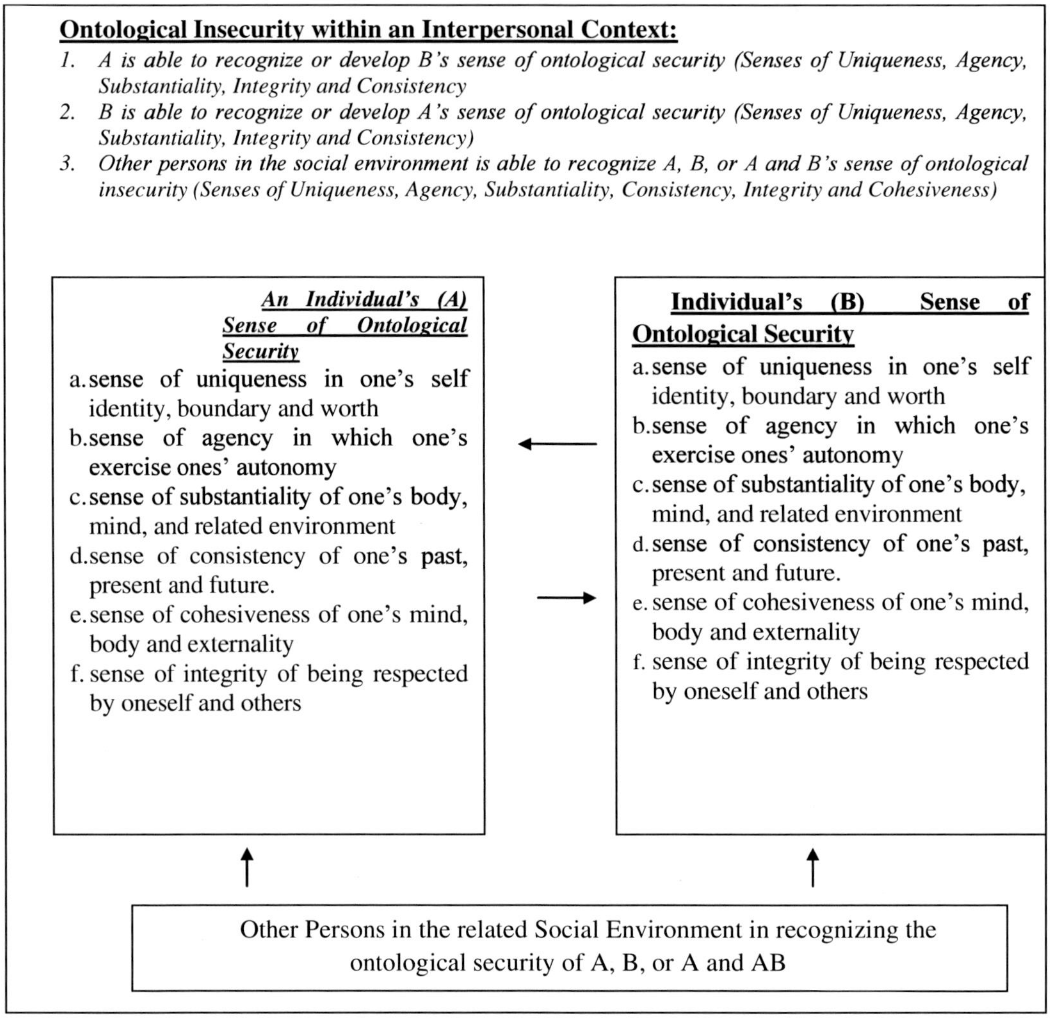

Figure 2. Full Sense of Ontological Insecurity within an Interpersonal Context in the Social Environment.

Full and Partial Ontological Security

Along Laing's line of thinking, a full sense of ontological insecurity can be regarded as an ideal condition aspired by the individual. In actual situation, various degrees of ontological security may occur. They can be roughly described in the following:

SA= Sense of ontological security owned by one individual (A). That includes SA1 (sense of uniqueness), SA2 (sense of agency), SA3 (sense of substantiality), SA4 (sense of consistency), SA5 (Sense of cohesiveness) and SA6 (Sense of Integrity)

SB= Sense of ontological security owned by another individual (B). That includes SB1 (sense of uniqueness), SB2 (sense of agency), SB3 (sense of substantiality), SB4 (sense of consistency), SB5 (sense of cohesiveness) and SB6 (Sense of Integrity)

ASB = Recognition of B's Sense of Ontological Security by A. That includes ASB1, ASB2, ASB3, ASB4, ASB5, & ASB6

BSA = Recognition of A's Sense of Ontological Security by B. That includes BSA1, BSA2, BSA3, BSA4, BSA5, & BSA6

OSAB= Recognition of A and B's sense of ontological insecurity by others. That includes OSAB1, OSB2, OSB3, OSB4, OSB5, & OSB6.

1. Full sense of Ontological Security in interpersonal context (Full SAB)

Full SAB = SA + SB + ASB + BSA + OSAB

It means that the individual can obtain a full sense of ontological security in interpersonal context, within which both his/her significant others (family members, peers, colleagues), as well as members in the community, all enable him/her to have a full sense of uniqueness, agency, substantiality, consistency and cohesiveness. In doing so, the individual also enable others to have a full sense of agency, substantiality, consistency and cohesiveness. This is an idealistic supportive social environment in which all related members are respectable, supportive and encouraging to one another.

2. Moderate sense of Ontological Security in interpersonal context (Substantial SAB)

Moderate SAB (without support by others) = SA+ SB + ASB + BSA

In actual reality, a full sense of ontological security can only be idealistic and temporary within certain situations; the individual can normally obtain a partial sense of ontological security within an interpersonal context. That means, the individual can have a full sense of uniqueness, agency, substantiality, cohesiveness and consistency.

In the same way, his/her significant others including his/her peers, family members, and colleagues can also give him/her a full sense of uniqueness, agency, substantiality, cohesiveness and consistency. In doing so, s/he can also enable his/her significant others a sense of uniqueness, agency, substantiality, cohesiveness and consistency. However, that sort of mutual support only occurs within the individual and his/her significant others but not with others in each interpersonal context. That means, while s/he has mutual support and ontological security with his most supportive colleague within his/her work context, s/he may not obtain similar support from other colleagues. In some cases, other colleagues may even be oppressive. Nevertheless, the mutual supportive relationship between him/her and his/her supportive colleague is sufficient enough for them to establish their own senses of uniqueness, agency, substantiality, cohesiveness and consistency.

3. Partial sense of ontological security in interpersonal context (Partial SAB)

Partial SAB (with no current support by other and significant others) = SA + SB + ASB/BSA

Within interpersonal context in interacting with one's significant others, there may be miscommunication, conflict and argument. Thus, at one time, one may try to forgive and accept another one. For example, A misunderstands B and then B forgives and accepts A. At the other time, s/he may need the other's acceptance and forgiveness. That means, B may have done something wrong and then A forgives and accepts B. Apart from his/her significant others, the individual does not have others to obtain his/her sense of ontological security, the individual's own senses of uniqueness, agency, substantiality, cohesiveness and consistency (SA or SB) may need to rely on prolonged memories and recall previous mutual supportive and intimate relationships with this significant others. So that one side (either A or B) can temporarily sacrifice his/her own current need of ontological security to provide support, acceptance and forgiveness to the other side with a hope that sooner or later, the mutual supportive relationship can be restored. Thus, a partial sense of ontological security implies a mildly unstable state of ontological security that needs to be strengthened to affirm a better sense of interpersonal ontological security and feeling of being.

4. *Thin Ontological security in intrapersonal context = SA/SB without support and recognition.*

This is a difficult situation, where no one trusts or supports the individual in related environments. That means, significant others may fail to provide the individual with senses of agency, uniqueness, substantiality, cohesiveness and consistency. Fortunately, the individual's significant others do not oppress, isolate, bully or neglect the individual. They simply cannot provide a sense of ontological insecurity for the individual. In other words, if two people are interacting with one another, they are interacting without mutual understanding, encouraging and supporting one another. They interact with one another for the sake of causal normal greetings or for a certain purpose, such as to accomplish a task or to perform some social functioning. Within this sort of social interaction, both parties' sense of ontological security is not facilitated. Instead, they interact with one another without warmth, genuineness and empathy. In the long run, a sense of thin ontological security is not a stable condition; the individual may feel uncomfortable interacting with a close friend, intimate family member, or a close working peer. Both parties within the interaction may expect better communication, understanding and support to one another. For various reasons, they cannot do so. In that case, both of them must sustain their own sense of ontological security rather than obtaining it from others. In fact, this would be an unstable state in which the individual strives for a partial sense or moderate sense of ontological security in interpersonal context with his/her significant others and other members in various social contexts.

Ontological Insecurity

Ontological insecurity implies that the individual's senses of uniqueness, agency, consistency, substantiality and cohesiveness are being threatened. It consists of several stages:

A. Poor condition and gradual loss of senses of uniqueness, agency, cohesiveness, consistency, integrity and substantiality.
B. Minimal levels of ontological security by sacrificing any one of the senses of uniqueness, agency, cohesiveness, consistency, integrity and substantiality to maintain the basic level of the other four senses in ontological security.

C. Risky level of ontological security by sacrificing any two of senses of uniqueness, agency, cohesiveness, consistency, integrity, and substantiality to maintain the basic level of the other three senses in ontological security.
D. Initial levels of ontological insecurity by sacrificing any three senses of uniqueness, agency, cohesiveness, consistency, integrity, and substantiality to maintain the basic level of the other two senses in ontological security (pre-morbid state in schizophrenia; development of the un-embodied self)
E. Moderate level of ontological insecurity by developing any one or two faulty/delusive senses of uniqueness, agency, cohesiveness, consistency, integrity and substantiality to substitute the actual loss of any one or two senses. As a result, the individual develops a delusive sense of ontological security. (Explicit state of divided self, prevailing manifestation of schizophrenia with clear self-splitting.)
F. Severe level of ontological insecurity by developing any three to four faulty/delusive senses of uniqueness, agency, cohesiveness, consistency, integrity and substantiality to substitute the actual loss of any three to four senses. As a consequence, the individual develops a severely delusive sense of ontological security (high manifestation of first rank symptoms, severe regressive negative symptoms in schizophrenia with complicated molar and molecular self-fragmentation)

The writer tries to elaborate these stages of ontological insecurity as follows:

A. Poor condition and gradual loss of senses of uniqueness, agency, cohesiveness, consistency and substantiality.

Laing (1960) defines ontological insecurity as follows:

`The individual in the ordinary circumstance of living may feel more unreal than real; in the literal sense, more dead than alive; precariously differentiated from the rest of the world, so that his identity and autonomy are always in question. He may lack the experience of his own temporary continuity. He may not possess an over-riding sense of personal consistency or cohesiveness. He may feel more insubstantial than substantial, and unable to assume that the stuff he is made of is genuine, good and valuable. He may also feel his self as being partially divorced from this body. (Laing, 1960: 42).

According to Laing (1960), a sense of ontological insecurity consists of the following:

a) feel unreal more that real (poor substantiality)
b) more dead than alive (poor integrity and agency)
c) questioning in identity and autonomy (loss of uniqueness)
d) lack of one's own experience (loss of agency and integrity)
e) temporary rather than continuity (loss of consistency)
f) lack of consistency and cohesiveness (loss of consistency and cohesiveness)
g) insubstantial more than substantial (loss of substantiality)
h) divorce self partially from body (loss of cohesiveness)
i) unable to assume genuineness, value and goodness in oneself (loss of sense of agency and integrity)

That means ontological insecurity begins with a gradual loss or poor condition of the following:

Gradual Loss and poor condition of ontological security in oppressive interpersonal context = Poor SA or SB being continuously oppressed, humiliated and isolated by others members. It is a:

Gradual loss and poor condition of sense of agency (Poor S1)
Gradual loss and poor condition of sense of uniqueness (Poor S2)
Gradual loss and poor condition of sense of cohesiveness (Poor S3)
Gradual loss and poor condition of sense of consistency (Poor S4)
Gradual loss and poor condition of sense of substantiality (Poor S5)
Gradual loss and poor condition of sense of integrity (Post S 6)

Facing all these losses, the individual faces an ontological threat that his/her sense of existence and being will be diminished. Thus, the individual will struggle for his/her survival. It is a kind of existential and phenomenological survival in which the individual has to safeguard his/her minimal state of existence as well as a spontaneous sense that s/he is still there without being diminished by others in the immediate environment. That means, the individual may try all means to obtain ontological security to preserve his/her sense of being and existence. Laing (1960) described the struggle for ontological sense of security as follows:

> `To anticipate, we can say that in the individual whose own being is secure in this primarily experiential sense, relatedness with other is potentially gratifying; whereas the ontologically insecure person is preoccupied with preserving rather than gratifying himself: the ordinary circumstances of living threaten his low threshold of security...If the individual cannot take the realness, aliveness, autonomy and identity of himself and others for granted, then he has to become absorbed in contriving ways of trying to be real, of keeping himself or others alive, of preserving his identity, in efforts, as he will often put it, to prevent himself from losing his self. What are to most everyday happenings, which are hardly noticed because they have no special significance, may become deeply significant in so far as they either contribute to the sustenance of the individual's being or threaten him with no-being' (Laing, 1960: 42-43)

B. Minimal level of ontological security by sacrificing any one of the senses of uniqueness, agency, cohesiveness, consistency and substantiality to maintain the basic level of the other four senses in ontological security.

In other words, facing the gradual loss and poor condition of senses of uniqueness, agency, consistency, substantiality as well as consistency, the individual tries every means to regain all these senses. In doing so, s/he may even sacrifice part of these senses to pretend further deterioration and losses of ontological insecurity. For example, a person may sacrifice his/her sense of agency in order to prevent further deterioration of senses of substantiality, consistency, uniqueness and cohesiveness. This can be illustrated in the following case.

`A was a personal secretary of a Chief Executive Officer in a large company. Her boss trusted her very much and delegated executive power for her to make important decisions while her boss was on holiday and on business trips. As she had been working in this company for more than a decade, A had a very good sense of ontological security in her work.

She could easily exercise her sense of agency by imposing order and command from her boss to other subordinates. She had very good sense of consistency as she had been in this position for many years and her boss respected and trusted her constantly. She also harbored a good sense of substantiality as her work and position could exert substantial influence on her colleagues and company. She had a very good sense of belonging to her company and her boss and she were really committed to the benefit and profit of the company. Thus she also embraced a good sense of cohesiveness.

Her happy, meaningful and committed working environment was recently threatened by the retirement of her boss. The new Chief Executive Officers was a young man who intended to change the whole company from a conservative team management style to a new innovative goal directed and competitive based management. A was no longer trusted by this new boss. Her sense of ontological security and sense of being in her company was deteriorating.

To regain her minimal sense of security, she sacrificed her sense of agency. Instead of asking for delegation of authority from her boss to impose command on others, she tried her very best to be submissive and obedient by asking her boss for every decision and command. She simply transferred her boss's memo or e-mail to others. She became a puppet of her boss. She hoped that all these could help her to secure a basic level of ontological security in terms of minimal level of senses of uniqueness (only she could follow her boss' command strictly), cohesiveness (she was very obedient and loyal to the boss and to the company), substantiality (she actually carried out every refined details given by her boss closely) and consistency (she was still an effective secretary in the past, present and in the future).'

In this case, it is clear that A tried to sacrifice her sense of agency so that she could safeguard her minimal level of sense of uniqueness, cohesiveness, substantiality, and consistency. That means the sense of ontological insecurity may begin with a gradual loss of sense of ontological security in terms of sense of being and existence. Then, it gradually reaches a state where the individual needs to keep a minimal level of sense of being in order to ensure the sense of existence and being can be sustained. It also ensures that individual self-system can be maintained in a low level of survival. As the external oppression, humiliation and isolation still prevails. Then the individual needs to sacrifice part of his/her sense of being to maintain this minimal level of survival.

Minimal level of ontological security in oppressive interpersonal context = Minimal SA/SB by sacrificing any one of the elements in sense of existence and being. It can be:

Minimal SA/SB by sacrificing S1 to maintain a survival level of S2, S3, S4, S5 and S6
Minimal SA/SB by sacrificing S2 to maintain a survival level of S1, S3, S4, S5 and S6
Minimal SA/SB by sacrificing S3 to maintain a survival level of S1, S2, S4, S5 and S6
Minimal SA/SB by sacrificing S4 to maintain a survival level of S1, S2, S3, S5 and S6
Minimal SA/SB by sacrificing S5 to maintain a survival level of S1, S2, S3, S4 and S6
Minimal SA/SB by sacrificing S6 to maintain a survival level of S1, S2, S3, S4 and S5

C. Risky level of ontological security by sacrificing any two of the senses of uniqueness, agency, cohesiveness, consistency, and substantiality to maintain the basic level of the other three senses in ontological security.

In the minimal level of ontological security in oppressive interpersonal context, the individual tries to sacrifice any two of the senses of uniqueness, agency, cohesiveness, consistency, and substantiality to maintain the basic level of the other three senses of ontological security. This can be represented by the following:

Risky level of ontological security in oppressive interpersonal context = Risky SA/SB by sacrificing any two elements in the sense of existence and being. It can be:

Risky SA/SB by sacrificing S1 & S2 to maintain a survival level to S3, S4, S5 & S6
Risky SA/SB by sacrificing S1 & S3 to maintain a survival level to S2, S4, S5 & S6
Risky SA/SB by sacrificing S2 & S3 to maintain a survival level to S1, S4, S5 & S6
Risky SA/SB by sacrificing S1 & S4 to maintain a survival level to S2, S3, S5 & S6
Risky SA/SB by sacrificing S3 & S4 to maintain a survival level to S1, S2, S5 & S6
Risky SA/SB by sacrificing S1 & S5 to maintain a survival level to S2, S3, S4 & S6
Risky SA/SB by sacrificing S2 & S4 to maintain a survival level to S1, S3, S5 & S6
Risky SA/SB by sacrificing S2 & S5 to maintain a survival level to S1, S3, S4 & S6
Risky SA/SB by sacrificing S3 & S5 to maintain a survival level to S1, S2, S4 & S6
Risky SA/SB by sacrificing S4 & S5 to maintain a survival level to S1, S2, S3 & S6
Risky SA/SB by sacrificing S1 & S6 to maintain a survival level to S2, S3, S4 & S5
Risky SA/SB by sacrificing S2 & S6 to maintain a survival level to S1, S3, S4 & S5
Risky SA/SB by sacrificing S3 & S6 to maintain a survival level to S1, S2, S4 & S5
Risky SA/SB by sacrificing S4 & S6 to maintain a survival level to S1, S2, S3 & S5
Risky SA/SB by sacrificing S5 & S6 to maintain a survival level to S1, S2, S3 & S4

At that level, the individual is actually in a highly risky situation to maintain a substantial, unique, consistent, cohesive and able sense of being and existence. S/he is caught in a dilemma. S/he is highly aspired for external recognition, support, comfort and care so that s/he can try his/her very best to increase his/her sense of ontological security. In doing so, s/he becomes highly vulnerable to external influence. That means, external oppression and condemnation can easily create intensive harm and hurt to the individual.

D. Initial level of ontological insecurity by sacrificing any three to four senses of uniqueness, agency, cohesiveness, consistency and substantiality to maintain the basic level of other two senses in ontological security (pre-morbid state in schizophrenia; development of un-embodied self).

In this stage, the individual actually enters an initial stage of ontological insecurity. His/her intense urge to connect and relate to others in the external environment so as to gain support and recognition makes him/her become highly vulnerable to external oppression. That means, while s/he is expecting support, recognition and comfort to restore his/her senses of uniqueness, agency, consistency and substantiality from others, the individual is actually encountering someone that is highly oppressive, humiliating and ignoring him/her. The more intimate the oppressive other is to the individual, the more destructive the relationship becomes and the more the individual feels ontologically insecure. Laing (1960) affirmed that oppressive interpersonal environment, which contributes to the sense of ontological insecurity, might consist of three important elements:

1. Engulfment (being swallowed and suffocated by oppressive others)
2. Implosion (Being provoked and suppressed by oppressive others)
3. Petrification and Depersonalization (Regarded as lifeless object and ....
   (Laing, 1960:43-47)

Engulfment, implosion, and depersonalization, in the sense of ontological insecurity, can be related to the above-mentioned six senses in ontological security. Briefly speaking, engulfment is the denial and deprivation of one's sense of uniqueness and consistency. Implosion is a denial and deprivation of one's sense of agency and cohesiveness. Depersonalization is a denial and deprivation of one's sense of substantiality and integrity. All of them have a crucial impact in putting one's sense of ontological security into risk and generating one's sense of ontological insecurity. They can be briefly described in figures below.

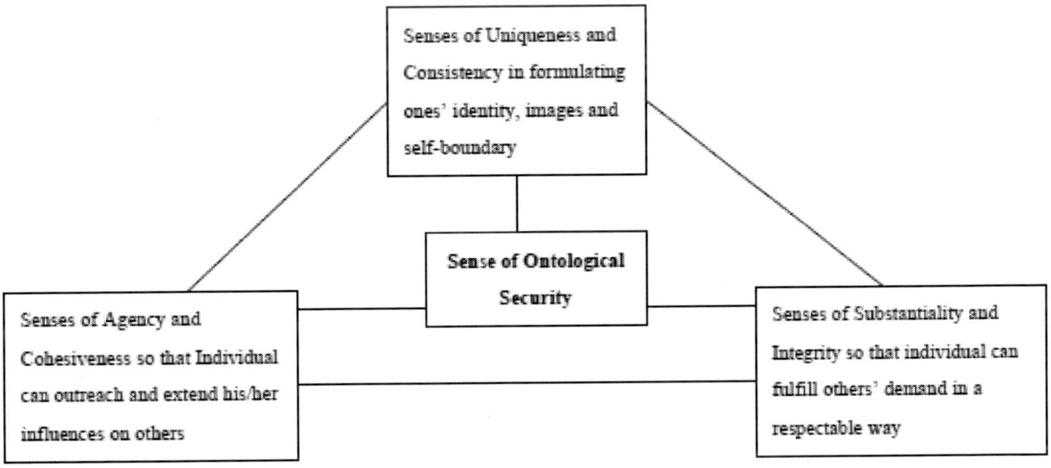

Figure 3. Elements of Ontological Security.

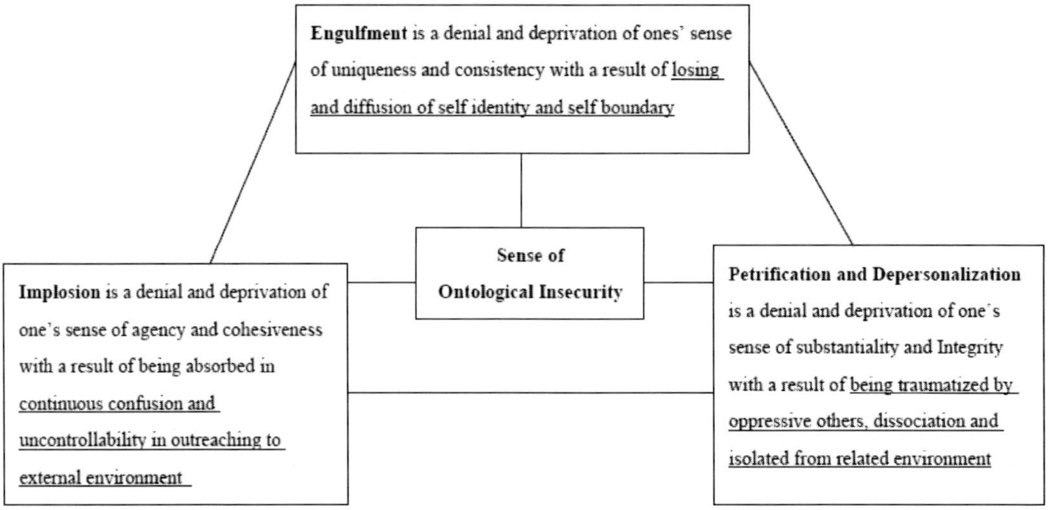

Figure 4. Elements of Sense of Ontological Insecurity.

Engulfment

Engulfment implies that the individual's sense of his/her own autonomy is taken away by intrusive, controlling, and manipulative others. In an actual situation, it can be an overwhelming mother, a highly oppressive boss, a bullying peer, or a humiliating teacher. All these significant others cannot provide any sense of uniqueness and consistency to the individual. That means, the individual's identity and self-boundary cannot be formulated, sustained or maintained by engulfing others. Instead, engulfment is a denial and deprivation of ones' sense of uniqueness and consistency. That means, the individual encounters highly oppressive significant others that do not allow him/her to demonstrate or exercise his/her own will, decision and behaviors. In doing so, the individual's image, identity, and autonomy is hindered and suppressed. Consequently, the individual's sense of uniqueness is suppressed and suffocated. In addition to that, his sense of consistency is also deeply affected. In fact, every individual has a strong urge to preserve his sense of uniqueness. S/he always harbored a strong urge that himself/herself could have a chance or opportunity to achieve a sense of uniqueness and distinctive identity in the future even though experiences in the past or the present are unfavorable. In other situations, unpleasant past experiences make the individual feel that the present pleasant experience is not realistic, s/he may still fixate in the unhappy past. To maintain a sense of consistency, the individual may tend to assume the following:

1. the past, the present and the future are unhappy and my sense of existence and being is denied
2. the past, the present and the future are unhappy and my sense of existence and being is preserved

In fact, in the normal situation, both assumptions are too optimistic or too pessimistic. Thus, a good sense of consistency should be the following:

1. Despite my unhappy past experience, there is still a chance to have a satisfactory present and a better future. Thus, I must try my best to attain it.

2. Despite my painful present moment, there are still good memories of past experiences that can sustain my pursuit for a better future.

Nevertheless, a highly engulfing significant other may tend to suffocate the individual's unique strength, will and power to actualize the above two assumptions. Instead, s/he tends to make the individual conclude that only with a total dependence on the significant other; s/he can ensure a good present and a good future.

Laing (1960) defined engulfment as follows:

> `A firm sense of one's own autonomous identity is required in order that one may be related as one human being to another, otherwise every relationship threatens the individual with loss of identity. One form this takes can be called engulfment. In this the individual dreads relatedness as such with anyone or anything, or indeed, even with himself, because of uncertainty about the stability of his autonomy and identity.

In other words, while one needs to validate and develop his/her sense of identity, autonomy by relating to others, his/her interpersonal interaction threatens his/her own sense of identity and autonomy.

Engulfment can exist in two ways. It can be engulfment by hate or by love.

> `Engulfment is felt as a risk in being understood (thus grasped, comprehended) in being loved, or even simply in being seen. To be hated may be feared for other reasons, but to be hated as such is often less disturbing than to be destroyed, as it is felt, through being engulfed by love. The main maneuvre is used to preserve identity under pressure from the dread of engulfment is isolation.

Engulfment by hate means that individual's significant others are highly critical and intrusive. No matter how hard the individual tries, and how much effort the individual has input in performing any task, s/he is still being criticized, teased and bullied by his/her significant others. Facing such highly critical and intrusive significant others, the individual may try all means to escape and isolate from them. However, because of various reasons, the engulfing others (parents, spouses, relatives, close peers) embraces ways to control and manipulate the individual (child, husband or wife, relative or peer) so that the individual must become closed and follow their command and instruction. That means the individual's sense of uniqueness in terms of unique identity, images, and boundaries are all defeated by intrusive and prevailing negative comments from his/her significant others. Also, his/her sense of good consistency is being threatened. From his/her intrusive and critical significant others, what s/he can obtain is only a negative sense of consistency. S/he may think that no matter how hard s/he tries; s/he will not be appreciated or even accepted by his/her significant others. Although s/he always harbors a wish that this time, or the other time, his/her performance will be uniquely accepted, respected and appreciated by his/her significant others, s/he failed every time in making him/her feel s/he is only inconsistently failed, his/her glimpse of hope of success is getting thinner and thinner as times goes by.

The second type of engulfment is by love in which the individual encounters important attachment figures in which, in fact, they care and love the individual. Nevertheless, they love and care the individual so much that emotionally, they are enmeshed with him/her. That means, unconsciously or consciously they use love to manipulate, control and even suffocate the individual. In terms of overwhelming love, they may prevailingly protect the individual from any decision, performance and actions in his/her own rights. The individual gradually loses his/her own senses of competence and experience in making his/her own decision, pursuing his/her own path, and actualizing his/her talents and performing his/her own attainment. Every time the individual intends to do so, s/he will be reminded by his/her significant others that s/he needs their help and assistance. The love engulfing significant others insist that their help is very necessary as they are struggling for the best of the individual. They justify and moralize that this is the only way to protect the individual from any harm and hurt from making the wrong decision, doing wrong things, getting along with unhealthy peers, and having a good future. In terms of intensive love and care, they remind the individual of every refined detail in doing anything. They feel intensely insecure and worry when the individual is alone, away or doing anything out of their control and experience. As a consequence, the individual is unable to develop a sufficient sense of uniqueness in terms of his/her unique self-image, self-identity and self-confidence. On the one hand, s/he harbors a strong urge to be autonomous and independent from his/her love-engulfing others. On the other hand, s/he does not have experiences, competence and encouragement to make his/her own decision, pursue his/her path, and attain his/her own achievement. S/he argues and struggles with his/her love-engulfing others for not being able to be autonomous and independent; however, s/he is psychologically, socially and mentally dependent on them. His/her good sense of consistency is deeply disturbed. Instead of thinking that s/he actually has the ability to make his/her decision, perform his/her own task and achieve his own autonomy, s/he may be trapped into the following thinking:

1. No matter how hard I try, I still need to be dependent on my beloved others in making decisions, performing tasks and achieving anything.
2. I do not like to be controlled by my beloved others, however, I cannot be alone as I need them to guide my way.
3. I earnestly hope to be autonomous in the present and in the future, but I am afraid I cannot do so. Also, I am not prepared to do so.

In extreme cases, *the engulfment can both be love and hate engulfment happening together to the individual.* That can occur in several forms.

a) One significant other is love engulfing to the individual and another significant others is hate engulfing to the individual. (For example, the father is love engulfing but the mother is hate engulfing to the individual.)
b) The significant other is at one time love engulfing to the individual and at another time, s/he is hate engulfing to the individual. (For example, the significant other is love engulfing to the individual while s/he is young and the significant other is hate engulfing to the individual while s/he is an adolescent. Also, the significant others can be highly fluctuating in their attitude towards the individual. At one time they are love engulfing. At another time, they are hate engulfing).
c) In interacting with the individual, the significant others may appear as love engulfing. However, underlying this is actually hate engulfing to the individual or vice versa. (For example, a stepmother may appear as highly loving engulfing to this stepson. Underlying her love engulfing is actually a hate-engulfing motive to

manipulate and to minimize the stepson's development of unique self-boundary, self-identity and self-image.)

In the actual situation, the love-hate engulfment is even more destructive than either hate or love engulfment. In hate engulfment, his/her significant other spontaneously criticizes the individual, where the individual's sense of uniqueness and consistency is ruined within the prevailing hate and criticism. In love engulfment, the individual is continuously enmeshed by the significant others to a stage or to an extent that s/he feels that s/he needs to depend on his/her significant others to accomplish any related tasks or performance or make any decisions. In both cases, the individual, despite being engulfed, still has a constant pattern in interacting with his/her significant others. In love engulfment, the individual is accustomed to be dependent on overwhelming love. Regardless of being engulfed by his/her significant others, s/he still knows that his/her significant others love him/her. To some extent, s/he still enjoys the feeling of being loved. In hate engulfment, the individual is used to being hated or severely criticized by others. Regardless of being hated, the individual still knows that s/he must struggle for his/her own survival and self-appreciation. However, in the love-hate engulfment, the individual, despite being engulfed, is deeply puzzled by the unstable and confused relationship with his/her significant others. On one side, s/he may feel that s/he is being loved. On the other side, s/he may feel that s/he is being hated. The love and hate dilemma makes the feeling of being engulfed and swallowed highly confused, complicated and dynamic. The senses of losing uniqueness and consistency can be easily expressed by the individual in love or hate-engulfment, since the attitude of significant others are clear and consistent. Instead of being fixated by thinking that s/he is not worthy of love or adequate enough to be independent, the individual fluctuates between these extremes. *As a consequence the individual becomes far more vulnerable to self-fragmentation and fracture in prolonged fluctuating extremes and polarization of self-images.*

Facing prolonged and prevailing experiences of being engulfed, in particular love-engulfing ones, individuals may easily be trapped within *a dilemma that s/he is either completely lost by being engulfed by others or completely isolated from others.*

> Thus, instead of the polarities of separateness and relatedness based on individual autonomy, there is the antithesis between complete loss of being by absorption into the other person (engulfment), and complete aloneness (isolation). There is no safe third possibility of a dialectical relationship between two persons, both sure of their own ground, and by this very basis, able to 'lose' themselves in each other. (Laing, 1960:42)

That means the individual, in facing prolonged engulfment by his/her significant others, no longer has confidence in building up his/her own sense of uniqueness and consistency constructively. S/he feels highly inadequate and powerless in negotiating with his/her engulfing others to develop his/her own sense of uniqueness and consistency. All s/he can do is either be completely engulfed or absorbed by others or be isolated from his/her love engulfing significant others. However, both cases are dreadful options for the individual. Being totally engulfed by others means that one would finally surround his/her sense of self-image, identity and boundary to others. Being isolated from others implies that s/he is unable to contact others in the actual reality so that s/he can obtain the necessary ingredients for his/her growth and development in formulating a decent self-image, identity and boundary.

> If a man hates himself, he may wish to lose himself in the other: then being engulfed by the other is an escape from himself. In the present case it is an ever-present possibility to be dreaded. (Laing, 1960: 44)

To avoid being engulfed or swallowed by others, individuals may use the technique of being detached and isolated from others. However, this self-isolation may lead to complete isolation with a dreadful feeling of dying inside, and a profound emptiness that is unbearable for the individual. Laing (1960) illustrated this by the case of James.

> 'Other people were necessary for his existence, said James. Another patient, with the same dilemma, behaved in the following way: he maintained himself in isolated detachment from the world for several months, living alone in a single room, existing frugally on low savings, daydreaming. But in doing this, he began to feel he was dying inside; he was becoming more and more empty, and observed a progressive impoverishment of my life mode.' (Laing, 1960: 53)

The dreadful feeling of emptiness and loneliness made James need to go outside his inner vacuum by relating to others. However, once he related with others, he might immediately feel trapped or engulfed by others again with immense feelings of frightened hopelessness, suspicion and shame. In other words, James was trapped within a vicious cycle of detachment with dreadful feelings of loneliness and emptiness, and engulfment with an intolerable sense of frightened hopelessness, suspicion and shame.

In other words, the *individual is trapped within a vicious cycle of the more s/he tries to compensate for his/her senses of autonomy and identity by relating and expecting others' recognition, support and appreciation, the more s/he becomes vulnerable and engulfed by others who are actually oppressive, humiliating and manipulative.* Since the individual may not be able to encounter supportive others, thus, even though s/he is being oppressed, humiliated, and manipulated by others, s/he still expects that his/her significant others can change from oppressive to supportive, from humiliating to appreciating as well as from manipulative to respective. However, all these are only individuals' unrealistic expectation with a result of becoming more dependent and more engulfed by his/her oppressive significant others. As a consequence, s/he may harbor a strong risk of being totally engulfed, swallowed, and intruded upon by others in a way, his sense of uniqueness (in terms of unique identity, position and autonomy) and the sense of consistency will be denied and lost.

> `Thus, the man who is frightened of his own subjectivity being swamped, impinged upon, or kill the other persons' subjectivity. The process involves a vicious cycle. The more the one attempts to preserve one's autonomy and identity by nullifying the specific human individuality of the other, the more it is felt to be necessary to continue to do so, because with each denial of the other person's ontological status, one's own ontological security is decreased, the threat to the self from the other is potentiated and hence has to be even more desperately negated.' (Laing, 1960: 52)

In many ways, these experiences are dreadful and inescapable. The individual may delusively felt or unconsciously disturbed by dreams in which *there are images representing the dread of being engulfed.* They are images of:

- being buried
- being drowned
- being caught
- being dragged down into quick sand
- fire recurs repeatedly
  (Laing, 1960: 42-45)

Laing (1960) further affirmed that all these images and dreams imply a deep suffocation of one's aliveness and uniqueness. Individuals with schizophrenia *`say in the acute phase that they are on fire and that their bodies are being burnt up'.* One describes himself/herself as cold and dry. S/he desperately looks for warmth or wetness. He will be engulfed by the fire of the water, and either way will be destroyed. (Laing, 1960). Medard Boss (1957) gives examples of several dream of psychosis. In one, the dreamer is engulfed by fire:

> `A women of hardly thirty years dreamt, at a time, when she still felt completely healthy, that she was on fire in the stables. Around her, the fire, an even large crust of lava was forming. Half from the outside and half from the inside of her body she could see how the fire was slowly becoming choked by this crust. ... Suddenly, she was entirely outside the fire, and, as if possessed, she beat the fire with a club to break into the crust and to let some air in. But the dreamer soon got tired and slowly she (the fire) became extinguished. Four days after this dream she suffered from acute schizophrenia. In the details of the dream the dreamer had exactly predicted the special course of her psychosis. She became rigid at first, and, in effect, encysted. Six weeks afterwards she defended herself once more with all her might against the choking of her life's fire, until finally she became completely extinguished both spiritually and mentally. (Boss, 1975: 62; Laing, 1960: 50).

In this case, it is clear that the woman faced a strong sense of being engulfed. Her whole body was on fire. Fire seemed to swallow her whole body. Together with this was a crust of lava that might imply she was being dissolved by the fire (the engulfment). She felt suffocated and choked by the over-whelming fire. It symbolized that she was taken over by engulfment. She tried to break into the crust to breathe in some air. However, no matter how hard she tried, she felt fatigued and tired. In other words, no matter how she tried to secure, restore and build up his/her sense of uniqueness, and consistency, she failed and the fire extinguished her implying that she was totally engulfed by her significant others. That was why four days later, she suffered from acute schizophrenia. Six weeks later, similar dreams occurred, in which she again defended herself from related choking with the fire. The putting off of fire meant that she was both spiritually and mentally engulfed with a total loss of psychic energy to struggle for the sense of ontological security in terms of maintaining her minimal sense of uniqueness and consistency.

To avoid the complete loss of being and engulfment by others, the individual may enter into a state of self-engulfment. That means, when she is engulfed by others s/he delusively thinks that no can control him/her, only s/he can control himself/herself (self-engulfment).

Also, when s/she is detached from others, s/he may delusively think that s/he still controls or manipulates others.

Constant self-engulfment and engulfing others makes the individual highly vulnerable to external threats and his/her self-identity and boundaries highly loose and diffused. In doing so, the individual may gradually become confused in his/her self-identity and boundary. That means, the individual may enter into a state of self confusion in terms of:

1. Ingredients (thought, feelings, body) inside the self system may flow outside and merge with external objects, events and persons (thought broadcasting, or merging one's identity and body part with the external environment or supernatural forces)
2. Ingredients (object, events, persons) in the environment crush in and merge with the inner self system (thought insertion and intense fear in facing external objects, or body parts being stolen by others)
3. External objects and internal self ingredients are in and out and mix together (two delusive voices, objects, or figures fighting with one another inside one's body.

All these can be shown in Figure 5.

Engulfment implies that individual's sense of own autonomy is taken away by intrusive, controlling and manipulative others

Engulfment by Hate	Engulfment by Love
Individual's significant others are highly critical and intrusive. No matter, how hard the individual tries and how much effort the individual has input in performing any task, s/he is still being criticized and oppressed	The individual's attachment figures love and care the individual so much that they enmeshed with him/her. They unconsciously or consciously they use love to manipulate and suffocate him/her

Difficulties in Developing Sense of Uniqueness and Sense of Consistency

The Engulfing Others (Hate or Love or both) take over individual's chance and experiences as well as competence to exercise his/her will and autonomy, build up or actualize his self image and identity, in the past, present and future

Struggle of Autonomy and Further Dependence The more the individual tries to compensate his/her senses of autonomy and identity by relating and expecting others' recognition, support and appreciation, the more s/he becomes vulnerable and being engulfed by others

↓

Dilemma of Complete Loss of Being Engulfed by Others or Completely Isolated from Others

The individual feels highly inadequate and powerless in negotiating with his/her engulfing others for developing his/her own senses of uniqueness and consistency. All s/he can do is either completely engulfed by others or isolate from his/her love-engulfing others

↓

Vicious Cycle of Detachment, Relating and Fear of Engulfment with Others

The dreadful feeling of emptiness and loneliness in self isolation make one needs to go outside his inner vacuum by relating to others. However, once s/he relates with others, he immediately feels being trapped or engulfed by others again with an immense feelings of frightened hopelessness, suspicion and shame. S/he is trapped within a vicious cycle of continuous detachment and engulfment

↓

Self Engulfment and Engulfing Others

To avoid the complete loss of being and engulfment by others, individual may enter into a state of self engulfment. That means, when she is engulfed by others s/he delusively thinks that no one can control him/her, only s/he can control himself/herself (self engulfment). Also, when s/she is detached from other, s/he may delusively think that s/he still controls or manipulates others

↓

Gradual Diffusion of Self Identity and Self Boundary

Constant self engulfment and engulfing others make the individual becomes highly vulnerable to external threat. His/her self identity and boundaries are highly loose and diffused. In doing so, the individual may become confused in his/her self identity and boundary. That means, individual may enter into a state of self confusion in terms of:

1. Ingredients (thought, feelings, body) inside self system flow outside and merge with external objects, events and persons (thought broadcasting, or merge one identity and body part with external environment or supernatural forces)
2. Ingredients (object, events, persons) in environment crush and merge with the inner self system (thought insertion and intense fear in facing external objects, or body part being stolen by others)
3. External objects and internal self ingredients are in and out and mix together (two delusive voices, objects, or figures fighting with one another inside one's body

Figure 5. Engulfment and Gradual Diffusion of Self-Identity and Self-Boundary.

Implosion

According to Laing (1960), apart from engulfment, ontological insecurity is also a result of implosion and depersonalization. Within existential and phenomenological articulation, engulfment should be a denial and deprivation of ones' sense of uniqueness and consistency with a result of losing and diffusion of self-identity and self-boundary. *Implosion is a denial and deprivation of one's sense of agency and cohesiveness with a result of being absorbed in continuous confusion and uncontrollability in outreaching to the external environment.* Implosion is a state of mind in which the individual feels that sooner or later, the whole external reality will be crashing in on him/her with a severe risk or threat that the individual's sense of existence will sooner or later be shattered. The individual tries to push back all these crushing forces, but s/he fails. Thus, his/her senses of agency and cohesiveness are under intensive challenge. *In normal threats or usual stress*, the individual may be able to exercise his/her psychic energy in pushing back, by a full fledge exercise of his/her sense of agency, in changing the adverse external environment or pushing back at least an external position and space for his/her own survival and existence. The more cohesive the individual is in perceiving himself/herself, the more focused the pushing force in facing the external threat and risks. Nevertheless, *in facing insurmountable, prevailing and overwhelming crushing in forces, the individual faces three difficulties.*

The first difficulty is that the crushing in forces comes from all directions. That means, the individual fails to focus his/her psychic energy to push back. The individual may at one time push back in one direction and at another time, another direction. No matter how hard s/he tries, s/he fails with a consequence that his/her own sense of cohesiveness is also deeply affected.

The second difficulty is that the crushing in forces are far too powerful for the individual to overcome. Instead of pushing these forces outwards, they crush in and penetrate deeply into individual's self-system. The sense of agency is deeply hindered and twisted to an extent that the self-system is unable to actualize and sustain its own shape and size. Its anchoring in the external reality is also confused and withering.

The third difficulty is that the crushing in forces are continuous and spontaneous for a very long period of time. If they can stop for a while, the individual can still take a rest, restore and accumulate his/her mental energy and push back strongly. However, for prolonged and continuous crushing in forces, the individual may use up all his/her internal psychic energy in pushing them back. Even in the beginning, s/he may possess enough energy to push back for a while, by the end of the day, s/he may feel dreadfully tired and fatigued in doing so. Finally, after prolonged pushing, s/he may lose not only his/her energy but also his/her will or belief that s/he can push back. Consequently, the crushing in forces deprives the individual's ability to push back. Ontologically, s/he loses his/her sense of being and power to deal with external threats and oppression.

Finally, because of these three sorts of difficulties, the individual gradually deprives his sense of cohesiveness and sense of agency in dealing with crushing forces in the actual reality. This is an impingement of reality. It is also an accumulation of individual anger; frustration and power that cannot be released as the prolonged crushing in forces suffocate their pushing back. *Instead, the accumulated anger, frustration, and power (pushing out forces) may accumulate to a maximum degree that leads to an explosion, internally, with a powerful fracture of the self system and sense of existence.*

> `Winnicott terms the impingement of reality. Impingement does not convey, however, the full terror of the experience of the world as liable at any moment to crash in and obliterate all identity as a gas will rush in and obliterate a vacuum. The individual feels that, like the vacuum, he is empty. But the emptiness is in him. Although in other ways he longs for the emptiness to be filled, he dreads the possibility of this happening because he has come to feel that all he can be is the awful nothingness of just his very vacuum. Any contact with reality is then in itself experienced as dreadful because reality, as experienced from this position, is necessarily implosive and thus, was related in engulfment, in itself a threat to what identity the individual supposes himself to have.' (Laing, 1960: 45)

According to Laing (1960), implosion contains the following elements:

a) impingement of reality
b) external world crash in
c) identity is exploded away
d) internal vacuum may result
e) a state of nothingness
f) struggle between emptiness to be filled as well as being taken away
g) internal explosion

That means, Laing (1960), in line with Winnicott's articulation, affirmed that implosion is based on an impingement of reality. That means, the individual is deeply threatened by the crashing in of the threatening reality. It is powerful, continuous, and overwhelming from all directions. The individual is caught within a dilemma. On the one hand, the crushing of oppressive reality deeply presses the self-system to a degree that the individual feels highly suffocated. On the other hand, prolonged but unable to be pushed back mental energy can be accumulated to a degree that cannot be resisted by the vulnerable self-system any more. As a consequence, implosion occurs in a form of inner explosion of the self-system. This sort of inner explosion cannot burst outward as it is suffocated and surrounded by the crushing in of oppressive reality. It only explodes inside the self-system making related elements in the self-system fracture and fragment with a prevailing feeling of emptiness and vacuum.

In facing the crashing in reality and result of implosion with an unbearable sense of emptiness and vacuum, the individual may have several ways to respond by being

- highly alert to external threat (developing paranoia and assuming others are bad)
- omnipotent and illusively powerful to resist external threats (extremely powerful self)
- shifting from one aspect of implosion to another aspect that is not so implosive until all aspects are being imploded by others

All these may be shown in Figure 6.

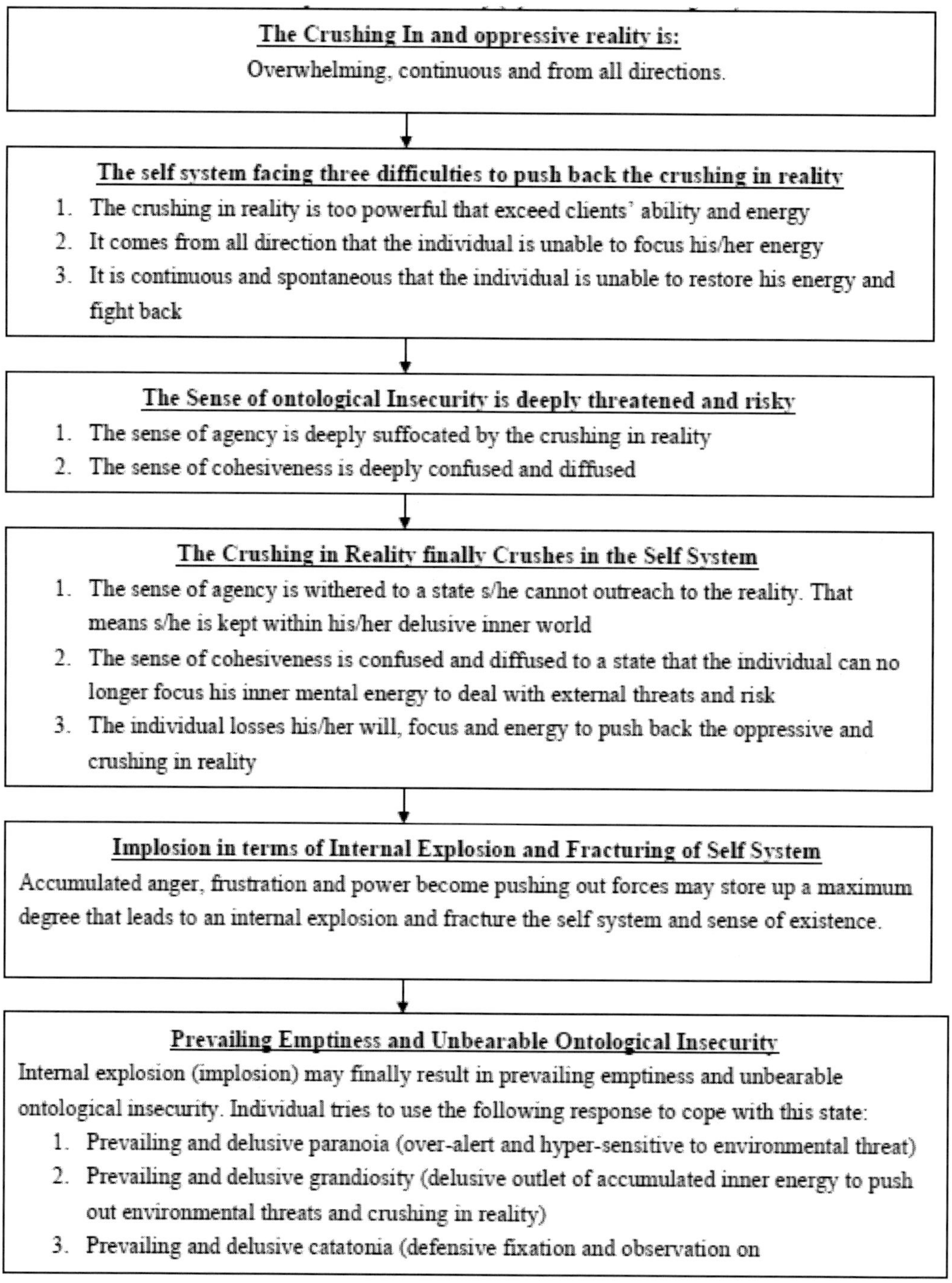

Figure 6. The Process of Implosion from Crashing in of Reality to Prevailing Emptiness.

Petrification and Depersonalizaton

According to Laing (1960), apart from engulfment, and implosion, ontological insecurity is also a result of petrification and depersonalization. Within existential and phenomenological articulation, engulfment should be a denial and deprivation of ones' sense of uniqueness and consistency with a result of losing and diffusion of self-identity and self-boundary. Implosion is a denial and deprivation of one's sense of agency and cohesiveness with a result of being absorbed in continuous confusion and uncontrollability in outreach to the external environment as well as the chronic state of internal emptiness and vacuum. *Depersonalization is a denial and deprivation of one's sense of substantiality and integrity with a result of being traumatized by oppressive others, dissociation and isolation from the related environment.*

The sense of substantiality is crucial in everyday life as one needs to feel that s/he himself/herself as well as things and persons within the related environment are substantially existing. It is a sense of body and flesh, actual existence and substantial changes as well as dynamics in the living world. Without a clear sense of substantiality, one may easily feel that s/he is not substantially present. For example, in a full sense of consciousness, one clearly feels that s/he actually exists with clear and concrete movements, thinking and interaction with related objects, things, and persons in the physical and social environment. Only by means of a feeling of substantiality from the environment, one can prove, actualize, and manifest his/her own substantiality in existence.

The sense of integrity is closely related to the sense of substantiality. While the individual needs the sense of substantiality in him/her and others from the environment to actualize his/her sense of substantial existence, *the sense of integrity implies substantial respect from others that the individual is worthwhile, individualistic, and concrete in the eyes of others*. That means, the sense of substantiality is perceived by the individual towards himself/herself and his/her surrounding world. However, the sense of integrity is originated from the perception of others towards the individual in regarding him/her as a substantial human being. *In doing so, the individual feels being respected, worthwhile, and individualistic. In other words, both the sense of substantiality and the sense of integrity exist together and reinforce each other.* The sense of uniqueness and the sense of consistency enable one to construct a clear and concrete sense of self-identity and boundary. The sense of agency and sense of cohesiveness enable one to have a successful and meaningful outreach in the related environment to anchor his/he position, to extend his/her influence, to exercise his/her will and actualize his/her functioning in the related environment. The sense of substantiality and the sense of integrity work together and enable the individual to fulfill others' demands, to adapt to the related environment, to gain others' respect, to interact with the related environment, and to carry out his/her obligation and roles smoothly.

However, in depersonalization and petrification, the individual's sense of integrity and sense of substantiality is deeply threatened. *The threat can occur in several ways.*

1. Individuals are not regarded as a lively human being. Instead, *they are regarded as lifeless objects.* Their feeling, cognition, will, individuality, and decisions are partially or totally ignored and neglected by others.
2. *Individuals are purposely isolated, detached, and excluded.* Individuals' significant others exclude them from participation in normal or crucial activities that are crucial for individual normal personal development in work, family and community. They may also purposely be isolated and detached by their colleagues, family members, and friends by labeling them as being unsuitable to join in these and any related social circles among family, work and peers.

3. *Individuals are unable to launch their request, cry for help, express his/her ideas, ventilate his/her feelings, ask for feedback and response, want to interact and cooperate with others.* Whenever they want to do so, they are rejected, expelled and belittled by others.
4. *Individuals are labeled and stigmatized by others as bad, nasty, incompetent, trouble making, weak, and inadequate or shameful to join in any external activities or linkage with others.* Thus, they should be excluded and isolated from all related activities and interactions.

Under these threats, the individual's senses of integrity and substantiality are gradually suppressed and withered by the individual's oppressive significant others. Laing (1960) affirmed that petrification and depersonalization is a dreadful form of taking the humanity and the `subject' of a person away, making him/her to become an object and even a lifeless thing with the following features:

> 1. A particular form of terror, whereby one is petrified, i.e., Turned to stone
> 2. The dread of this happening: the dread, that is, of the possibility of turning, or being turned, from a live person into a dead thing, into a stone, a robot, an automation, without personal autonomy of action, and without subjectivity.
> 3. The magical act whereby one may attempt to turn someone else into stone, by petrifying him, and by extension, the act whereby one negates the other person's autonomy, ignores his feelings, regards him as a thing, and kills the life in him. In this sense one may perhaps better say that one depersonalizes him, or reifies him. One treats him not as a person, as a free agent, but as an 'it'. (Laing, 1960: 46)

Being depersonalized and petrified is a painful dehumanization. The individual feels his own livelihood is being gradually taken away. It is one of most dehumanizing ways to nurture various mental illnesses, in particular schizophrenia. Below is such a dehumanized feeling of a person with schizophrenia, as described by Laing (1960):

> `Some of the above points are illustrated in the life of James, a chemist, aged twenty-eight. The complaints he made all along were that he could become a person. He had no self. I am only a response to other people; I have no identity of my own. He felt he was becoming a mythical person. He felt he had no weight, no substance of his own. I am only a cork floating on the ocean. This man was very concerned about not having become a person; he reproached his mother for his failure. "I was merely her emblem. She never recognized my identity". (Laing, 1960: 51)

It is clear that in James' situation, he felt that he was totally neglected by his mother. His mother did not care about his feelings, cognition, decisions and being. His sense of integrity, as well as his sense of substantiality, was deeply impaired. He felt that he was not a living being in front of others. He had no self. He was just a lifeless thing, such as:

a) a cork floating on the ocean
b) a response to other people
c) a mythical person

d) no self
e) no identity
f) no weight
g) no substance

James' self-narration showed that his sense of substantiality was totally denied, which was why he felt that he had no weight and no substance. His sense of integrity was also neglected by others, which was why he had no self, no identity. The loss of sense of substantiality and integrity made him become deeply petrified and depersonalized in becoming a lifeless thing and not a person. That was why he claimed himself as a cork floating on the ocean, a response to other people, and a mythical person. Similar feelings of being petrified and depersonalized by others can appear in dreams.

Facing that sort of threat and being petrified and depersonalized by others is highly painful and unbearable. *The best way to cope with this is that instead of being petrified by others, it is better for the individual to petrify (turning others into stone) or depersonalize others (regarding others as lifeless objects).* By doing so, the individual is able to disregard others' petrification and depersonalization. That means, as the others in the external reality are turned into stone, their power of petrification and depersonalization is depowered and ignored. In doing so, it leads to denial of the need and actualization of the sense of integrity and substantiality. The individual claims that s/he can be alone, and isolated from others. S/he withdrew from social interaction. However, prolonged turning of others into stones and depersonalizing objects implied that the whole psychosocial and physical environment may also turn into a lifeless place without actual `humans' and `lives'. Following this will be a dreadful sense of loneliness and emptiness that may also be unbearable, painful and intolerable for the individual.

To avoid this, s/he prefers to stop this loneliness and emptiness by stopping this petrification and depersonalization of others. To cope with this, he may involve self-petrification and self-depersonalization before others can petrify and depersonalize him. Nevertheless, self-petrification and depersonalization are also unbearable and intolerable. As a consequence, s/he may constantly shifting between self-depersonalization and petrification; depersonalizing and petrifying others; as well as depersonalization and petrification by others. The whole shifting process is highly complicated and ambivalent. Frequent shifting between self-petrification and petrification by others fixates the individual in a chronic state of internal and external petrification of depersonalization with a prolonged paralysis of a sense of integrity and substantiality. It can appear in forms of:

1. Blunt affect (internal and external petrification and depersonalization of emotional response and emotional reception)
2. Anhedonia (internal and external petrification and depersonalization of positive and enlightening life experiences)
3. Alogia (internal and external petrification and depersonalization of expression and communication with others)
4. Avolition (internal and external petrification and depersonalization of meaningful activities and performance)

This process can be summarized into several stages as shown in Figure 7.

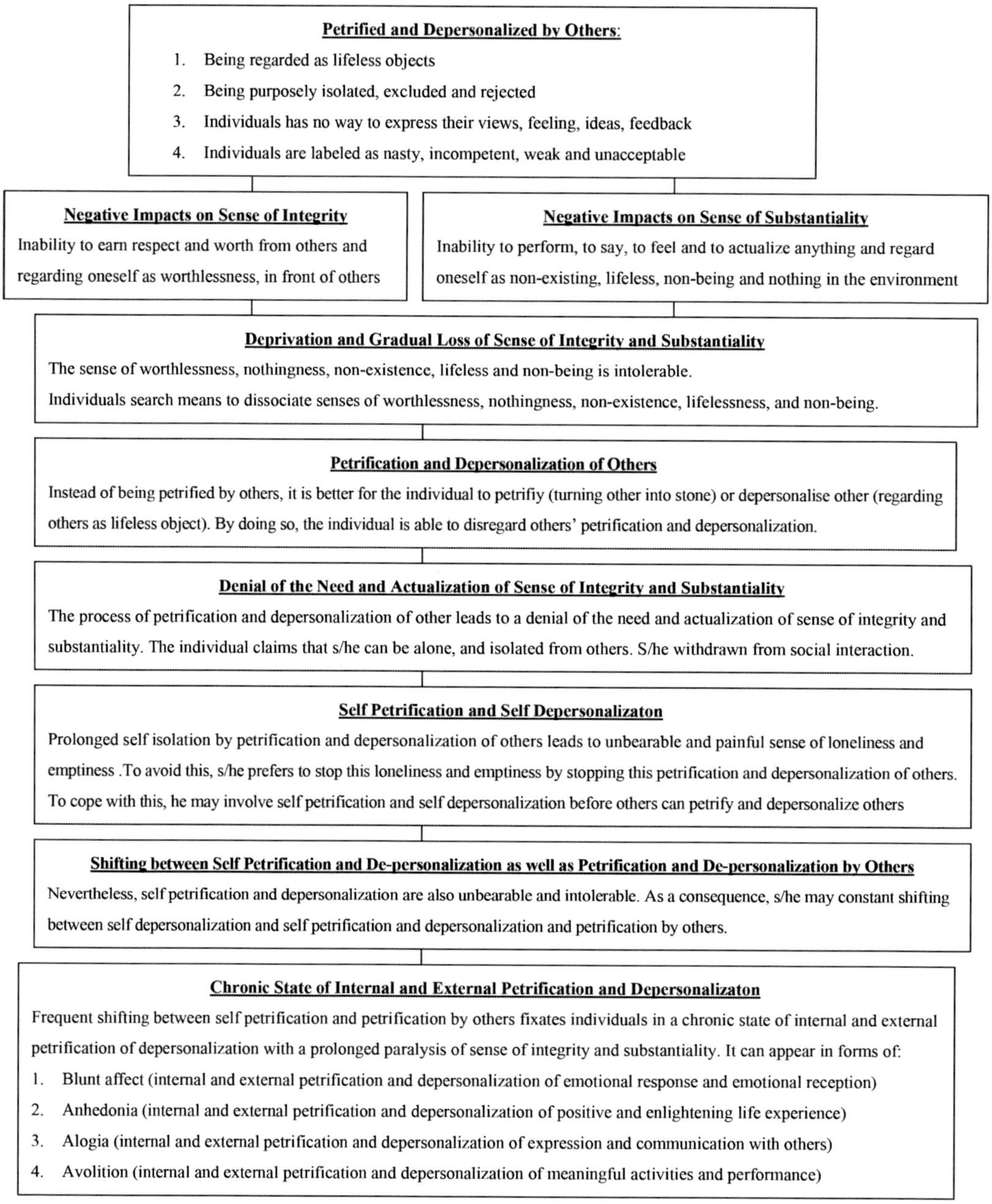

Figure 7. The Prolonged Process of Petrification and Depersonalization in Ontological Insecurity.

The dreadful sense of turning others into stones and objects can also appear in dreams and fantasies, which can be an unconscious signal of psychotic breakdown. Laing (1960) illustrates this in the following case.

> `A girl of twenty-five years dreamt that she had cooked dinner for her family of five...she called her parents and her brother and sister to dinner. Nobody replied...She found the sudden emptiness of the house uncanny. She rushed upstairs to look for her family...In the first bedroom, she could see her two sisters sitting on two beds.....

> Suddenly she noticed that they were stone sisters. She escaped in horror and rushed into her mother's room. Her mother too had turned into stone and was sitting inertly in her armchair staring into the air with glazed eyes. The dream escaped into the room of her father… But he too was made of stone … . The same horrible dream was dreamt by the patient on successive occasions within a few days. …Ten days after the fourth repetition of the dream, the patient was taken ill with an acute form of schizophrenia displaying severe catatonic schizophrenia. She fell into a stone, which was remarkably similar to the physical petrification of her family that she had dreamt about. She was now overpowered in waking life by a behavior pattern that in her dreams was merely observed in another person. (Laing, 1960: 51)

In this dream, it is clear that the girl had unconsciously petrified and depersonalized her whole family into stone including her mother, father and sister. In fact, she prepared to have a warm dinner with them. However, they had all turned into stones. They were in the family, however, they could not move, speak, interact and communicate. That means, deep down in her heart, she looked for a warm and genuine family. However, in reality, her family members, despite their close relationship with her, might be highly petrifying and depersonalizing to her. Or she might transfer the depersonalizing and petrifying relationship with others into her family. Turning them into stones might mean a total release for her to turn away from petrification and depersonalization by others. However, in doing so, her family became a highly apathetic and lifeless place where she felt dreadfully fearful, lonely and empty. All these dreadful feelings are intolerable and painful; the individual intended to get rid of these feelings. She might be self-petrifying and depersonalizing in actual reality but petrifying others in dreams.

The spontaneous struggle and vigorous shifting between self-petrification and depersonalization as well as petrifying and depersonalizing others implied a highly vulnerable mental state that is prone to onset of psychosis.

E. Different levels of ontological insecurity in terms of different degrees of engulfment, implosion, and depersonalizaton.

In the above-mentioned elements of ontological insecurity including engulfment, implosion and depersonalization, there may be various ways and combinations in articulating the levels of ontological insecurity. The first way may be changes in the forms of engulfment, implosion and depersonalization. It can be:

Level 1: Engulfment by others (oE), Implosion by others (oP), and/or Depersonalization (oD) by others. (mild degree of ontological insecurity)

Level 2: Engulfing other (Eo), Imploding other (Io) and/or Depersonalizing other (Do) (moderate degree of ontological insecurity)

Level 3: Self Engulfment (sE), Self Implosion (sI), and /or Self Depersonalization (sD) (severe degree of ontological insecurity)

Level 4: Shifting between Eo & sE, Io & sI, and/or Do & sD (very severe degree of ontological insecurity)

As mentioned above, level one is the mildest level of ontological insecurity in which one's sense of uniqueness, consistency, agency and cohesiveness, as well as integrity and substantiality are all affected. All these important senses of self are being threatened, to protect one from prolonged and intensive engulfment, implosion and depersonalization, *one needs to come to the second level. That should be a moderate level of sense of ontological insecurity in which the individual begins to engulf, to implode and/or to depersonalize others.* However, in reality, s/he is actually being engulfed, imploded and depersonalized by others. Thus, this form of engulfing, imploding and depersonalizing others are actually delusive manifestations of individual's urges and ideas with passive distortions of reality.

Facing the continuous overwhelming crushing in of reality that comes from all directions, in which the individual has no way to push back, the only way available is to stay within his/her inner world, deluding oneself that there is no such crushing of reality or s/he is actually pushing back the crushing in reality. These two purposes can be attained simply by the delusion that s/he is controlling/oppressing others rather than being controlled/oppressed by others. S/he may think that if s/he likes, s/he can continuously control/oppress others in all directions whereas others have no way to escape.

An example is a man, oppressed by others, and the individual is unable to fight back and control the prevailing oppression. He either has no ability to fight back or cannot focus his energy to fight back. His sense of agency and sense of cohesiveness is threatened. The only way that can temporarily lessen his intolerable mental pain is to imagine that the individual is not controlling/oppressing him or that s/he has an imaginative or delusive power to decrease the oppression or to control the oppressors. That means the individual tries to compensate for his gradual loss of senses of self by delusive senses of uniqueness, consistency, agency, cohesiveness, integrity and substantiality. In doing so, he tries to compensate for the gradual increase of ontological insecurity by a gradual increase of delusive ontological security. However, the more s/he engages in that sort of delusive ontological insecurity, the more s/he is vulnerable to external engulfment, implosion and depersonalization and the more s/he feels that the external environment is threatening and fearful.

Thus, s/he needs to go into the third level with a severe degree of ontological insecurity. Instead of being engulfed, imploded and depersonalized by others, the individual enters into a state of self engulfment, self implosion and self depersonalization as well as self petrification. It is similar to the situation of killing oneself so that other cannot kill him/her. Certainly, it is an extremely passive and negative way to take back one's senses of self. In doing so, one senses of self enters into a state of delusive distortion. In self-engulfment, one's senses of uniqueness and consistency are not swallowed away by other (engulfment) nor do they become delusive thinking that one has the power to oppress or manipulate others (engulfment of others). Instead, one engages in a delusive assertion, one does not need any sense of uniqueness and consistency in reality, since s/he is already highly unique and consistent in his/her delusive inner world. In self-implosion, one's sense of agency and cohesiveness do not need to actualize in the reality. Instead, the individual deludes that s/he can fully reach out to others and master others. In the reality, s/he may be a subordinate being oppressed by others in which s/he has no way to fight back. In his/her fantasy, the individual may believe that no one can oppress him/her.

For example, an adult male is oppressed by his boss with continuous manipulation in every detail of his job. He has no way to come out from this oppression and manipulation. In a form of engulfment of another, he is deluded in thinking that he actually manipulates his boss. In fact, he has many ways to manipulate his boss even though he does not fight back. In self-engulfment, his delusion becomes even more complicated. He deludes that no one can manipulate or control him; only he himself can do so. In that sense, his delusion is far more complicated than he can control with his boss. He controls himself to avoid being controlled by others. In doing so, he is in a complete vacuum with total isolation from others, which is unbearable. Also, in reality, his boss is still controlling him. *Thus, the only way to tackle engulfment by others is the combination and shifting between engulfment of others and self-engulfment. This is the fourth level of ontological insecurity in which the individual has a very severe sense of ontological insecurity.*

The individual deludes himself into thinking that he actually controls his boss to control him. In doing so, he can accept the fact that he is being controlled by his boss. However, this control is actually further manipulated by him. That means he replaces the loss of his sense of uniqueness and consistency by a totally deluded sense of uniqueness and consistency. As a consequence, his self-identity and self-boundary as well as the sense of reality become highly diffused. He feels puzzled whether he is controlling himself or his boss is controlling him. To anchor or clarify his diffusion, he may even further develop his idea that he is actually the super boss in the company but he needs to disguise his identity to investigate a scandal or corruption in the company. By means this delusive grandiosity he can fully justify that he is controlling his boss to control him. In rapid shifting of self-engulfment and engulfing of others, the individual's self-boundary is so diffused that the individual's inner ingredients in the self-system tend to be thrown out. At the same time, external object, events or persons may flow inside the self-system. That can appear in a form of thought insertion (external ideas being inserted by others) or thought broadcasting (individual's ideas can influence other minds). In some cases, individuals may engage in a constant fear that part of his body or mind can merge with external objects, persons and events in the immediate environment. All these are the manifestation of first rank symptoms in schizophrenia.

Similar things happen in self-implosion and self-depersonalization in which the individual needs to shift between self-implosion and implosion of others as well as shifting between self-depersonalization and depersonalization of others. In the shifting of self-implosion and imploding others, the individual may suffer from highly confused senses of agency and cohesiveness in which the individual fails to adapt to external demands in the immediate reality. When s/he engages in self-implosion, s/he believes that no one, except himself/herself can control the external reality. With rapid shifting between self-implosion and imploding others, the individual gets confused whether the crushing reality is actually present; only him/her can actually construct and create the crushing reality for others (imploding other); no one can construct the crushing reality except him/her; or crushing reality imposed on him by others is actually constructed by him/her and he possesses the omnipotent power to do so. As a result, s/he tends to construct prevailing paranoid, grandiose, or catatonic delusions and hallucinations in defending his/her authentic inner self from the crushing reality. They are actually the manifestation of the positive symptoms in schizophrenia.

In the same pattern, the shifting between self-depersonalization and depersonalizing others has an intensive confusion of the individual's sense of integrity and substantiality. In depersonalizing others, the individual is deluded that others cannot depersonalize him/her, only he himself/herself can delude others. In doing so, s/he compensates for his gradual loss of senses of integrity and substantiality by delusive senses of integrity and substantiality. In self-depersonalization, an individual in a highly delusive idea assumes that no one can depersonalize him/her, but that only s/he can depersonalize himself/herself. In doing so, s/he can avoid being depersonalized by others. However in the shifting of self-depersonalization and depersonalizing others, the individual is kept with a dilemma that s/he depersonalizes other to depersonalize himself/herself. In other words, his/her sense of integrity and substantiality is both delusive and self constructing. By doing that s/he either turns other stone or turns himself/herself into a stone. In both ways, it intensifies individual's inertness towards himself/herself and others. That means the whole world becomes stagnant, apathetic and motionless. S/he may have no emotional involvement and response towards others as well as towards himself/herself. Within this mental state, the individual has no affective response towards others (blunt affect). S/he has no sense of happiness or enlightenment (anhedonia). S/he harbors an entire inertness to express his/her ideas or thinking (alogia). S/he is not clear about the direction/goal of his/her own actions (avolition). All these can be regarded as manifestation of negative symptoms.

Different levels and degrees of ontological insecurity can be represented in Figures 8.

Mild Degree of Ontological Insecurity Engulfment by others (oE), Implosion by others (oP), and/or Depersonalization (oD) by others. The individual feels higher insecure in the engulfing, implosing and depersonalizating environment.	**Initial Gradual Loss of Senses of Self including:** Initial and Graudal loss of sense of uniqueness and consistency Initial and Gradual loss of senses of agency and cohesiveness Initial and Gradual loss of senses of integrity and substantiality Senses of self are threatened by oppressive other. The individual becomes more and more intolerable to external engulfment, implosion and depersonalization
Moderate Degree of Ontological Insecurity Engulfing other (Eo), Implosing other (Io) and/or Depersonalizing other (Do). Individual delusively thinks that s/he is engulfing, implosing and depersonalizing others	**The Loss of Senses of Self is Compensated by a Delusive Senses of Self:** Delusive senses of uniqueness and consistency by delusively engulfing others Delusive senses of agency and cohesiveness by delusively implosing others Delusive senses of integrity and substantiality by delusively depersonalizing others. However, the engulfing, implosing and depersonalizing others are still there. Thus, the individual becomes more and more detached from the actual reality. S/he also becomes more and more vulnerable to external oppression.
Severe Degree of Ontological Insecurity Self Engulfment (sE), Self Implosion (sI), and /or Self Depersonalisation (sD). Individual deludes that s/he is self engulfing, implosing and depersonalizing	**The Delusive Senses of Self is Transformed to Self Defeating so that Others can not Defeated the Individuals** Denial of the Need of uniqueness and consistency by Self Engulfment Denial of the Need of agency and cohesiveness by Self Implosion Denial of the Need of integrity and substantiality by Self Depersonalization (In doing so, the individual's sense of existence is diminishing and his/her sense of sense is also deteriorating to a critical state for the struggle of minimal and confusion of survival)
Very Severe Degree of Ontological Insecurity Shifting between engulfing other and self engulfment (Eo & sE), implosing other and self implosion (Io & sI), and depersonalizing other and self depersonalization (Do & sD)	**Shifting between Delusive Sense of Self and Self Defeating** Highly confused senses of uniqueness and consistency due to shifting of self engulfment and engulfing other with a result of diffusion of self boundary and self identity (**Manifestation of First Rank Symptoms with** external objects, events and persons merging with one's self) Highly confused senses of agency and cohesiveness due to shifting of self implosion and implosing others. It results in a highly delusive sense of reality and decrease of one's ability and social functioning (**Manifestation of Positive Symptoms**, paranoid, grandiose and catatonic delusion) Highly confused senses of integrity and substantiality due to shifting of self depersonalization and depersonalizing others with a result of a highly detached sense of reality and sense of onself. (**Manifestation of Negative Symptoms**, blunt affect, anhedonia, alogia, avolition) (The individual uses self engulfment to cope with negative effects of engulfing other and vice versa, similar patterns happen in self implosion and implosing other as well as self depersonalization and depersonalizing others)

Figure 8. Various Degrees of Ontological Insecurity of Engulfment, Implosion, and Depersonalization.

Implications to Mental Health Recovery for Clients with Schizophrenia

It is clear that according to Laing (1960), schizophrenia is formed by an intensive sense of ontological insecurity in which the individual undergoes a vigorous process of self fragmentation by an intensive but delusive engulfment, implosion, and depersonalization towards self to escape from the engulfment, implosion, and depersonalization by oppressive others in the painful reality. All these can be shown in the following case illustration. Related parties' consensus to use their own stories for academic purposes was sought. For the sake of confidentiality, their personal identity and information were properly disguised.

The Endless Struggle of P

P was born into a middle class family in China with a highly engulfing mother with whom he had to struggle for his own existence. His father was a high official in the government. Because of fulfilling official duties and obligations, he had to travel around China and other countries in the world, frequently leaving P and his mother at home. Even if he returned home, he was far too busy engaging in various types of social activities with high officials from other governmental department as well as directors of various companies. P tried to relate with his father but he simply neglected him. Occasionally, he promised P to buy him anything he wanted. But he never had sufficient intention, time, and space to interact with and love P.

P's mother was a highly anxious person. She tried all manipulations with P to fulfill his needs. In fact, as her husband was always away, unconsciously she regarded P as her substitute husband. Emotionally, she was enmeshed with P. From the time P was born, she embraced P and slept with him every night. She also took baths together with P until P was ten years old. She also took tight control on everything in P's daily life, including his schooling, recreational and social activities. In doing so, it was very hard for P to construct his own sense of self and ontological security. Despite this, he tried hard to struggle to have his sense of self, under the severe detachment from his father and severe engulfment from his mother; his sense of self and ontological security could never be developed. Instead, he had poor sense of ontological insecurity. His senses of uniqueness, consistency, agency, cohesiveness, integrity, and substantiality could never develop. Below was his self-narration in describing his hard struggle in gaining his own sense of self and ontological security in life.

P said: throughout my childhood and adolescence, I could never have my own sense of being. Whenever, I wanted to make my decision or have my own way (sense of agency), my mother would decide for me. I wanted to be a unique human being with my own interests and my own sports. I wanted to choose my own clothes, choose my own hobbies, and develop my own potentials (sense of uniqueness). However, my mother forced me to play football, to wear the clothes she liked and to learn piano. In fact, I did not like to play football. I preferred marital arts. I hated piano and liked to play guitar. My mother governed everything in my life. Neither my father nor my mother respected me as an adult with my own ideas and preferences. Every time I tried to speak up my view and be respected as a mature human being (sense of respect), they simply regarded my view as childish and unnecessary. Once, my father said, I was a useless adolescent knowing only how to play and enjoy life. In fact, I was not. I wanted to live a substantial life (sense of substantiality). I intended to do volunteer work to serve the elderly but my parents thought this was only a waste of time. Every time, when someone, including my friends and relatives, asked my view, my mother told them that they could neglect mine and her view was far better than that. I wanted to express my own view and actualize it in practice (sense of cohesiveness) but my parents always said all my views were crazy and impractical. Frankly speaking, I did not exist in this world. I was my mother's baby existing in the world. My hope to be a unique human being in the past, present, and future (sense of consistence) could never be actualized.

From the above case illustration, it was clear that P's sense of ontological security in terms of senses of uniqueness, consistency, agency, cohesion, substantiality, and integrity were diminished by P's mother's intensive engulfment and his father's depersonalization. These were also the explicit causes making P gradually develop schizophrenic symptoms and undergo a process of self-fragmentation. All these happened in P's adolescence. That means, the onset of schizophrenia was fueled by P's self-engulfing, self-implosion and self-depersonalization.

P's mother's engulfment and his father's depersonalization continued into his childhood. They intensified in P's adolescence. At that time, P's father had an extra-marital relationship with another female. Then, he rarely returned home. P's mother was furious about that but she could do nothing to stop that. Later, they divorced. Consequently, she regarded P as the substituted object for her divorced husband. She engulfed P more seriously. At that moment, P was in the process of self-fragmentation. He suffered from intensive engulfment from her mother. Since his father abandoned him, he suffered from serious depersonalization. In addition, at school his classmates bullied him. They called him `useless dump shit'. Whenever P intended to fight back, they laughed and ran away, making P furious but he had no way to release his anger. Instead, this intense rage turned inwards and caused an internal implosion. Under that sort of condition, P began to develop psychotic symptoms. He embraced a severe sense of ontological insecurity in which he was totally being engulfed, imploded and depersonalized from his mother, father, and classmates. To cope with this painful reality, he had to develop delusions and hallucinations in which he could engulf, implode, and depersonalize others.

From that time onwards, P harbored a strong delusional thought that his mother was not his real mother. Instead, she was a seductive woman. She seduced many handsome men around. Occasionally, he heard people around gossiping about his mother's immoral relationship with other men. P was actually a prince from a foreign country. Someone in his own mother country stole him, and smuggled him into this city and brought him to his father. As his father was a high official in this city, he used a great sum of money to buy P as his son because of P's noble blood, hoping that one day, P would return to his mother country and inherit the throne as a king. Then it would be a great profit for P's father.

Once such delusions and hallucinations were formulated, P was no longer a submissive or quiet person subjected to his mother's continuous engulfment, his classmates' bullying, and implosion as well as his father's depersonalization. Instead, he fought back. He cursed his mother as an immoral and unethical woman. When his mother cursed back, he even slapped his mother on her face. He also sent some strange, odd, and bizarre e-mails and letters to his father telling him that his mother was immoral. He frankly blamed his father, as an irresponsible stepfather that failed to recognize his noble blood and did not fulfill his promise to bring him back to his mother country. If his father continued doing so, when he became a king, he would punish his father. For any classmate in the school who bullied him, he would fight back. Once, a classmate called him chicken, and he broke this classmate's nose.

From that time onwards, P became aggressive and confused. Apart from engulfing, imploding, and depersonalizing others, he also engulfed, imploded, and depersonalized himself by forming related hallucinations and delusions. On one hand, he affirmed that he harbored noble blood. On the other hand, he felt that people around him questioned his noble blood. They watched him everywhere. They tried to steal his noble blood away. P felt he was being controlled by them (self-engulfment). Even though he tried to neglect them, they were everywhere. To deal with them, P was deluded into thinking that the king (his deluded father) from his own mother country had already sent someone to rescue P and would take him back. However, they could not find him (self-depersonalization and petrification). To help them find him, P tried to stir up issues around him. He let others insult, bully, and humiliate him (self implosion). In order to tolerate of all these, he affirmed that one day those rescuers might finally appear. As a consequence of self-engulfment, implosion, and depersonalization, P became very anxious and mentally unstable.

When his assumed rescuers did not appear; when others' humiliation became intolerable; and when delusive control by others was too painful, he would shift back into engulfing others by overtly pronouncing that he actually could diminish the delusive and oppressive others; imploding others by cursing delusive and oppressive others loudly; and petrifying the delusive others by saying that he did not care about all these delusive others. Under all these conditions, P's mental state was highly confused. His sense of reality was poor. Not only with odd and bizarre behaviors, but also with confusing self talk, he was taken into a nearby mental hospital. The psychiatrist affirmed that he suffered from acute psychosis.

From P's case, it was clear that P's process of self-fragmentation underwent the following stages of development:

Stage 1: Being engulfed, imploded, and depersonalized by his significant others including his father, mother and classmates (precipitating stage of schizophrenia)

Stage 2: P began to develop delusions and hallucinations *(his mother was a seductive women and P was a prince in a foreign country)* to engulf his mother *(curse his mother)*, to depersonalize his father *(label his father as controlling and manipulative)* and to implode his classmates *(fight back on any one bullied him)* (pre-morbid stage of schizophrenia)

Stage 3: Related delusions and hallucinations *(people from his country searched around him)* were further developed into being engulfed, imploded and depersonalized by delusive others (morbid stage in schizophrenia)

Stage 4: Continuous conflict and dilemmas of engulfing and being engulfed, imploding and being imploded, depersonalizing and being depersonalized in confused delusions and hallucinations *(shifting around, being followed by rescuers from his mother country as well as being humiliated or maltreated by others so that the rescuers could find him)* (acute stage of schizophrenia)

In fact, in all these stages, morbid, pre-morbid and acute stages of schizophrenia, the individual clients' sense of ontological security, including senses of uniqueness, consistence, cohesiveness, agency, substantiality and integrity are being disturbed. Individuals with schizophrenia can only get all these senses within their self-constructed delusive reality. In other words, mental health recovery should mean that related professionals should help clients with schizophrenia to have their sense of ontological security within an actual supportive reality. That means, related concepts or components of mental health recovery should be closely related to a reconstruction of all these senses of ontological security. In the following section, the writer described related components of mental health recovery that relate to different senses of ontological security.

The Ten Principles of Recovery and Sense of Ontological Security

Recovery has been a concept ever since the 1990s in the U.S.A. After a decade of discussion and advocacy, related parties finally reached a national consensus as a crucial guideline in mental health practice and service. Related parties included the following:

1. The Substance Abuse and Mental Health Services Administration within the U.S. Department of Health and Human Services
2. The Interagency Committee on Disability Research
3. Six other Federal agencies
4. 110 expert panelists consist of:
   i. mental health consumers,
   ii. family members,
   iii. providers,
   iv. advocates,
   v. researchers,
   vi. academicians,
   vii. managed care representatives,
   viii. accreditation organization representatives,
   ix. State and local public officials and others.

All these parties participated in the National Consensus Conference on Mental Health Recovery and Mental Health Systems Transformation on December 16-17, 2004. They had successfully formulated the National Consensus Statement of Mental Health Recovery (U.S. Department of Health and Health Services, 2004).

The Consensus statement consists of ten components in recovery. These ten components can be regarded as ten fundamental principles for mental health recovery. They are self-direction, individual and person centered, empowerment, holistic, non-linear, strength based, peer support, respect, responsibility and hope. The definition of each component is discussed and their relationship with senses of ontological insecurity is discussed as follows:

Principle One: Self Direction

It is defined by the Consensus Statement, as follows:

> `Self-Direction: Consumers lead, control, exercise choice over, and determine their own path of recovery by optimizing autonomy, independence, and control of resources to achieve a self-determined life. By definition, the recovery process must be self-directed by the individual, who defines his or her own life goals and designs a unique path towards those goals. (U.S. Department of Health and Human Services, 2004.)
>
> In application to mental health recovery for clients with schizophrenia, self-direction should mean developing clients' sense of uniqueness. Their path and pace of recovery should not be merely designed by related professionals or caregivers. Rather, every client should define his/her own path, pace and way of recovery. While one client assumes that recovery as a fulfillment of social roles as a parent or child, another client may define his/her mental health recovery as having a stable job and good income. Self-direction also

implies individuals with schizophrenia can regain their sense of autonomy in designing their own path of recovery.

Principle Two: Individualized and Person-Centered

The second principle proposed by the consensus statement is individualized and person centered in the process of recovery.

> Individualized and Person-Centered: There are multiple pathways to recovery based on an individual's unique strengths and resiliencies as well as his or her needs, preferences, experiences (including past trauma), and cultural background in all of its diverse representations. Individuals also identify recovery as an ongoing journey and result, as well as an overall paradigm for achieving wellness and optimal mental health. (U.S. Department of Health and Human Services, 2004)

Individualized and person centered means that an individual's strengths, resilience and potentials, preferences, and experiences are being respected and considered in related interventions and psychosocial environments. In terms of ontological security, individualized, and person-centered recovery implies that clients' senses of integrity and substantiality are respected and re-established in the recovery process. It is clear that development of clients' potentials, strengths, experiences, and preferences certainly make clients' lives more substantial and meaningful. For clients with psychotic delusions, the more substantial and meaningful their living is, the less they rely on self constructed delusions and hallucinations to gratify their unfulfilled needs and aspirations. In doing so, the individuals' sense of integrity is also enhanced. Through manifestation of their strengths, potentials and preferences, they certainly feel that they are individuals with integrity, respect, and worth.

Principle Three: Empowerment

The third component and principle in recovery is empowerment. It implies that individuals gain control and join with other consumers together to advocate and ensure their rights, dignity, and needs in their process of recovery.

> `Empowerment: Consumers have the authority to choose from a range of options and to participate in all decisions—including the allocation of resources—that will affect their lives, and are educated and supported in so doing. They have the ability to join with other consumers to collectively and effectively speak for themselves about their needs, wants, desires, and aspirations. Through empowerment, an individual gains control of his or her own destiny and influences the organizational and societal structures in his or her life.' (U.S. Department of Health and Human Services, 2004)

For clients with schizophrenia, the manifestation of power in the process of recovery certainly enables clients' sense of agency fully. As mentioned above, delusions and hallucinations constructed by clients with psychosis are ways to empower themselves within a highly oppressive and depowering reality. The process of empowerment within an actual and supportive reality certainly gives them a full sense of agency. In doing so, they are no longer objects to be controlled by the oppressive. Instead, they can exercise their influence on others. What s/he thinks can be actualized. When s/he speaks can be performed. What s/he aspires to can be fulfilled. It is an active process of construction of clients' sense of cohesiveness

(cohesiveness between word and deeds, thinking and implementation, as well as aspiration and reality) and sense of agency (ability to control, to influence and to help others).

Principle Four: Holistic

The fourth component in recovery is holistic orientation in the process of recovery for persons with mental illness.

> Holistic: Recovery encompasses an individual's whole life, including mind, body, spirit, and community. Recovery embraces all aspects of life, including housing, employment, education, mental health, and healthcare treatment and services, complementary and naturalistic services, addiction treatments, spirituality, creativity, social networks, community participation, and family supports as determined by the person. Families, providers, organizations, systems, communities, and society all play crucial roles in creating and maintaining meaningful opportunities for consumer access to these supports. (U.S. Department of Health and Human Services, 2004)

Taking a holistic view on our clients is necessary in helping clients with schizophrenia. It means that we have to consider their life history including their past, present and future of our clients. Helping clients to feel and achieve wholeness mean that s/he can feel consistent in the past, present and future. Enabling a client with schizophrenia with good housing, good accommodation, good education, good religion and meaning of life certainly increases his/her sense of being respected, sense of substantiality, and sense of integrity.

Principle Five: Non-Linear

The fifth component is `non-liner' in the process of recovery. That means persons with mental illness are not recovered in a linear way. Instead, their recovery can be fluctuating.

> `Non-Linear: Recovery is not a step-by-step process but one based on continual growth, occasional setbacks, and learning from experience. Recovery begins with an initial stage of awareness in which a person recognizes that positive change is possible. This awareness enables the consumer to move on to fully engage in the work of recovery. (U.S. Department of Health and Human Services, 2004)'

A full articulation that the process of recovery is non-linear as well as self-directedness implies that clients with schizophrenia, in the process of recovery should be regarded as unique and consistent. Everyone should have his/her own pace and rhythm of recovery. Their pace of recovery is fully determined by their own background, needs, readiness, and contextual restraints. In doing so, the individual senses of uniqueness and consistency is being re-established.

Principle Six: Strengths Based

The sixth component is strengths-based orientation. As mentioned above, it means that the recovery process should be an actualization of individual capabilities, strengths, resiliencies, talents, coping abilities and inherent worth of persons with mental illness. They should embrace full opportunities in exercising their new normal life roles as friends, caregivers, students or employees within their normal community.

`Strengths-Based: Recovery focuses on valuing and building on the multiple capacities, resiliencies, talents, coping abilities, and the inherent worth of individuals. By building on these strengths, consumers leave stymied life roles behind and engage in new life roles (e.g., partner, caregiver, friend, student and employee). The process of recovery moves forward through interaction with others in supportive, trust-based relationships. (U.S. Department of Health and Human Services, 2004)

Recognition and development of client's strengths certainly has a crucial influence on clients' sense of agency, uniqueness, consistency and cohesiveness, integrity and substantiality. When clients' talents and strengths are recognized, they certainly feel that they are unique and special in comparing with others. In the process of being appreciated by others, they certainly feel that they are being respected and integrated. In proper manifestation and exercising their strengths, they certainly feel they have their own autonomy as well as good influence on others as well as good contribution to the society. Thus, their sense of agency is actualized.

Principle Seven: Peer Support

The seventh component is peer support. That means that persons with mental illness should support each other mutually, especially in sharing their experiences and wisdom in the process of discovery. They should mutually encourage one another in providing a sense of belongings, supportive relationships, and community integration in the process of recovery in self-help groups; locality-based supportive networks, clients' social clubs, family mutual supportive networks, and day-to-day friendships.

Peer Support: Mutual support—including the sharing of experiential knowledge and skills and social learning—plays an invaluable role in recovery. Consumers encourage and engage with other consumers in recovery and provide each other with a sense of belonging, supportive relationships, valued roles, and community. (U.S. Department of Health and Human Services, 2004)

In having good peer support, individuals with schizophrenia feel highly respected, with a good feeling of having a substantial life. Also, in rendering support to others as a peer helper, individuals with schizophrenia can regain their senses of worth, uniqueness and agency (with good influence and contribution to others in various social circles).

Principle Eight: Respect

The eighth element in recovery is respect. That means that others should adequately respect people with mental illness, including persons in the workplace, community, and society. Their consumer rights and personal rights to receive equal opportunities and treatment in society should be fully respected. Persons with mental illness should be facilitated, encouraged, and respected to develop their normal self acceptance and self competence in living a normal life with full participation of community activities in all aspects of life.

Respect: Community, systems, societal acceptance, and appreciation of consumers —including protecting their rights and eliminating discrimination and stigma—are crucial in achieving recovery. Self-acceptance and regaining belief in one's self are

> particularly vital. Respect ensures the inclusion and full participation of consumers in all aspects of their lives. (U.S. Department of Health and Human Services, 2004)

Gaining good respect from others, in particular ones' family members, peers, friends, and colleagues are crucial in human life. For clients with schizophrenia, indeed, it is important that they can regain their sense of worth and importance in real life situations rather than in their delusions and hallucinations. With respect from others, one's sense of integrity is fully attained. Also, being respected by others also means that one can exercise their sense of agency smoothly in various social circles and social contexts.

Principle Nine: Responsibility

The ninth element in recovery is responsibility. That means, persons with mental illness should have a personal responsibility for their own recovery, including proper self-care, social activities, and determination to live a normal life. Related professionals should take positive steps to facilitate persons with mental illness to understand and give meaning to their unique experiences and healing process.

> Responsibility: Consumers have a personal responsibility for their own self-care and journeys of recovery. Taking steps towards their goals may require great courage. Consumers must strive to understand and give meaning to their experiences and identify coping strategies and healing processes to promote their own wellness. (U.S. Department of Health and Human Services, 2004)

Full mental health recovery for clients with schizophrenia should include a full actualization of one's responsibility and obligations in various aspects of life. They can be responsible and committed children for their parents, diligent and good colleagues for their bosses in their work, brilliant students in their school performance as well as good and supportive friends for their peers. Helping clients to resume their responsibility in life also facilitates them to rebuild meaningful and constructive relationships with their significant others.

Principle Ten: Hope

The tenth component of recovery is 'hope'. That means, in the process of recovery, people with mental illness should be able to nurture hope in their life so that they can have a bright future in their work, education, and their community life. Their hope and recovery not only benefits themselves but also their families, communities, societies, and countries.

> Hope: Recovery provides the essential and motivating message of a better future — that people can and do overcome the barriers and obstacles that confront them. Hope is internalized; but can be fostered by peers, families, friends, providers, and others. Hope is the catalyst of the recovery process. Mental health recovery not only benefits individuals with mental health disabilities by focusing on their abilities to live, work, learn, and fully participate in our society, but also enriches the texture of American community life. America reaps the benefits of the contributions individuals with mental disabilities can make, ultimately becoming a stronger and healthier Nation. (U.S. Department of Health and Human Services, 2004)

As what Deegan (1996) mentioned, hope is the most important ingredient in a full mental health recovery. Without hope, everything in the present and future is stagnant, fixated and frozen. With hope for a better future, with hope for a better environment, with hope to have supportive significant others, and with hope to live a normal life; all spark one's psychic, mental and physical energy to recover from self-fragmentation. In fact, with hope, all senses of ontological security are being activated. With hope, one can regain his own worth and dignity (sense of integrity). With hope, one can develop strengths and talents (sense of substantiality and sense of uniqueness). With hope, one can have a continuity of past, present, and future in a hopeful way (sense of consistency). With hope, one finally knows that one day s/he can unite with his/her significant others in a meaningful and mutually supportive way (sense of integrity and sense of substantiality).

Recovery of P by Regaining His Sense of Ontological Security

All the above-mentioned components in mental health recovery can be shown in P's case.

> P was hospitalized for around three months and then he was discharged home. After that, he still harbored a strong delusion that his mother was immoral, and his neighbors tried to steal his noble blood so that his father, the king, and those who rescued him could not find him to inherit his father's kingdom. He refused to return home to live with his mother. Upon the advice of the medical social worker there, he was thus admitted into a psychiatric half way house, where the writer was the clinical consultant. Under the clinical supervision of the writer, the responsible social worker tried to develop P's sense of ontological security in his recovery process
>
> Instead of focusing on P's deficit and symptoms, the responsible social worker K, identified P's strengths and talents and manifested it in the half way house. He had a long chat with P and his mother. From their narration, he knew that K was very interested in playing football. Apart from that, P was also gifted in drawing lovely cartoons. In addition to that, P enjoyed singing popular songs. Based on all these, the social worker K encouraged P to manifest all these in the half way house.
>
> First, P was encouraged to draw a set of cartoon pictures as a wall decoration in the half way house. Residents in the halfway house really appreciated P's drawings. With the appreciation process, P's sense of uniqueness (being the only one who could draw cartoons in the half way house), sense of integrity (being respected by others), sense of substantiality (doing something substantial for the house), and sense of consistency (in the past and present, he could draw good cartoon pictures) was attained.
>
> Secondly, because of such beautiful cartoon drawings, P was invited by the worker in the sheltered workshop to draw interesting cartoons and print it on commercial products. P was really excited by it. He focused all his attention in drawing cartoons. He enjoyed being appreciated by others. He tried his best to draw and produce a high level product. By doing that, he successfully regained a sense of integrity (being deeply respect by others as well as having a feeling of being trustworthy and honest.). As he had to discuss and negotiate with others in drawing suitable cartoons for the commercial product, P became very sociable, and his sense and connection with reality was greatly strengthened. He did not need to use hallucinations and delusions to gratify his unfulfilled needs and regain his sense of ontological security. Under this condition, P's mental state became very stable. His self-confidence and social functioning was restored. One year later, he found a stable job as a cartoon illustrator in a marketing company. To further improve his competence in this area, he enrolled in a diploma course of design and marketing in a post-secondary institution. From that time onward, P's career and social life was highly normalized and healthy. His sense of ontological security was restored.

He rented a flat and lived with his colleagues. As his sense of ontological security was fully achieved, he was fully recovered from schizophrenia. He stopped his medication and had no sign of symptoms of schizophrenia any more.

Psychodynamic Internal Causes of Self-Fragmentation

From External Cause to Developmental Internal Cause of Self-Fragmentation

Critically speaking, social construction of mental illness, including Foucault and Glass's orientation, can be regarded as external causes of self-fragmentation of schizophrenia. Both of them focus on the destruction of power in the self-system of the individual. While Foucault focused on the overwhelming power from the external environment, Glass talked more on the destructive power of psychotic times in which the self-system of persons with schizophrenia needs to be empowered delusively in terms of self-image, times, space, resources and ego functioning. It is clear that the overwhelmingly powerful external environment by culture, civilization, circulatory network, as well as related institutions, and related professionals in terms of language, power and discourse depower the individual to an extent that s/he needs to be internally or delusively self-empowered so as to maintain his/her minimal survival of meaning, self-image, boundary and existence. In doing so, it is clear that psychosis being constructed is not only a social labeling and constructed madness; it is also an internal self-fragmentation on self-image, boundary, and ego functioning because of prevailing external oppression. However, both Foucault and Glass did not make this point clearly. Instead, Laing (1960) made this point well in terms of the divided self-system due to external implosion, engulfment, and depersonalization from the individual's significant others. Laing's orientation, as he claimed, is existential and phenomenological. In another book, Sanity, Madness, and Families, Laing and Estersen (1970) affirmed that schizophrenia is also related to parental manipulation and oppression in an individual's adolescence. In other words, implosion, engulfment, and depersonalization are done within a family context in terms of parent child interaction. Nevertheless, Laing (1960) did not go in detail on that. He just took an existential and phenomenological stance by a full description of the individual's current situation with a glimpse of possible parental oppression in childhood and adolescence within his case illustration. Thus, the developmental process of the individual's pre-psychotic state should be described by another orientation, the psychodynamic perspective in this section.

Arieti's Development Pre-Psychotic Personality

Arieti (1974), based on related literature in the psychodynamic approach, affirmed that persons with schizophrenia embraced a pre-morbid childhood and pre-psychotic personality.

Psychodynamic Development of Childhood of Persons with Schizophrenia

1. Avoid the Lonely External World and Focus on the Inner World

Artieti (1974) described that persons with schizophrenia may possess a childhood that is lonely, unattached, and introversive. The unpleasant external environment makes the individual child turn inwards, accustomed to being absorbed in his/her inner world.

'He tends to be by himself, and thus aloofness favors an over-development fantasy or life or images. The child escapes from the external life and lives preponderantly in his inner life. He finds himself having to relate to a mother who, because of her perfectionism, excessive anxiety, or hostility, exposes him to overwhelming scolding, criticism, and nagging. At other times, a detached attitude makes the mother appear remote, inaccessible, ungiving, and perhaps inimical.' (Artieti, 1974: 89)

From the Artieti (1974) orientation, it is clear that the child is deeply troubled by a highly anxious mother that is highly critical, or by a detached mother. Both of them make the external world intolerable for the child.

2. Intolerable Inner World and Escape

In facing severe criticism and hostility, the child feels highly uncomfortable and his/her self-identity, his/her self-image and self-boundary is severely threatened. In facing intensive detachment by his/her parent/s, the individual child feels lonely and boring. In both ways, external objects and the external world are not acceptable and tolerable. The individual child tends to withdraw within his inner world. S/hc tends to be self-stimulating and absorbed in his/her inner world. Under this condition, s/he may be accustomed to a self-triggered internal image and self talk. However, being trapped within this inner world, the individual, in no way feels happy. Instead, s/he is also in an unpleasant internal state full of dilemmas.

'The child escapes from the external life, and lives, preponderantly, in his inner life. But the inner life is not pleasant either. A certain number of children perhaps succeed in escaping this dilemma, and eventually in escaping psychosis, too, by reverting to the antecedent sensorimotor level of development. They become hyperkinetic. They indulge in actions, even if not very coordinated or goal directed, rather than inner life. Only a minority of children can avail themselves of this defense…these hyper kinetic children had undergone minimal brain damage at birth and the psychological factors only accentuated the pathology' (Arieti, 1974: 89).

3. Poor Maternal Image and Inner Object of Mother

Arieti (1974) affirmed that the child with a highly critical or highly detached parent would engage in a dilemma of involving a highly lonely and empty inner world or in a highly unpleasant outer world. Only some children can escape from this dilemma by engaging in meaningless and repetitive external activities. While other normal children can build up an inmate attachment with their parents in particular mothers, children who are at risk of schizophrenia can only have a poor maternal image because of the thin inner object of mother.

`We have seen that in normal circumstances, or even when the disturbance was only of moderate intensity, the child tends to build a positive or benevolent image of the mother. The future schizophrenic, however, does not build this benevolent maternal image in early childhood. … Even though the mother may have positive characteristics and may even love the child and try her best, the future patient becomes particularly sensitized to one or all of four fundamental negative characteristics: anxiety, hostility, detachment and unpredictability. The child becomes particularly aware of these negative characteristics because they are the parts of mother that hurt and to which he responds deeply. He ignores others. His use of the primary process cognition makes it possible and perpetuates this partial awareness, this original part object relationship…. The patient who responds mainly to the negative parts of mother will make a whole image of the

> mother out of these negative parts of the resulting whole, which will be a monstrous transformation of the mother. (Arieti, 1974: 90)

Despite the mother of a potentially schizophrenic child still possesses positive characteristics, her negative aspects in terms of hostility, detachment, anxiety and unpredictability are so strong in a way, they create a permanent and negative influence to the child.

4. Negative Image of Self and Others

Along Arieti's (1974) description, the negative image of the mother is so powerful in a way that it distorts the individual child's formation of self-image and perception. S/he may both internalize such images and criticism as well as projecting them outside. In internalizing such maternal hostility, anxiety, and unpredictability, s/he may also regard himself/herself as inferior, lonely and worthless. In projecting this maternal hostility, anxiety, and unpredictability outside, s/he may also regard others as hostile, anxious and unpredictable.

> `Thus the image of the mother as an inner structure is radically difference from that built by the child raised in normal circumstances. Later, this negative image may attract other negative aspects of the other members of the family or of the family constellation as a whole, so that the mother image will be intensified in her negative aspect....Her image becomes a malevolent image, an inner structure that, in a latent or conscious way, may persist for the lifetime of the patients. (Arieti, 1974: 90)

5. Projection of Negative Image to Other

The negative image of the mother within the child's mind can be gradually transferred or generalized to become the image and memories of others. Arieti (1974) regarded it as an I-Thou relationship in which the individual child is `I' and the other as `Thou'

> 'If at this time, the child could possess the vocabulary of the adult, he would call the mother barbarous, bitter, bloodthirsty, brutal, callous...hateful, hellish, ill disposed, ill-natured, ...inhuman, ...the mother image, as the representative of the other - that is, of any other human being and of the interpersonal world - becomes a negative Thou. A normal I-Thou relationship, in Buber's sense, cannot exist. The child will have difficulty in accepting the others, whom he models after the mother. The Thou is too threatening and is a carrier of too much anxiety. This is the beginning of schizophrenic cleavage, this never complete acceptance and integration of the Thou, of that part of the self that originates from others. Unless deprived of its emotional import of potentiality, this Thou tends to remain un-integrated or become dissociated, like a foreign body that is easily externalized later in life in forms of projection and hallucination (Arireti, 1974: 90)

Due to the influence of bad image of the mother, the individual child, in his/her developmental process may have difficulty in accepting others. S/he may project his/her feelings and experiences with his/her highly critical or disengaged parents towards others. On the one hand, s/he may model his/her mother, being highly critical with others or being highly disengaged and detached from his/her mother. On the other hand, being continuously rejected, disapproved and disengaged from his/her mother, s/he himself/herself may have no confidence in meeting the appreciation, approval and even acceptance from others. Within his/her mind, this is also an internalization of his mother's criticism and disengagement that s/he is actually unacceptable to others. Nevertheless, it is highly painful for the child to conclude that s/he is never acceptable by others. Following the thinking of Kelin's (1935) schizoid position, the child may split his `bad self' (the part of self being unacceptable and rejected by others) and project it outward on others, concluding that others are unacceptable, hostile and critical as well as anxious. All these can contribute to his/her pre-psychotic poor I –Thou relationship.

6. Negative Response of the Mother and the Father

> `The vision of the mother is somewhat understood by the mother, who responds to the child with more anxiety. The mother expresses her anxiety in the form of hostility towards the child, who in his turn, will be even more adversely affected. He will respond with behavior that will be more objectionable to the parent. Furthermore, the mother most of the time feels guilty for her hostility and this guilt feeling increases her anxiety. A circular process of ominous proportions originates, which produces intense distortions and maladaptations.... In the majority of the cases, the inner object of the father also consists of negative, although less intense, characteristics. The future schizophrenic feels that both parents, in different ways or in similar ways, have failed him. In a minority of cases, the parental roles are inversed, what we have described in reference to the maternal image patients to the paternal and vice versa. We have seen that in only approximately 25 percent of the cases does this inner image correspond to the real mother. Why is 75 percent of schizophrenia transforming the image into a worse one?' (Arieti, 1974: 90-91)

According to Arieti (1974), there is a vicious circular process. The anxious mother expresses her anxiety as well as hostility towards her child. The child, in response, will become more and more rebellious and objecting to the parents. In result, the child's negative response will also make the mother become more and more anxious and hostile. Apart from the negative maternal image, the father image can also be negative to the child with potential schizophrenia. In a few cases, the father image can be positive. That means, if the mother image is negative but the father image is positive, the child's internal negative object and inner world absorption can be much lessened. S/he will have less chance to develop schizophrenia. However, if the mother image is negative and the father image is negative or slightly negative, the child is more likely to have self-absorption and negative internal objects. Thus, s/he is more likely to develop schizophrenia in the future. Interestingly, as Arieti's (1974) pointed out, only 25% of cases his/her mother image correspond to the real mother, 75% of cases do not. In other words, the negative image of the mother, in the form of a negative internal object, is formed by the child within the vicious circular process in which the anxiety and hostility of the mother, as well as the rejecting attitude of the child, increases drastically far beyond their original expectation, actual personality, and demand. The negative mother image is being constructed with this vicious circular process rather than the actual mother-child connection and attachment.

7. Underdeveloped Inner Object: Poor Self Image, Body Image and Gender Identity

The problem in I-Thou relationship in pre-psychotic childhood will result in an under-developed inner object in terms of poor self-image, body image, and gender identity.

> `The child does not respond equally to all appraisal and roles attributed to him. Those elements hurt him more than stand out as salient elements and are integrated disproportionally. **The self image**, thus, although related to the external appraisal, is not a reproduction of them, but a caricature of them. The grotesque representation of the self of the future patients already from this early age would stupefy their parents if they were aware of it. ....' (Arieti, 1974: 92)

Being spontaneously criticized, rejected, and disengaged by parents; the pre-psychotic child internalizes all these and regards himself/herself as inferior and worthless. These feelings may manifest in a self-deflating way, such as self-teasing and a caricature of others' rejection and comment. Certainly, all these may finally result in construction of poor self-identity and self esteem. The pre-psychotic child internalizes that s/he is rejected and unwanted by others. They perceive themselves as being bad, a bad child for their parents.

> `Self identity and self-esteem in the age period that we are considering are difficult to study. Future schizophrenics at this age do not see themselves as occupying a definite role within the family. *They perceive themselves as being unliked and unwanted. Some of these children have a definite feeling of being bad,* but others are not even sure of being bad; because they may change and improve. Paradoxically, they would feel less insecure if they could see themselves consistently bad, without any uncertainty about their role or image.' (Arieti, 1974: 93)

The feeling of being bad is better than feeling good in reducing the child's sense of insecurity. Facing parental rejection, criticism, as well as disengagement, a positive self-image and good feelings may arouse intensive inner conflict or endless struggle. The individual child may feel trapped within an intensive struggle of being good to win back parental acceptance and love and minimize criticism. Nevertheless, if it does not work, it creates further intensified senses of hopelessness and insecurity. Thus, it would be more secure for the individual child to regard himself/herself as bad in the eyes of their parents. In doing so, s/he can regard his/her parents' critical comment, hostility and detachment as predictable and even reasonable. However, regarding one as bad, in no way feels comfortable, and s/he still feels angry with their parent's hostile or disengaged response. As a consequence, the child keeps himself/herself within a dilemma. On the one hand, s/he tries to ensure that s/he is bad and punishable by parental hostility and detachment. On the other hand, s/he regards her parents are unreasonable, uncaring and rejecting that s/he is simply a victim of these attitudes.

That sort of negative perception not only confines to self-identity but also prevails in body image. As the child perceives himself/herself, despite his/her actual body size and appearance, s/he regards himself/herself as little, feeble, helpless, and distorted.

> `The body image does not generally correspond to the actual physical appearance. The child may perceive him as little, feeble, helpless and distorted. In children who tend to become schizophrenic in adult life, the uncertainty about sexuality is of a different nature.' (Arieti, 1974: 92)

Body figure and self-identity can even diffuse to gender identity in which the child's feelings of hatred towards his/her parents are gradually absorbed and transferred into his/her own gender identity.

> `It concerns sex, gender and identity. Some of these children do not know what their sex is going to be. Although they know that they are boys or girls, they are not sure that they will maintain their sex throughout their lives…in the pre-schizophrenic they assume the form of serious and disturbing thoughts. *In many cases, the doubts are related to the fact that children connect a sense of hostility coming from others that belong to a given sex. If they were girls instead of boys; or boys instead of girls, they think their parents would be more pleased with them. If the most disturbing parent is the opposite sex, the child would like to be of the same sex as this parent, so that he could resist him or her better.*' (Arieti, 1974: 93)

The disturbance of gender identity, according to Artieti, merely comes from the poor image as well as hostile feelings towards their parents that reject, criticize, or detach from them. If the child is of same sex as the rejecting parent, s/he may think that the opposite sex may be able to gain more parental acceptance. If the child is of the opposite sex of the rejecting parent, s/he may think that being the same sex as the parent may help in gaining the love and concern of their parent. However, if both parents are rejecting, the child becomes more vulnerable to onset of psychosis.

> `The most common cause of sexual or gender uncertainty is the fact that the child who feels rejected by both parents tends to reject both parents and therefore has difficulties in identifying with either one of them. I have found fear of castration to be an important or frequent cause of the anxiety that leads to schizophrenia. …in families or cultural environments where sex is strongly expressed or repressed, the Oedipal situation may, in certain cases, increase the already existing anxiety and make the occurrence of schizophrenia more probable. The child attributes his sexual desires to his being bad.' (Arieti, 1974: 93).

The child with both rejecting parents may fail to identity with them, including their gender identity. Following this fear of castration, Oedipal complex, and increasing anxiety inhibit the child's sexual desires. All these become important ingredients leading to schizophrenia.

8. Development of Pre-schizophrenic Defense System: Unresolved Conflict between Good and Bad Parental Image

In early childhood, the individual needs to connect with a good parent in forms of irreplaceable parent-child attachment, bonding, and modeling. Thus, despite the rejecting attitudes of the parents and his/her hostile and rejecting response towards his/her parents, particularly the mother, deep down in his/her mind, s/he still harbors an intensive urge that his/her parents are good or can be good in the future. This sort of urge is necessary for the child to affirm his/her bonding and attachment with his/her parents.

> `the child who is raised in this environment and wants to maintain the image of the mother as a benevolent person tends therefore to accept the negative appraisal of him. By accepting this negative appraisal, he develops the self-image of the bad child. That is, he considered himself inadequate and bad and has little self-esteem. The preservation of the good image of the parent is made possible by the removal from the consciousness of the most unpleasant traits of the parents. Thus, the child will have two images of the parents: the good image, which is conscious, and the bad image, which will remain unconscious. The good parental image appears is myths, legends, and dreams as God, the fairy, the

> magic helper, or the protector. The bad parental image appears as the witch, the stepmother, the bad man, and so forth. (Arieti, 1974: 95)

Maintaining a good parental image is by being unconscious of the negative traits of individual parental images. He may have two parental images, one is bad, and one is good. No doubt, it can be conflicting. To resolve this, the child has to make one image being unconscious and the other one being conscious. In that case, there can be several alternatives, which can be shown by the following:

a) Being conscious of good parental image and being unconscious of bad parental image (Cg + Ub)
b) Being conscious of bad parental image and being unconscious of good parental image (Cb+ Ug)

Arieti (1974) affirmed that Cg + Ub is the most common way to keep a good parental image, in particular the mother image, so that the child can secure his/her affective bond and attachment with his mother. Furthermore, the good maternal image also represents Thou in the interpersonal relationship. The child must accept her in order to fulfill his socialization as well as generalizing her satisfactory interpersonal relationship with others.

> `She is the Thou, the representative of the interpersonal world. The child must accept her in order to fulfill his inborn potentialities for full maturation and socialization. ...It is more tolerable for the child to think the good parent punishes him because he deserves to be punished than to think that he is unfairly punished. If he is punished although he is not bad, he will have a feeling of despair; the situation will seem to him beyond remedy, hopeless ...(Arieti, 1974: 95)

In doing so, the bad parental image is being suppressed. However, that sort of suppression cannot be long lasting, as in reality, the parents, in particular the mother, is hostile, critical, and disengaged. Whenever this occurs to a prevailing extent, the child's suppressed bad parental image will become conscious and the good parental image will be suppressed. That means he shifts back to the state of Cb + Ug.

> `In the majority of the cases where schizophrenia will eventually occur, the transformation of the parental image into a benevolent one does not take place. At a conscious level, the Thou remains distressing, although not malevolent. The child, however, remains hostile towards the parents. Moreover, the characteristics of the internalized parents are generalized to some extent to all women or to adults. (Arieti, 1974: 95)

Although Arieti (1974) mentioned further about the stability of the state of Cb + Ug, it can be understandable that being conscious about the bad image of the mother but being unconscious about good image of the mother (Cb + Ug) can lessen the harmful impact on the self-esteem of the child but it also threatens the necessary emotional bonding and attachment with his/her mother. Thus, s/he may need to shift back to the state of Cg + Ub, being conscious of the good image of her mother and being unconscious of the bad image of her mother so as to temporarily regain the parental attachment and bonding of the mother. As time goes on, s/he may be kept within a dilemma of constant shifting between Cg + Ub and

Cb + Ug to maintain a fragile and but minimal survival of self-image and attachment bonding in the developmental process. In no way, is this constant shifting beneficial to the individual in childhood development. It exhausts all his/her inner psychic and ego energy. It hinders the normal development of ego image, identity, and boundary. It weakens his/her competence in relating to others. As a consequence, the overall ego functioning is deeply burdened and retarded. The child develops a weak sense of self, but is not only bad but highly ambivalent. His sense of self is weak so that the external distress and hostility will not have a very strong destructive effect on him/her. However, the weak self also carries a strong risk that the individual cannot develop a full and cohesive ego in dealing with and coping with adversity and hardship in the external environment.

> 'The 'I', which is the self-image, is also altered. The negative attributes of the self are, to a large extent, repressed. Also, the child no longer sees himself as hated, falsely accused, or the target of hostility. He continues, however, to see himself as weak. The 'bad' me is transformed into the 'weak' me. The child will see himself as a weakling in a world of strong and distressing adults. (Arieti, 1974: 95)

This process of change in the defense mechanism contains the following stages within a constantly and continuously distressing parent in terms of hostility, disengagement, and criticism.

i. Being conscious of a good parental image and being unconscious of a bad parental image so as to accept parents' attitude and secure parental attachment (Pa) but with a bad self image (Sb) (Cg + Ub = Pa + Sb)
ii. Being conscious of a bad parental image and being unconscious of a good parental image so as to get rid of the intolerable sense of a bad self image (-Sb) but bears a risk of losing parental attachment (-Pa) (Cb + Ug = -Pa + -Sb)
iii. Constant shifting between these two stages (Cg + Ub / Cb + Ug) so that the parental attachment and self image has minimal survival in the developmental process but with a consequence of poor self development, a weak sense of self (Sp) and poor ability to deal with external distress from others (Op) (Cg + Ub / Cb + Ug = Sp + Op)

Apart from a weak me, a minority of cases of future schizophrenia may develop intensive regressive behavior with total reliance on their mothers.

> `In a minority of cases of schizophrenia, the child is able to retain the good maternal image that he built before the end of the second year of life, when the mother could still relate to him with care and some devotion. In these cases, the child tends to continue to act like a baby or to manifest strong regressive tendency towards babyhood. He learns to remain a dependent person. If he is completely taken care of and has no will of his own, the mother will be good to him. The mother then will appear again not only as good, but also as omnipotent and competent, and the child will tend to maintain a parasitic attitude. Any separation from the mother is capable of producing great anxiety even much later in life. (Arieti, 1974: 95-96)

That means, according to Arieti (1974), a few cases of future schizophrenia fail to shift to a state of being unconscious of good parental image and being conscious of bad parental image (Cb + Ug). In other words, these cases have no room to build up their own self-image and self-uniqueness. As a consequence, they are regressive and dependent on their mother in everything. All the stages in developing a pre-psychotic child can be shown in Figure 9.

1. Highly Critical or Highly Disengaged Mother:

The child relates to a mother who is very hostile and anxious or detached or disengaged and inaccessible

↓

2. Intolerable External Reality and Painful Inner World

Self identity, image and boundary is severely threatened by maternal criticism. Dreadfully lonely and boring in facing maternal detachment. Intolerable external reality intensifies withdrawn, self stimulating and absorption in his/her inner world. Absorption in self triggering, internal image and self talk. Trap within empty and painful inner world.

↓

3. Poor Permanent and internalized Negative Maternal Image

a. Over-sensitized mothers' hostility and detachment and undermine mothers' love and other good natures.
b. Being accustomed to respond to the negative features of the mothers rather than the holistic features

↓

4. Negative Image of Self and Another

Negative image of mother distorts formation of self image and perception of others.
Internalizes maternal hostility and disenagement and generates inferior, lonely and worthless feeling.
Projecting of maternal hostility, disengagement and regard others as hostile and unacceptable.

↓

5. Poor I-Thou Relationship

Models mother's hostility and disengagement and be highly critical and disenaged with others
Being disengaged from mother, losses self confidence in gaining others' appreciation and approval
Internalizes his mother's criticism and disengagement and think that s/he is actually unacceptable to others.
Split `bad self' and projects it outward on others and conclude that others are hostile and critical.

↓

6. The Negative and Vicious Circular Response of the Mother and the Father

a. The anxious mother expresses her anxiety as well as hostility towards her child.
b. The child, in response will become more and more rebellious and objecting to the parents.
c. The child's negative response will also make the mother becomes more and more anxious and hostile.
d. If the father can be positive, it can compensates the negative image of mother
e. It is the destructive effect of the projected negative maternal image rather than the actual one
f. 25% of cases are affected. 75% can be free from negative effects because of other positive factors

↓

7. Negative Self Image, Body Image Gender Identity and Early Defense System

a. Assuming self `bad' and unliked by parents. b. Rejected one's own gender identity as a way to reject parent. c. The child may perceive him as little, feeble, helpless and distorted in body image. d. Problems in sex identity. e. Development of pre-psychotic defense mechanism with a result of weak sense of self

Figure 9. Pre-psychotic Development of Mother-Child Relationship in Childhood.

Development of Pre-psychotic Personality

Arieti (1974) further elaborates that under the prolonged influence of a highly hostile, critical, and/or disengaged parent, pre-psychotic children may be inclined to develop two types of pre-psychotic personality, the schizoid and the stormy one.

1. Schizoid personality

> `The schizoid personality is a character armor that will protect the child in his increasing contacts with the world. The schizoid personality will continue to transform the malevolent Thou into a less disturbing agent, the distressing Thou, or to be more correct, the distressing other. The designated other in the third person implies distance. The schizoid personality defends the self from the distressing other who constitutes the family and the world. It is a set of defenses built as a reaction to chronic danger, not to immediate fear; it provides tepid responses to poorly expressed states of anxiety and anger. (Arieti, 1974: 103)

Arieti (1974) affirmed that the individual child with a pre-psychotic nature might try all means to lessen the destructive effective of others, in particular her hostile or disengaged mother. In doing so, the individual is able to alleviate his/her *sense of anxiety and anger towards himself/herself as well as towards the distressing others.*

> 'By detaching himself emotionally the patient will avoid the pain connected with the attacks on his self-esteem. Furthermore, it will be easier for him to tolerate the inner images, which, although not as unpleasant as those of the previous period, are still disturbing... and to the image of himself as the weak me. The hostility for the parents produces less guilt feelings, and the image of the self, at least at first, produces less decrease in self-esteem. The intense relatedness among members of the family, which was often present during the first period, is now in many instances replaced by distance and coldness' (Arieti, 1974: 103)

The most effective way to lessen the destructive effect of the distressing others on the individual child is to keep a physical distance, and being emotionally repressed and numbed to hostility and disengagement of his/her parent.

> `The schizoid appears aloof, detached, and less emotional than the average person, less concerned and less involved. Actually, at an unconscious level, he continues to be very sensitive, but he has learned to avoid anxiety and anger in two ways (1) by putting a physical distance between himself and situations that are apt to arouse these feelings, and (2) by repressing all emotion. This physical distance is maintained by avoiding interpersonal relations of refraining from actions that will evoke an unpleasant reaction of the other people. Often when the schizoid person is in the latter stages of his childhood, he would like to be a participant or a doer, but he still remembers from early childhood that action does not pay because it provokes a storm of intense and threatening emotional responses in the surrounding adults.' (Arieti, 1974: 104)

The physical distance is maintained by avoiding interpersonal relation. For a pre-psychotic child, this can be attained by several ways.

a) Avoid physical contact with any persons by keeping oneself in social isolation
b) In actual physical contact, they may avoid interpersonal interaction, eye contact, and verbal contact with others
c) Even in verbal contact, they try to keep quiet, avoid expressing their own view or be submissive to others' wording

Together with this is a total repression of all related emotions in interpersonal interaction. It is a repression of deep-seated emotion such as anger, guilt, and loneliness in facing prolonged hostility and/or disengagement of their mothers or fathers. It is a repression of related emotions in interpersonal interaction. It is also a repression of emotional response from others' criticism, hostility, disengagement, exclusion, and ignorance. As a consequence of emotional repression and being distant from others, *in later childhood, the child becomes underactive or even inactive in action.*

> `Anticipation of action means anticipation of a repetition of these emotional storms. The patients themselves become underactive. In some cases, the patients have actually encouraged him not to do things; doing nothing meant being a good child, because what the child did was always bad. The patient grows older with a deeply rooted pessimism as an outcome of his actions (Arieti, 1974: 105).

That means, the pre-psychotic child gradually become highly pessimistic in interpersonal interactions and in participating and doing anything with others. S/he will be preoccupied with a pessimistic idea that no matter how hard s/he does anything, s/he will be criticized or rejected by others. The state of being inactive, of being a non-doer, and being withdrawn is the best way for survival. *S/he loses his/her self-confidence in interacting with others to a degree, even in avoiding looking into others' eyes.*

> `A characteristic of the schizoid person is the difficulty he has in looking into the eyes of the person who is with him. The schizoid child, and even more so later on, in the schizoid adolescent and young adults, may look elsewhere or make fleeting eye contact. Eye contact not only makes him aware that another person is there, but that person looks at him, as long as the other person may be experienced as an object. (Arieti, 1974: 105)

The avoidance of eye contact serves several important functions. The first function is that the individual tries to avoid being criticized, attacked, or even looked through by others. The second function is that s/he is actually keeping not only a physical distance but also a psychological and social distance from the others. That sort of distance makes him/her feel safe and secure. The third function is that that the individual with safe distance allows him/her to have his/her autonomy in thinking, action, and even imagination. Without looking into others' eyes, and without being looked at by others, the individual can be free to imagine or involve in his/her own fantasy. *S/he can even assume that the other persons are actually lifeless objects* that can be avoided or ignored rather than being controlled, manipulated or humiliated by them.

> `Contrary to what the compliant person does under parental pressure, the child who has developed a schizoid personality prefers not to comply. And yet, to the observer, he quite often gives the impression of being extremely complaint. Actually, he complies in a

> perfunctory way. He goes through the motions of the imposed act, but without being emotionally involved. In order to avoid anxiety, he becomes a person uncommitted to what he is doing or to what he is participating in. We must remember that if the patient succeeds in experiencing himself as being emotionally uninvolved, it is because his resentment and hostility are deeply repressed. Should he later becomes schizophrenic, the resentment and the hostility may be displaced towards non-parental figures, who may become persecutors. (Arieti, 1974: 105)

In facing the profound and continuous hostile and critical or disengaged parents, the pre-psychotic child intends to keep a physical and emotional distance. However, s/he needs to rely on their parents' attachment, care, and bonding. In doing so, s/he needs to comply with their views, interactions, and even command. However, this type of compliance is not a real compliance. According to Arieti (1974), in schizoid personality, *it is a kind of compliance in a perfunctory way. That means, the individual child/adolescent does it as a duty but without care, interest, and emotion. S*/he becomes a person without real emotional involvement. S/he repressed all his/her emotions including his/her resentment and hostility towards his/her parents. Instead, s/he may displace all these to others and label them as persecutors.

The child/adolescent may need to have some insight towards his/her schizoid personality. S/he knows that detachment is a very unsatisfactory solution in interpersonal interaction. However, s/he does not have any way out. S/he needs to be compliant instead of being aggressive to get as least some kind of substitute s/he wants. However, in doing so, s/he pays a great price by suppressing all his/her emotions into a particular hostility towards others. That means, consciously, s/he is a person with good compliance but great emotional and physical detachment from others. Unconsciously, s/he becomes more and more aggressive and hostile. S/he also harbors a secret wish to be reconnected with others. In others words, the child/adolescent faces *two types of inner conflicts:*

a. a conflict between conscious compliance and unconscious hostile and aggression
b. a conflict between being detached from others covertly but a wish to reconnect with others latently.

These conflicts prevail making the individual child/adolescent's mental state become highly unstable, and anxious with poor sense of reality. In fact, they are highly unbearable. All these *repressed emotions, together with the wish to be connected with their parents usually may get their release in dreams and fantasies.*

> `The sensitivity still exists at an unconscious or preconscious level. The dreams or fantasies of the schizoid often reveal great emotional potentialities; they are very dramatic and have great intensity of feelings and vivacity of actions. They transport the patient into an adventurous life, and often into storms of affect. With this action, on the other hand, the schizoid person tries to be as static as possible. Often, if he acts, he will be very impersonal and will try to avoid communication by direct contact. (Arieti, 1974: 105)

Children/adolescents with pre-psychotic tendencies may even choose some unrealistic or detached ways to express their repressed emotions and suppressed urges to connect with their hostile and/or disengaged parents.

> 'A 9 years old schizoid girl used to write letters to her parents in which she would explain what she did not dare not tell them directly. Even when they are older, schizoid patients prefer to write letters, rather than make telephone calls, and even when they write, they do so in a cold, formal, businesslike manner. In schoolwork, the schizoid learns much more from a book than from the direct presentation of the teacher. Written materials convey meaning to him much more than spoken material, because a direct interpersonal interaction is eliminated.' (Arieti, 1974: 106)

All these mechanisms are done to preserve the child from related danger from his/her distressing significant others. All these distressing others are not only substantial external objects. They penetrate into the mind of pre-psychotic child and become his/her distressing inner objects. Being detached and distant to other is the only way for him/her to maintain a fragile balance in his/her self-development and interpersonal interaction.

> `the schizoid persons...later in life appears to others as ... being detached, cold, peculiar, suspicious, arrogant, condescending, and cocky. Thus, the interpersonal world will not be able to interact with ease with schizoid persons. A state of tension, distance, mistrust, and misinterpretation is likely to occur that will reinforce in the patient his schizoid attitude. That is, he will continue to envision his being with others as a chronic, unspoken, moderate state of danger or surrounding hostility from which he has to continue to defend himself.' (Arieti, 1974: 106)

2. Stormy Personality

Apart from the schizoid personality, pre-psychotic children may also develop a stormy personality in which they are highly fluctuating between detachment and hostility towards distressing others. Comparing with those with schizoid personality, children/adolescents with stormy personality are accustomed to rapid change in dealing with external distressing others. Their `I-Thou' relationship is different from those with schizoid personality. *Their distressing others are distressing not in a stable manner, instead they are highly fluctuating and unstable.* At one time, these distressing others may be supportive and kind. At the other time, these distressing others can be prevailingly hostile and critical. All these changes can be highly unpredictable and rapid. Thus, the children/adolescents are used to rapid changes. They can be suddenly become highly aggressive and hostile, so as to defend themselves from the hostility and severe criticism of their distressing others. In fact, a child with a stormy personality is even more difficult than a schizoid personality in forming their sense of self.

> 'He was uncertain about the role that the parents, not siblings, assigned to him in the family. He could not make out what he meant to each of the surrounding persons, especially adults, but also siblings. He felt inconsistently unwanted, the meaning to this identity or presence in the home remaining not well established, unless connected with overt rejection. As we have seen, no general attitude towards others (either of compliance, aggressiveness, or detachment) could become well established. This uncertainty about the role attributed to him is due not only to the fact that the parents were inconsistent and torn by opposite feelings, like hostility and a sense of duty. It is due also, and perhaps predominantly, to the fact that the child tried to deny the role he felt the parents were attributing to him. He was too frightened to become aware of something that was presumably bad. (Arieti, 1974: 107-108)

Facing the rapid changes of the their parents, pre-psychotic children with stormy personality embrace intensive uncertainty and inconsistency in which they are highly anxious and frightened to accept the fact that their parents are hostile or they are unacceptable and bad to their parents. The spontaneous uncertainty and inconsistency may make their personality and mental state highly fluctuating and unstable to an extent that they are unable to formulate their own self worth as well as self-esteem.

> 'He vacillated between all possible views. He saved some self-esteem, but at the expense of a stable sense of self-identity…. He harbored serious doubts about his personal significance and self worth. But at least he succeeded in preserving his self as an entity, as a unity… .The family members, too, consider the patient unpredictable and respond with varying behaviors, which reinforces the child's inner images of the family members' (Arieti, 1974: 108)

Pre-Psychotic Personality in Adolescence and Early Adulthood

1. Extensive Detachment and Rebellion from Parents

Both children with stormy and schizoid personality have difficulties in constructing their own self-esteem and self-identity. It is even worse than those with stormy personality. For those with schizoid personality, they are detached and stayed with their self-image as 'bad child'. However, for those with stormy personality, they are still searching related roles that are suitable for them. Despite having a wide social circle, they fail because of their own instability and rapid changes that are intolerable for others. (Arieti, 1974: 112-3).

For adolescents with schizoid personality, they are more inclined to retain their prolonged and continuous detachment as ways to avoid hostility and disengagement by others. They are emotionally detached followers in groups, particularly in some peculiar groups such as an army, religious group, or even some marginalized society. They may be particularly interested in attachment to a supreme God to whom s/he regards as substituted good and protective parents (Arieti, 1974). S/he may try every means to attach to groups or organizations that are different or even deviant from his/her parents as a way to escape from his/her parents' engulfment. However, s/he will never be successful in doing so, as his/her continuous detachment defense mechanism still prevails in fearing that others may still be hostile and hypocritical to him/her. S/he is accustomed to repression of feelings and detachment from intimate contact and relationship. All these repressions and detachments, on the one hand, protect him/her from being hurt by others. On the other hand, they are also highly intolerable and uncomfortable for a lively and drastic growing adolescent. To get rid of these uncomfortable feelings, they may occasionally be involved in the abuse of drugs and alcohol.

2. Unavoidable stressful involvement in competitive life and self-injury

If the psychosocial condition is fairly stable, and the stormy and schizoid defense mechanism is effective in coping with stress and frustration in daily life, the pre-psychotic adolescents may never develop schizophrenia. Nevertheless, if environmental conditions are far too stressful, there may be significant injury of the self that continues the development of schizophrenia. There may be some pre-conditions in self-injury, which lead to onset of schizophrenia.

> `In many cases, the schizoid or stormy character structure eventually no longer constitutes adequate protection. The difficulties become more apparent the more the patient proceeds towards adulthood, for several reasons. The school situation, the increase of sexual desires, and the search for a position in a competitive world plus his character armor are serious strains. The defenses that the patient was able to mobilize earlier in life used to be fairly efficient when he had to contain extensively or predominantly with his family. Now he feels he has to deal with the world at large. In spite of his emotional detachment the schizoid person resents that fact that both the family and society demand that he relinquish his detachment and withdrawal - a request he cannot fulfill; his schizoid defense not only does not protect him, but also actually handicaps him when social pressure compels him to do things in his withdrawal. (Arieti, 1974: 115).

Arieti (1974) affirmed that the schizoid and stormy coping mechanism, despite their effectiveness in dealing with highly hostile, unstable, or disengaged parents in childhood, may fail to cope with the increasing demand from various psychosocial contexts in the fast growing adolescence and demanding adulthood. Facing all these huge external and competitive demands, withdrawal, detachment, or being ignored from external environment can no longer work efficiently. Individuals with a pre-psychotic personality are forced to face all these involuntarily and unwillingly. All these are out of the coping capacity of the individual with a result of possible injury to the individual.

3. Poor Conceptual Thinking and Self Image

The individual may become highly sensitive in interaction with others with a presumption that others may resemble his/her parents' hostility, criticism, and disengagement. As a consequence, his/her own schizoid detachment mechanism prevails to a degree that s/he fails to establish a good and integrated self esteem and identity. Arieti (1974) asserted this in terms that the conceptual life of the individual is deeply disturbed.

> `The conceptual-feeling of personal significance, of self identity, of one's role in life, of self esteem, now constitutes a great part of self..... Because of these adverse experiences, the pre-schizophrenic continues to change in a negative way the image of the self. We have seen that in spite of his detachment, the schizoid person has maintained and reinforced the image of himself as the bad child. But at a certain age, to be bad acquires the meaning of being incapable, inadequate, worthless, and even guilty for being so. The stormy person, in spite of his desperate attempts, will never find a reliable meaning for his existence. He will reach a point where he can no longer trust life as a possible source of pleasure or self-fulfillment. The worsening of the self-image is largely determined by the patient's new orientation towards time. (Arieti, 1974: 116-7)

Arieti (1974) affirmed that the pre-schizophrenic individual is unable to establish a substantial and good self-image as s/he is kept within a conceptual thinking, image, and memories of incapability, inadequacy, worthlessness, and guilt. S/he fails to harbor hope towards life in the future. S/he keeps thinking that life is bad and pessimistic. His/her life is bad and worthless as s/he is bad and worthless. That sort of negative thinking is different from persons with depression. Their sadness and sense of worthlessness usually occurs when their beloved object is lost and disappeared. However, in persons with pre-schizophrenia, the beloved object never appears. Instead, s/he only faces continuous bad and highly hostile and disengaged objects. S/he may conclude, even though good objects are available; s/he will never be worthwhile to attach to it.

> `Eventually he may conclude that his life is going to be bad because he is bad or worthless. He feels that if he has always done wrong, it is because there is something wrong with him; if he has not been loved, it is not because loves does not exist in this world, but because he is not lovable.... He hates himself more that any one hates him... (Artiei, 1974: 116)

Psychosexual Conflict

The pre-psychotic children fail to establish their successful sex identity because of the prevailing hostility, criticism, and disengagement of their parents. In childhood and early adolescence, such failure is hidden and concealed properly. However, in adolescence especially, in the puberty state, this unresolved and uncertainty in sexual identity manifests and prevails. Such sex difficulties may appear in different forms such as homosexuality, difficulties in sexual performance, and inability to seek pleasure (anhedonia) including sex. Regarding homosexuality, Freud's Schreber case (Freud, 1911) was a clear example showing that homosexuality is intermingled with psychotic paranoia, morbid jealousy, and envy. However, latent homosexuality is not a must for pre-psychotic adolescents. The most common form of the phenomenon is that they fail to regard sex as a source of pleasure, personal involvement, or as a link of a lovable object.

> `He feels even more inadequate as a sexual partner and a love object. Feeling undesired sexually and unloved are experiences injurious to the self, but feeling unlovable and undesirable is even a more devastating emotion. In other words, what is particularly damaging is not the idea that the patient does not obtain love or sexual gratification now. It is the idea that his constitution and personality make it impossible for him ever to elicit love or sexual desire.' (Arieti, 1974: 119)

The weak and inadequate self image, the prolonged detachment from the distressing others, the inadequacy of formulating a clear sexual identity from hostile and critical parents, all contribute to the individual's sense of indifference to his/her heterosexual partner or boyfriend/girlfriend. They have severe difficulties in finding pleasure in sex, to feel loving or being loved by others. It seems that his/her sexual identity, desires, sex and courtship ability, and sensitivity is deeply repressed by an injurious self image and self identity. In some cases, the individual may engage in sexual masturbation and frequent sexual intercourse to stimulate his/her sense of being.

> `In relation to the psychodynamics of schizophrenia, sexual life is not important in itself, but only insofar it may affect injurious self image. Since the patient sees himself as a sexually inadequate person, or a homosexual, or an undesirable sexual partner, or lacking sexual self-control, or having no definite sexual identity, he may develop a devastating concept of himself. Moreover, in the case of lacking definite sexual identity, there is continual draining of the resources of the person who strives towards self-identity. (Arieti, 1974: 120).

Pre-psychotic Panic

Despite that the individual has spent all his efforts in detachment and coping with the distressing others, s/he will still be in a difficult situation in facing all developmental challenges and frustrations, and from the social environment to an extent that his/her fragile self system can no longer tolerate any more. Finally, before the onset of psychosis, the individual usually suffers from a state of pre-psychotic panic outbreak in which s/he is deeply threatened by a 'jungle' of threat to his/her already weak and inadequate self-image.

> 'It is when the patient comes to believe that the future has no hope, that the promise of life will not be fulfilled, and the future may be even more desolate than the present that the psychological decline characteristic of this third period reaches it culmination. He feels threatened from all sides, as if he were in a jungle…a jungle of concepts where the threat is not to survival, but to the self-image. The dangers are conceptual feelings such as that of being unwanted, unloved, unlovable, inadequate, unacceptable, inferior, awkward, clumsy, not belonging, peculiar, different, rejected, humiliated, guilty, unable to find his own way among the different paths of life, disgraced, discriminated against, kept at a distance, suspected, and so on. (Arieti, 1974: 120).

Before the onset of schizophrenia, individuals are overwhelmed with the threats from surrounding distressing others. They are highly sensitive to being rejected, excluded, neglected, undermined, unloved, and humiliated by others to an extent that they have no way to escape in their path of life. That means, even if they try their best, they fail to detach and ignore them. Similarly, Sullivan (1953) described this as a stage of dreadful disorganization, terror, and perception of danger in which the individual cannot escape or cannot dissociate. Sullivan (1953) affirmed that as the failure of dissociation mechanism. The horrifying feeling comes from the individuals' of senses of uncertainty, loss of control, and unpredictability. They retreat to their primary process of regression and they fail to face their distressing others in a sensible and rational way.

> `In the totality of his human existence, and through the depth of all his feelings, the individuals now sees himself as totally defeated, without any worth or possibility of redemption. In the past, he had undergone similar experiences, but they were faint; now they are vivid. They are vivid even though they are verbalized and occur in a nonrepresentational, almost abstract form. They include experiences that cannot be analyzed or broken down into pieces of information, and yet they are accompanied by increasingly lugubrious feelings…everything seems useless, meaningless, or frightening. He cannot accept life or himself anymore. He does not dare express these feelings in words. In many cases, he would not able to do so. Nevertheless, in some circumstances he tried to appeal for help… (Arieti, 1974: 121)

The individual before the onset of schizophrenia is surrounded by the dreadful sense of horror from overwhelming distressing others. S/he is being totally defeated without any sense of worth and redemption. S/he cannot accept himself/herself any more. S/he is so frightened that s/he dares not to express any words. S/he is in a plight of breaking down in which s/he is totally confused, threatened, worthless, and helpless in a way that s/he is going to break down mentally.

The Period of Psychosis

Psychosis starts when the individual is totally uncontrollable to external threats with a loss of conceptual feeling on self-image and self-identity.

> 'The psychosis starts not only when these concept-feelings are projected to the external world, but also when they become specific and concrete. The indefinite feelings become finite, the imperceptible become perceptible, and the vague menace is transformed into a specific threat. It is no longer the whole horrible world that is against the patients: they are against him. He no longer has a feeling of being under scrutiny, under the eyes of the world; s/he no longer has a mild sense of suspiciousness toward his unfriendly neighbors. The sense of his/her suspiciousness becomes the conviction that they follow, watch, influence, or even control him. The conceptual and abstract are reduced to the concrete, the specific. (Arieti, 1974: 123)

That means, psychosis starts when all these conceptual and perceptual over-whelming fears from distress others reach an intolerable state. They turn into concrete and specific fears in forms of distinguished and well-organized paranoia and/or grandiose delusions and hallucinations. It can be one of the following examples:

a) changing the sense of suspiciousness of neighbor to a concrete sense of being closely watched by the neighbors
b) turning a distressing and hostile father and mother image into a highly powerful and mighty fairy and king that can govern one's life and fortune
c) changing the hostility and criticism of distressing others into other alienated controlling forces such as powerful and over-whelming electronic and microwave control and detection from others, such as FBI agents or spies from certain countries.
d) attributing individuals' misfortunes, hardships, and suffering in life to the control of supernatural powers in the form of evil spirits, ghosts and bad fairies

All these paranoid hallucinations and delusions are well organized to an extent that the individual become the center and victim of a well-organized persecution by others.

> 'The patient often experiences some phenomena that convinces him that something is done or ordained against him. He is the victim of a plot. He is accused of being a spy, a murderer, a traitor, or a homosexual. He hears hallucinatory voices that repeat these accusations. He is unhappy, fearful, and often indignant. (Arieti, 1974: 123)

On the one hand, the individual suffers a lot from the self constructed persecutory delusions and hallucinations. Comparing this with the pre-psychotic state, the individuals' conceptual fear turns into a substantial and concrete one. However, in doing so, the individual's weak and fragile self-image is delusively strengthened. The sense of guilt is also appropriately eliminated. The negative part of the self-image is being projected and symbolized.

> 'The externalization (or projection), and the reduction (or concretization) of some psychodynamic conflicts into these psychotic symptoms....The projected feeling of being a failure, but the feeling of being a failure does not appear as a belief of being accused of being a failure, but of being a spy or a murderer.... The delusion of persecution is not just

> a projection and a concretization. As the unpleasant part of the self image is reinstituted, brought back to symbolic equivalents of the people who originally appraised the patient in a way that was rightly or wrongly experienced as destructive and undermining.' (Arieti, 1974: 124)

The mechanism of projection, as well as symbolization, is an abnormal adaption to the unfavorable environment so that the harm of the oppressive environment can be reduced to a minimum. That means, the individual, in facing the highly distressing others, projects and symbolizes his/her negative self-image outward. S/he develops a highly powerful but delusive detector of possible persecutors. All these measures serve a vital function in restoring a minimal survival of his/her weak, fragile, and even split self-image.

Implications to Mental Health Recovery for People with Schizophrenia

It is clear that Arieti (1974) described a clear and detail developmental process in the formulation of schizophrenia from childhood, adolescence to early adulthood. It can be summarized into the following stages;

1. highly critical or highly disengaged mother
2. intolerable external reality and painful inner world
3. poor permanent and internalized negative maternal image
4. negative self image and others
5. poor I-Thou relationship
6. the negative and vicious circular response of the mother and father
7. negative self image, body image, gender identity and early defense system
8. development of pre-schizophrenia defense system-unresolved conflict between good and parental image
9. development of pre-psychotic personality
    a. extensive detachment and rebellion from parents
    b. unavoidable stressful involvement in competitive life and self injury
10. pre-psychotic panic
11. the period of psychosis.

Similar to Laing (1960), the development of schizophrenia is directly related to a highly stressful and oppressive psychosocial environment, in particular the family context in which parents consciously and unconsciously become oppressors. In forms of criticism, rejection, isolation, and detachment, parents hinder their children's normal development of healthy self-image and identity. Instead, they internalize their mothers' negative comments and hostility and develop negative self-images and perceptions towards others with a consequence of poor I-Thou relationship. Based on this, the individual gradually nurtures a stormy or a schizoid personality, which finally leads to the onset of schizophrenia. All these have the following implications on intervention for the clients' mental health recovery.

1. Related professionals should accept and understand clients' confusion in the mental state of psychosis

2. Clients within the psychotic panic should be understood in terms of facing intolerable internal conflicts within their relationship with others. They may be highly confused in good and bad others, as well as good and bad self.
3. It is important that related interventions in recovery of schizophrenia should be found in a highly supportive and caring psychosocial environment in which positive I-Thou relationships can be developed and nurtured
4. Within the highly supportive and caring psychosocial environment, related professionals should facilitate clients with schizophrenia to reformulate a positive self-image as well as a positive perception of others.
5. The development of positive self-image and perception of others within a positive I-Thou relationship should initiate from a positive worker-client relationship and among clients in various service contexts and gradually transfer to other social circles such as peers and colleagues.
6. For those clients' parents who are still highly rejecting, criticizing and even oppressive, related professionals should understand their demands, needs, emotions, and frustrations. Based on this, related professionals should facilitate them to build a positive parent-child relationship with clients.

All these can be demonstrated in the following case illustration. Related parties' consensus in using their stories for academic purposes was sought. For the sake of confidentiality, their personal identities and personal information were properly disguised.

H was a client with schizophrenia residing in a psychiatric half way house. He was born in a middle class family in which his father was a busy merchant. His mother was a beautiful woman who spent most of her time in keeping own beauty. In fact, her pregnancy with H was just an accident entirely out of the expectation of his mother. When H was small, he was entirely under the care of his grandmother. H's mother did have some in-law problems with H's grandmother. She did not want H's grandmother to stay in her house with an excuse of taking care of H. Thus, by various reasons, when H was only two years old, she purposefully expelled H's grandmother.

From that time onwards, H was taken care by a Filipino maid. H's mother was obsessive and critical in parenting H. She rarely embraced H but she required H to follow every detail of her comment in family life, school life, and social life. When H was small, he cried bitterly and required the togetherness of his grandmother. But his mother refused. Instead, she hit him to stop his crying. When H was older, he was required to follow a very tight and strict schedule in everyday life. If he failed to do so, he would be closely watched and controlled by the maid under the tight supervision of his mother.

In no way, could H have a positive mother image. He hated his mother's control. But whenever he tried to fight back, his mother exerted even stronger control, criticism, and physical punishment upon him. Gradually, H became accustomed to keeping quiet, internalizing his anger and suppressing all his negative feelings. As a consequence, H became inferior, inert, withdrawn, and passive. He did not have the competence to relate to others. Because of his weak and inert appearance, his classmates frequently bullied him. They simply called him the 'dead monkey'. Some even pushed him and dumped his lunch box. H was deeply frustrated by that, but instead of fighting back, he simply absorbed it.

To face this painful reality, H gradually developed a schizoid personality in which he tried to detach himself from both family and school. At home, his detachment from his mother's critical comments appeared in a form of rebellious behaviors. He seemed not to follow his mother's instruction or showed no emotional response to his mother's dialogue. He simply appeared as inert, passive and shut his ears from his mother. All this made his mother become highly furious. She hit him hard but H only tolerated it quietly and passively. Once, he ran away home for a whole day to avoid being seriously beaten by his mother.

At school, H was absorbed in his daydreaming. Gradually, he developed related delusions and hallucinations. He imagined his parents were not his real parents. Instead, his real father was in fact, an army general in China. Instead of being inert, passive, and withdrawn, he became overtly aggressive, annoying, and irritable. Once, a classmate bullied him as a dead monkey, he became furious and chased around the bullies. At first, the bullies felt happy about that. However, as H turned into a panic state with a very large voice yelling that his father was the General of the Army in China, he came to defeat all enemies. He grasped a long stick, and chased around the bullies making them fearful and they ran away.

Related teachers called the police and took H to an emergency unit. He was immediately hospitalized in a nearby mental hospital. His psychiatrist diagnosed him as suffering from schizophrenia. He stayed there for six months and was later discharged home. At that time, H was only 16 years old. To ensure his recovery, everyday H had to attend a day center in a rehabilitation service agency in which the writer was the professional consultant. Under the supervision of the writer, they induced proper psychosocial intervention for the mental health recovery of H.

From the above case illustration, it was clear H had a highly critical mother giving H a poor self-image as well as a poor I-Thou relationship. Gradually H developed a schizoid personality in which he tried his best to detach himself from the painful and oppressive reality. Prolonged detachment and self-isolation made him develop related hallucinations and delusions. His psychosis finally outburst after a period of pre-psychotic panic triggered by the bullies from his schoolmates. Below was the self-narration of the social worker, Z, in the day center in describing how he induced proper psychosocial intervention for the mental health recovery of H.

Z: 'When H first came to the day center, his mother accompanied him. Indeed, she was a powerful woman. She demanded us to take good care of his son. Whether his son wanted to express anything, she simply came in aggressively saying that H was not mature. We should follow her instruction solely. H seemed to be angry at his mother's dominance. However, to avoid being further oppressed by his mother, he simply kept deadly quiet in front of his mother. In his mother's eye, it seemed that he was an inadequate person. But he tried to neglect, ignore, and detach from his mother's negative comment and dominance. He tried to prove that he was good and competent. It was clear that Z was confused about his own self-image in facing the mother's highly oppressive dominance.

Under the advice of our professional consultant, I tried to separate H from his mother so that he could have his own personal space in developing his positive self-image and relationship with others. In fact, H voiced that he did not want to live with his mother. Under that sort of condition, I tried to apply for residence in one of our psychiatric halfway houses for H. At first, his mother strongly opposed that decision. However, since it was suggested by H's psychiatrist, she accepted it. Two months later, H was admitted into our psychiatric half way house. In the daytime, he came to the day center to join various activities and programs. At the nighttime, he stayed in the psychiatric half way house.

From the above self-narration by Z, it was clear that related psychosocial intervention began with a deep understanding of H's deep confusion of self-image and perception of others, in particular in relating to his mother. It was crucial that H should be free from his mother's dominance and oppression before he could recover. Under the supervision of the writer, Z tried to establish a supportive and caring psychosocial environment for H. In the day care center, Z tried to formulate a group for several young male adults with him. They were all clients with a past record of schizophrenia. Z facilitated them to enjoy interesting social and recreational activities. Within these activities, Z enabled them to support one another. Under these conditions, H was very happy and enlightened. The following was H's self-narration about his feelings towards interaction and activities in this group.

> H: I liked this group. It really enlightened me. In the past, I had no friends. I was just bullied, isolated, and oppressed by others. However, in this group, thanks to the work of social worker Z, all members in this group were very supportive. They were all young clients with schizophrenic record. Interestingly, all of them had a powerful and dominant father or mother. We shared our experiences frankly and comfortably. We supported one another in related social and recreational activities. Once, I was sick and had a fever, they all comforted me. Whenever, I felt sad about my past experiences, they cheered me up. They were kind and empathetic. I got a feeling the whole group turned into a caring family. Z seemed to be our good mother and all other young guys in the group were my good brothers. I felt being deeply respected and cared. Indeed, it was a very good feeling.

From H's self-narration, it was clear that Z arranged a highly supportive social environment so that H could develop a good I-Thou relationship. In addition to that, Z continuously engaged in constructive activities so that H could develop a positive self-image and relationship. Z described this in the following details

> Z: H felt happy and supportive in the half way house. As his mental state was stable and related hallucinations and delusions decreased accordingly, we tried to encourage him to receive proper vocational training so that he could develop his own potentials and construct his career life. In fact, H had a strong interest in computer programming. Apart from playing computer games, he drew very good computer cartoons, and was very keen in designing new computer games. On that condition, we encouraged H to enroll in a certificate course in computer programming.
>
> At first, H did not show much interest in it, as he was still afraid of connecting with strangers within a new environment. In that condition, we arranged another two clients to accompany him to enroll in this course. With these two clients, H was much more stable psychologically and mentally. Gradually, he was stable to develop a strong interest in the course. He finally graduated with a good result, and was immediately recruited by a famous computer games firm as a game designer. His creativity and talents were able to develop and manifest in an appropriate way.
>
> Two years later, H was promoted to be a senior pregame designer. From that time onwards, H was no longer a client with schizophrenia. He was free from anti-psychotic medication. Occasionally, he might still think that his real father was the general of the Chinese army; however, he knew that it was just his own imagination and fantasy. He no longer had a poor self-image and a poor I-Thou relationship. Instead, he was a normal person with good talents and a career path. Because of his achievement, he was able to rent his own flat and lived with two of his colleagues in his company. They were a remarkable team in designing profitable and attractive computer games.

Regarding H's mother, since H no longer lived with her, she could not dominate, criticize, and control him. Also, as long as long H had a good career path, she came to have better respect towards him.

It was clear that under the good arrangement of Z, H was able to develop his potential and talents in computer programming. By means of this, he was able to construct his self-image and self-identity. Based on this, H had a speedy recovery. He was no longer a client with schizophrenia. Instead, he became a remarkable young person with a brilliant career path as a computer game designer.

From Trauma and Dissociation to Schizophrenia

Several forces cause self-fragmentation of persons with schizophrenia. The first force is external oppression coming from a highly oppressive environment with overwhelming of power and control on the individual. The social construction view is best described by Foucault's concept of power and civilization of madness. According to Glass (1995), external oppressive power is gradually transformed into internal self-destructive power in the formation of regressive delusion and hallucination. However, within this process of transformation, the individual feels highly insecure. S/he suffers from a process of ontological insecurity and emptiness. The process of turning from an ontological security position to an ontological insecurity position, within the onset of psychotic fragmentation, is best described by Laing's (1960) forces of engulfment, implosion, and petrification. Arieti (1974) further elaborated that this process occurs within the individual's childhood and adolescence in pre-psychotic development. All these concepts demonstrate that psychotic self-fragmentation is caused by highly destructive events happening within the overwhelming oppressive social environment. These destructive events have a traumatic impact on the individual making her/him become schizophrenic. In this section, the writer describes how related studies show that trauma is one of major causes of self-fragmentation in persons with schizophrenia. There are three major groups of concepts and studies describing how individuals' self system can be fractured by traumatic experiences:

1. Breaking down of one's ego system in traumatic experiences and recall (Individual's weak and fragile ego system is gradually or abruptly broken down by traumatic experiences and related recall) (Garland, 1991).
2. Failure of dissociation mechanism (Dissociation of traumatic experiences protects the individual from traumatic recall and allows the individual to absorb the negative impact of the traumatic experience gradually. However, the failure of the dissociation mechanism implies an overwhelmingly negative impact on the individual. The loss of the protective mechanism leads to a final fracture of the individual self system) (Sullivan, 1956)
3. Spontaneous evidence and co-morbidity between traumatic experiences (child abuse, bullying, victimization) and psychosis (Morrison et al., 2006). (There are numerous studies in this decade showing that trauma is one of the major psychosocial causes leading to psychosis in which positive symptoms, negative symptoms, and first rank symptoms, are closely related to process, details, contents of traumatic experiences, individual experiences in abuse, victimization, bullying, and disasters, in particular those happening in childhood and adolescence.)

Breaking Down of Ego System in Post-trauma Fear

For many individuals who embrace a weak ego system in his/her developmental process, a traumatic event may make him/her risk a breakdown of his/her ego system. The break down process may start with the discriminatory, filtering, and denial process in facing one's traumatic experiences, in particular over-whelming fear in recalling all these traumatic experiences.

> `By creating links of what is already there, by joining up who enters with exciting features or functions of the mind, the ego is attempting to create once more structures of some permanence in which ego functioning is possible…The central difficulty with a disaster lies, I believe, right here: the very intensity of the struggle to deal with the flood of unmanageable material in the absence of the apparatus for thinking itself locks that material powerfully and precisely to whatever has been released by the breakdown of internal barriers and structures.' (Garland, 1991:45)

The individual, without an integrated and cohesive ego system, in facing the traumatic event, is unable to deal with the adverse stimuli constructively. S/he is lacking an internal apparatus to contain, to interpret, and to incorporate all these negative stimuli into the ego system. Instead, the overwhelming negative stimuli may be intensive and strong enough to break the already fragile and loose ego system. The impacts of powerful negative stimuli from traumatic events stir up the early phantasies of devastation and cruelty of the individual.

> `In other words, the traumatic influx of stimulation from the present stirs up the early fantasies of devastation and cruelty, and paranoid views of relations between objects, which then get bound up with the present events in a way which is hard to undo. It seems that the more intense and long lasting the traumatic event, the greater and the more lasting the emotional load that it carries, which makes it still harder to disengage from the newly-released and highly charged material to which it gets attached.' (Garland, 1991: 19)

The more long lasting traumatic experiences are, the greater and long lasting is the emotional loading to the individual, and the more vulnerable s/he becomes in facing both external and internal adverse demands and stimuli. Very often, it is not the actual traumatic experiences that matter, rather it is how the individual contains, selects, interprets, recalls, and filters the traumatic experiences. In fact, the breaking down of the individual's ego system in traumatic events is based on four groups of related factors.

Group A: Destructive effects of the traumatic experiences (intensity, duration, and frequency of harm created)

Group B: Durability of the ego system in facing external threat (stability and integrity of the ego system, unsettled and unresolved emotional complex)

Group C: Related support from external environment (support, care, comfort, and acceptance from others. Or rejection, isolation, stigmatization, exclusion and punishment from others)

Group D: Inner processing of traumatic experience (filtering, containing, interpreting, repressing, and recalling of traumatic experiences

(Yip, 2013)

Following Freud's line of thinking, Garland (1998) described the breaking down process after traumatic experiences in detail.

> `The mind is flooded with a kind and degree of stimulation that is far more than it can make sense of or manage. Something very violent feels as though it has happened internally, and this violence is felt to have happened, or indeed has actually happened, in the external world. This is a massive disruption in functioning, amounting to a kind of breakdown. It is a breakdown of an established way of going about one's life, of established beliefs about the predictability of established mental structures, of an established defensive organization. It leaves the individual vulnerable to intensive and overwhelming anxieties from internal sources as well as from the actual external events. Primitive fears, impulses, and anxieties are given fresh life. Trust in the fundamental goodness of one's objects, that is to say the world itself, is shattered....Loss of a belief in the predictability of the world, and in the protective function of good objects, both internal and external, will inevitably mean a resurgence of fears about the cruelty and strength of the bad object. There is a rapid slide into primitive paranoid beliefs about one's status in the world. Crucially, the anxieties coincide; the external events is perceived as confirming the worst of the internal fears and fantasies – in particular the reality and imminence of death, or personal annihilation, through the failure of those good objects (internal and external) to provide protection from the worst.' (Garland, 1998: 10)

Following the line of thinking of the individual protective shield in facing an external threat, Garland (1998) described that there is a breakdown of one's normal ego functioning and defense mechanism in life in facing traumatic experiences. Yip (2013) concluded that the breakdown of the ego system includes the following:

1. a breakdown of an established way of going about one's life,
2. a breakdown of established beliefs
3. a breakdown about the predictability of established mental structures
4. a breakdown of established defensive organization.
5. a breakdown of the trust in the fundamental goodness of one's objects,
6. a breakdown of protective function of the good objects
7. a breakdown of the world itself, is shattered
   (Garland, 1998: 10)

Following this initial breakdown is a chronic fear and paranoid belief about one's status in the world. That means, the individual's substantiality, cohesiveness, and integrity is gradually shattered. Externally, s/he becomes over-sensitive, over-responsive, and inappropriately reacts to external threat and difficulties. Internally, s/he loses his/her defense, competence, beliefs, trust, and predictability in facing frustration in reality. In other words, apart from the fear of breakdown, the individual's fear is generally transformed into a primitive paranoia towards the external world as well as his/her ability and life. That is a constant validation of external events by internal fears and fantasies in which the individual is spontaneously threatened or even diminished by external others. Facing this sort of ontological fear, the individual has nowhere to go, as his/her internal and external good objects are unable to provide any protection to him/her. Together with the traumatic loss of the beloved object, it may end up with a splitting of the ego system.

`The recognition that the ego could, by dividing itself into parts, take a part of itself as its own object, opened up the possibility of an internal world populated by objects in the dynamic relations with each other. Moreover, understanding that parts of the ego could become identified with objects was revelatory when it came to recognizing what was happening when mourning went wrong. The processes of mourning, and its pathological counterpart, melancholia, have particular significance for the final outcome of trauma for the individual. So often, the long-term outcome presents a state of chronic melancholia. In this case, the identification with the lost object becomes a way of avoiding unbearable guilt - ultimately the guilt of having survived at all, sometimes compounded by the survivor's feeling in some way being responsible for the death.' (Garland, 1998: 19)

Within Garland's formulation, the ego system is not only breaking, but can split into various parts. The individual's ego takes a part of it and transfers it into the lost objects. The transformation is completed by a full identification of the lost objects. According to Yip (2013), within this transformation, the individual actually undergoes several inner psychic processes such as the following:

1. splitting the ego into at least two parts (one part represents the ego itself, one part represents the lost object. In some case, according to Klein, the splitting can be further. The part representing the ego itself can further split into the good and bad self. The part representing the lost object can further split into the good and bad other)
2. strong and unconscious identification with the lost object.
3. fantasy that the part of ego has actually become the lost object

In doing so, the more intensive the identification of the lost object is, the more the individual can deny the actual occurrence of the traumatic experiences. Unconsciously, the individual, with the transformation of his/her part of ego as the lost object, can totally deny the loss of the beloved object by embracing the lost object mentally and spiritually. Not only is traumatic fear replaced, the intensive sense of guilt in attributing the traumatic loss and death of the beloved one is also alleviated or even diminished. Within this process, several mechanisms occurred. They were listed as follows:

1. Loss of beloved object
2. Over-whelming traumatic fear in facing the loss of beloved object
3. Prevailing guilt in the traumatic fear of beloved object
4. Symbolization of the beloved object
5. Introjection of the symbol of the beloved object
6. Splitting of the ego into parts
7. Part of the ego (the split ego) fully identifies with the symbol of the lost object
8. Denial about the loss of the beloved object
9. Dissociation and repression of fear and guilt due to the loss of the beloved object. (Yip, 2013)

This is a complicated process. Firstly, the individual avoids the fear of breaking the ego system by sealing up this fear by related dissociation of mind, body, and external perception. Secondly, the individual tries to deny the related loss in the trauma by splitting part of ego and identifying with the lost object. These three mechanisms are closely related and reinforce one another. It is a combination of three crucial mental processes that occur in schizophrenia, depression, and trauma.

1. Self-splitting in the schizoid self-fragmentation (schizophrenia)
2. Identification of lost object in the depressive self introjection (depression)
3. Dissociation of body, mind, or memory in the traumatic experience and recall (trauma).

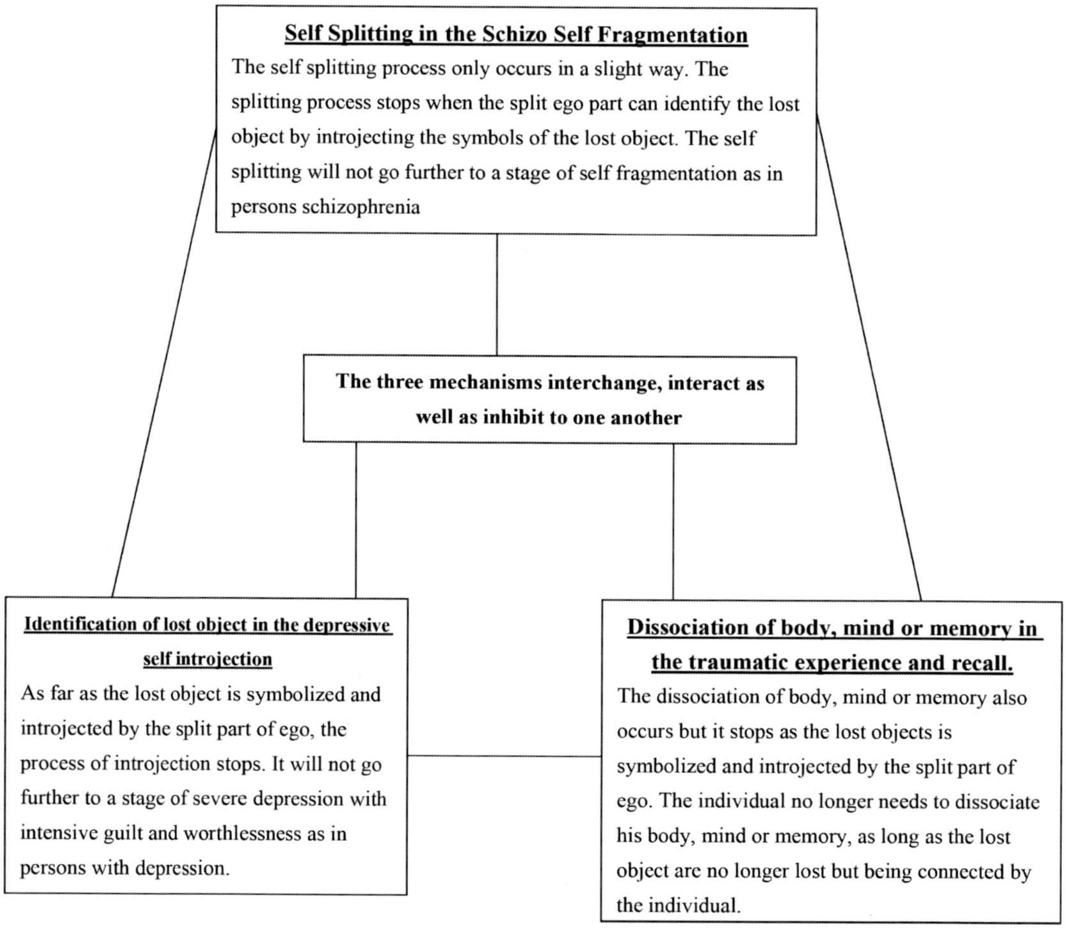

Figure 10. Self-Fragmentation, Dissociation, and Introjection in Facing Traumatic Loss (Yip, 2013).

However, all these mental processes are only in an initial stage. The self-splitting process only occurs in a slight way. The splitting process stops when the split ego part can identify the lost object by introjecting the symbols of the lost object. The self-splitting will not go further to a stage of self-fragmentation as in persons with schizophrenia. The identification and introjection of the lost object occurs. It only occurs in an initial stage. As far as the lost object is symbolized and introjected by the split part of ego, the process of introjection stops. It will not go further to a stage of severe depression with intensive guilt and worthlessness as in persons with depression. The dissociation of body, mind, or memory also occurs but it stops as the lost objects are symbolized and introjected by the split part of the ego. The individual no longer needs to dissociate from his body, mind, or memory, as long as the lost objects are no longer lost but being connected by the individual. The individual needs to not further the dissociation process in forms of severe malfunctioning of bodily and ego functioning (Yip, 2013). In other words, these three mechanisms interact with one another. They cope with one another as well as inhibit one another until the individual reaches a somatic and mental equilibrium. All these may be shown in the following diagram.

In other words, if the individual can use these three mechanisms together, s/he is able to avoid being fixated on any one of them. That means, if either the dissociation mechanism or the introjection mechanism fails, the individual is doomed to involve fully in the self-breaking mechanism that may finally lead to the onset of schizophrenia. In the following, the writer is going to describe how H. J. Sullivan (1956) described the failure of dissociation that leads to the onset of schizophrenia.

Sullivan's Dissociation Dynamism

Definition and Function of Dissociation Dynamism

Sullivan (1956) defined dissociation as a dynamism, which does not require disturbance of the contents of consciousness, and which does not act as an impediment to the conduct of life, in which there is no dissociation (Sullivan, 1956: 169). He further described dissociation as being used for the sake of giving the individual partial impulse to the external stimuli in which the individual wants to cover up. It also enables the individual to suppress or repress related stimuli that arouses conflicts and inconsistency in self-image and identity. In doing so, s/he easily rationalizes his/her ignorance, neglect, and indifference to all these external stimuli. In other words, it is a crucial mechanism of self-integration. Sullivan (1956) attributed this in detail:

> `A client with dissociated impulse will experience special cognitive distortions about anyone whose combination of positive values horribly moves the patient to integrate his dissociated impulse. The patient then endows these positively valued people with the negative of the feelings that would accompany this integration, so that one literally, suavely, and automatically misidentifies the meaning of such a person. In other words, in order for the dissociated tendency to never disturb awareness, it will not provoke anxiety - because if it did, one would be anxious so much of the time that one could not do things that are necessary to life - the security system has come to include very elaborate pseudo memories, revere processes, and so on, which amount to a wonderfully thorough piece of fantasy that nearly and very adequately excludes any of the ordinary ways by which one would become aware of something.' (Sullivan, 1956: 174)

According to Sullivan (1956), the dissociation mechanism is used to maintain the integration of the self-organization. The individual tends to separate those unpleasant or traumatic experience and memories from awareness to ensure normal ego functioning. However, in encountering any external stimuli and clues such as related objects, events, persons, or even smell, touch, or visual images and voices that can trigger the recall of these experiences and memories, the individual engages a security system by avoiding further stimulation so that the individual's ego functioning can be integrated without disturbance. If the avoidance is not powerful enough to separate the reception of related stimuli, the individual may also generate pseudo memories and fantasies that can reverse the arousal of the stimulation. All these are a highly complicated self-process going smoothly out of individual's awareness in normal daily life and social interaction. However, the self-process of dissociation consumes his/her inner psychic energy. Thus, if the individual needs to focus his/her full attention on certain matters, the self-process of dissociation will be upset.

> `We will get clear evidence of the magnitude of the self-processes concerned in maintaining dissociation, only at times when the person is engaged in such a complex task that practically all his abilities are called upon - when he is under considerable pressure from a task requiring microscopic attention, swift placing of many factors, and so on. If, under those circumstances, he encounters another person who awakens the dissociated tendency, and who makes his presence felt to any of the sense organs – by his speech, for instance – then there will be certain evidence of the dissociative process. This evidence will appear in the fact that the presence of this person will disturb the concentration necessary for the difficult task, but if the person notices it, it will be immediately rationalized, often by means of a pseudo recollection, which is the easier thing in this culture that a person can build in himself to resist the capacity of interesting people to disturb awareness.' (Sullivan, 1956:175)

Attention and Inner Psychic Energy Spent on Dissociation Dynamism

That means, the individual may need to spend his/her inner psychic energy to maintain his/her dissociation mechanism. But, at the same time, s/he has to play full attention to certain affairs. Then, any presence of external stimuli will lead to either or both of the following result:

1. Upset of the dissociation mechanism
2. Disturbance of attention on the object/affairs that requires his/her attention

Either of these two results is not tolerable for the individual. To restore the dissociation mechanism as well as to regain full attention to the object/affair, the individual will immediately try to rationalize his/her distraction and avoid further stimulus that relates to his/her covered-up drive, unpleasant prior experiences, and traumatic memories. As a consequence, to ensure the proper functioning of the dissociation mechanism, the individual needs to decrease his/her external awareness to prevent further disturbance or triggers by related stimuli (Yip, 2013).

Vicious Cycle of Dissociation Dynamism and Deep Ego Disturbance

As dissociation dynamism is only a continuous repression of unwanted but highly powerful impulses. *Prolonged repression implies a vicious cycle of over-sensitivity to external stimuli, intensive repression, and avoidance.* As a result, the individual is living a wear and tear life, spending most of his/her psychic energy and effort to cut off, from awareness, the related stimuli that trigger his/her traumatic memories or covered desires.

> `When the material easily accessible to awareness - that is, the self - has artifacts which neatly cut off any reasonable prospect of one's noticing a tendency to become integrated in a type of situation the impulse for which is dissociated. In the self, one gets unquestionable evidence of the wear and tear of life that is brought about by the dissociated system only when there is the right sort of person around for the integration

> and the subject person is troublesome, and goes way. Thus, people with major systems in dissociation are often singularly at the mercy of troubles of one kind or another; a good many things annoy them dreadfully, and they go away, get out of the annoying situation, with some excellent rationalization. They have no anxiety in the situation, but have just found it such a nuisance that they could not get their work done. This is particularly pathognomonic of dissociation. (Sullivan, 1956: 177)

That means, the whole life of the individual will gradually become limited or restrained by continuous fear and avoidance of related triggering objects, events, and persons to achieve equilibrium and ego functioning maintained by the dissociation dynamism. *S/he enters in an endless cycle of being triggered, getting away, and using rationalization to justify these actions of avoidance.* Gradually, his/her daily activity and concentration in achieving normal activities becomes more and more disturbed by the dissociation dynamism. This is a kind of deep disturbance to the ego system where the intensive but dissociated impulses continuously interrupt the individuals in various aspects of life with a profound effect on his/her personality and interpersonal interaction.

> `In other words, if you find yourself disturbed by another person, but by the most minute investigation convince yourself that he does not stir anxiety, then you can be quite sure that the other person is of great significance to some dissociated impulse in the personality. It shows that way because there is such an elaborate pseudo or artifact organization in the self that anxiety simply is not going to be called out by anything short of a cataclysmic collision with this other person. (Sullivan, 1956:177)

Symbolization and Fantasy in Prolonged Dissociation Dynamism

Sullivan (1956) further affirmed that the dissociation mechanism embraces a highly powerful and dangerous impulse that if it comes to consciousness, it would mean extreme disturbance and anxiety. In the operation process of dissociation, it can be highly symbolic and involves certain use of fantasy.

> And since the tendency system in dissociation must be a powerful one - for it includes an impulse that is so extremely dangerous that it must even be permitted to stir anxiety, which is the formula that leads to dissociation - quite obviously symbolic operations with imaginary people are not going to be very deeply satisfying. Thus, we expect in the total personality that there will be an extraordinary sensitivity to anything that touches upon the dissociation system....Impulses in dissociation have lots of experience, they grow, and they grow at a not so terribly different rate or degree from that of any impulse system... (Sullivan, 1956:178)

Within the dissociation dynamism, the individual may reach a state that the triggering from related objects, events, and persons in actual reality become more and more symbolic and delusive. That means, the individual is not actually responsive or being triggered by directly related objects, events and persons. Instead, *s/he becomes highly sensitive even to symbolic meanings, and imaginative or even delusive images aroused by unrelated objects, events, and persons*. In extreme cases, these unrelated objects, events, and persons do not substantially exist but are delusively constructed by the individual himself/herself. For example, words, pictures, or even hidden symbols would create anxiety and disturbance to one's ego system (Yip, 2013). That means, if the individual has a traumatic experience of being bitten by a dog, then the barking of a dog, the word 'dog', or even any object similar to the shape of a dog may immediately arouse his fear and create intensive anxiety and disturbance to one's ego system.

Failure of Dissociation Dynamism: Tremendous Symbolization, Fantasy and Psychotic Breakdown

As the symbolization and fantasy mechanism grows tremendously, the individual may finally come to a psychotic break down.

> `The schizophrenic patient, for instance, is often a person who has in the past persistently shown the dynamism, which we call dissociation, as a means of resolving the conflict between powerful needs and the restrictions that the self imposes upon the satisfaction of these needs. That is, people who have dissociation anything as powerful as lust, for example, are in great danger of schizophrenic collapse' (Sullivan, 1956: 6)

As the primitive impulse increases tremendously, the dissociation dynamism may fail. That means the conflict between the powerful need to satisfy and to restrict this primitive impulse prevails with a high risk of schizophrenic breakdown. That means the self-system is torn by this conflict to a state of breakage.

> `*The schizophrenic change, I believe, is quite generally due to an inability to maintain dissociation*. Now in order for there to be dissociation, a rather elaborate body of processes must be built into the self to maintain it, and so when one is unable to maintain the dissociation, it does not mean that all this invention in the self totally vanishes. This invention still remains, and things that do not have simple and uncomplicated access to awareness collide with it and suffer as a result of it. *Thus, the schizophrenic has an unsure mental state, in which he is clearly aware of activity of the dissociative system but unable to get the thing into clear personal focus*. It is from this continued activity of an inadequate dissociating system that the profound puzzlement arises, which characterizes long reaches of some schizophrenics' lives. *And from the stress of being unable to maintain a system of dissociation comes the loss of control of the contents of consciousness*. (Sullivan, 1956:1987)

In other words, schizophrenia is originated from the failure of the dissociation dynamism. In fact, the dissociation dynamism is maintained by an elaborated mechanism with the self-system. The failure of this dynamism means that the individual fails to keep his/her self-system into a cohesive system, in which s/he is unable to keep those unwanted stimuli from the physical environment away from his/her consciousness. That means, s/he still tries their best to keep them out but the unwanted stimuli still rushes in. Intense anxiety continues and increases drastically. In other words, s/he still bears both the dissociation dynamism and/or the attempt to operate it fully but in vain. His/her mental state is highly ambivalent and confusing. His/her inner conflict of restricting as well as satisfying his/her primitive impulse prevails and becomes uncontrollable. Consequently, s/he fails to get external things into his/her own personal track. Those s/he does not want to keep focusing on are in a stage of intensive awareness. Those s/he wants to be conscious and clearly aware of may be ambivalent. The loss control of dissociation making the individual's sense of self and sense of agency fails. Instead, s/he is kept within a highly confused and ambivalent state of psychotic confusion.

`What ensures is that there are highly referential processes along with much more primitive and general referential processes, coupled with observational data, which one cannot treat to anything like one's satisfaction, partly because they are primitive and deal in rather cosmic terms, with things that are essentially impersonal, and partly because there is interference from remaining effective parts of the self system which were carefully *organized to cut off recall of things that would imply awareness of the dissociated tendency*. Thus, the schizophrenic picture is not only somewhat complicated by the large amount of autistic referential knowing operations. It is also complicated by a continuance of obstruction to recognize a part of life which came into being to maintain the dissociation - and yet the dissociation is no longer anything like complete, but tends actually to get into behavior… (Sullivan, 1956:188)

In terms of dissociation, Sullivan (1956) affirmed that the psychotic state is a diffused and ineffective dissociation dynamism with the following natures (Yip, 2013):

1. autistic referential process with gradual decreases of consciousness in environment (avoidance of continuous triggering by a wide range of objects, persons and events in environment constructed by delusive symbolization)
2. highly restricted daily life due to the over-involvement in maintaining the deteriorating dissociation dynamism and avoiding delusive and symbolic triggering
3. deep interference of the remaining parts of the self system to maintain normal ego functioning,

From Dissociation to Schizophrenia

According to Sullivan (1956), the total failure of dissociation dynamism, as summarized by Yip (2013) consists of the following stages of development:

1. Unpleasant/traumatic past experiences or covered desire/drive that needs to be covered up and avoid coming to consciousness.
2. Individual needs to turn all these out of his/her consciousness to maintain the integration and normal functioning of his/her self system
3. Any encounter of related objects, events and persons that possibly trigger his/her well concealed desires and traumatic past experience may arouse anxiety.
4. The feeling of anxiety and uneasiness is an unconscious warning signal that the dissociation mechanism may come to a point of fracture that needs to take immediate action.
5. The individual will consciously or unconsciously try all means to avoid or separate himself/herself from related object/s, event/s and person/s that possibly trigger his/her well concealed desires and traumatic past experience to maintain his/her deteriorating dissociation dynamism and eliminate his/her sense of anxiety.
6. All these avoidance acts are well justified by rationalized excuses, personalized reasons, and preferences that appear as normal and natural in interpersonal interaction. That means, his/her unpleasant/traumatic past experiences or covered desire/drive can be further covered up and come into his/her consciousness.
7. The whole life of the individual will gradually become limited or restrained by continuous fear and avoidance of related triggering objects, events and persons to

achieve equilibrium and ego functioning maintained by the deteriorating dissociation dynamism.

8. S/he enters in an endless cycle of being triggered, getting away, and using rationalization to justify these actions of avoidance. Gradually, his/her daily activity and concentration in achieving normal and important duties may be more and more disturbed by the deteriorating dissociation dynamism.
9. As the deteriorating dissociation dynamism becomes more and more fragile and the individual's ego disturbance is more and more serious, the individual may reach a state that s/he is not only disturbed by substantial existence of related objects, events, and persons in the actual environment but are also disturbed by unrelated objects, events, and persons imaginatively or even delusively constructed. In doing so, the deteriorating dissociation dynamism is complicated by the individual's use of symbolization and fantasy.

Prolonged and increasing symbolization and fantasy implies that the individual completely loses control of repression of consciousness of unwanted impulses. S/he may be in a stage of confusion of consciousness. Those objects or external clues s/he does not want to be aware of may be in clear awareness. Those s/he wants or needs to be aware of in reality may be disturbed by his/her ambivalent consciousness. Furthermore, prevailing symbolization and fantasy may serve as ingredients for the construction of delusions and hallucinations in schizophrenia (Yip, 2013)

Trauma, Abuse, Victimization and Psychosis

In recent years, there are plenty research evidences showing that psychosis is closely related to trauma (Larkin & Morrison, 2006) in the following ways:

a. Child abuse, victimization experiences and psychosis
b. Post-traumatic Stress Disorder (PTSD) in response to acute psychosis
c. Psychosis with co morbidity of PTSD
d. Internal process from traumatic memories, emotions and negative self to psychosis

In this section, the writer is going to describe every one of them in detail:

Child Abuse, Victimization and Experiences in Psychosis

Holowka's (et al., 2003) study showed that among adult outpatients with schizophrenia, 35% of them suffered from emotional abuse, 42% with physical neglect and 73% of them had emotional neglect by their parents during their childhood. Similarly, Lipschitz's (1996) study showed that among adolescent patients with schizophrenia, 52% of them experienced emotional abuse, 61% of them had physical neglect, and 31% of them had emotional neglect from their caregivers.

Bebbington (et al. 2004), based on the findings of the second British National Survey of psychiatric morbidity, explored the relationship between psychosis and victimization in childhood. Victimization experiences include sexual abuse, bullying, being taken into local authority care, violence in the home, running away from home, being kept in a children's institution, being expelled from school, being homeless, being a victim of serious injury, illness or assault as well as violence at work. Percentages of respondents with psychotic disorders with all such victimization experiences were summed up in Tablel 1.

Related studies also show that there is a strong relationship between child abuse and specific psychotic symptoms, particularly positive symptoms of hallucination and delusion. The onset of auditory hallucinations is found to be preceded by either a traumatic event or an event triggering memories from previous traumas (Honing et al. 1998). Many studies showed that there was a high correlation between child abuse and hallucination. Read and Argyle (1999) showed that for those subjects with former child sex abuse experiences, 53% of them demonstrated some forms of hallucination. For those with physical abuse experiences in childhood, 58% of them showed some forms of auditory hallucinations. For subjects with both types of experiences, 71% of them exhibited auditory hallucinations. Also, hallucinations are particularly common in incest survivors (Ellenson, 1985: Ensink, 1992: Heins et al., 1990; Read and Argyle, 1999).

Table 4. Percentage of Respondents with Psychotic Disorders Experiencing Different Types of Victimization (Source: Bebbington et al. 2004)

Victimization Experience in Childhood	Percentage of Respondents with Psychotic Disorder
Sexual Abuse	34.5%
Bullying	46.4 %
Taken into local authority care	17.9%
Violence in home	38.1%
Running away from home	34.5%
Time in a children's institution	20.2%
Being expelled from school	1.2%
Being homeless	27.4%
Victim of serious injury, illness and assault	64.3%
Violence at work	11.9%

Regarding the content of hallucination, many studies showed that clients with sexual abuse or physical abuse history in childhood might harbor hallucinations with refined details of such experiences. In some cases, clients may even harbor a highly symbolized delusive hallucination (Famularo et al., 1992; Sansonnet-Hayden et al., 1987; Heins et al., 1990). Below are some extracts described by related clients with sex abuse experiences:

1. 'I saw sperm in my foot and my drink' (Raune et al., 1990: 124)
2. 'One believed that her body was covered with ejaculate and another that had sexual relations with public figures (Beck & Van der Kolk, 1987:1475)
3. One client who had been raped by others several times hallucinated that: 'being tortured by people getting into the body, for example, the Devil and the Beast… at one stage had bleeding secondary to inserting a bathroom hose into self, stating wanting to wash... people are trying to put aliens into my body....
(Read et al., 2003: 12).

All these contents clearly showed that child abuse experiences were so traumatic to an extent that it had a strong breaking force making the individual become psychotic with highly delusive configurations and diffusion of their previous traumatic abusive experiences. That means, in the developmental process, all these traumatic experiences, coupled with other adversities in life may gradually nurture the first onset of psychosis. Jackson and Birchwood (2006) argued that there is no simple cause and effect relationship between trauma and psychosis, especially the first onset of psychosis. Early trauma (sexual, physical, emotional abuse) in childhood and adolescence, become a complicated array with interacting psycho biosocial factors including emotional dysfunction that arises because of disruption to a person's development trajectory. Whether or not the individual becomes psychotic, it also depends on individuals' coping style to his/her traumatic experiences in his/her childhood as well as his/her ability to recover from the first appearance of psychotic-like experiences (Birchwood, 2003; Jackson & Birchwood, 2006). Its complexity may be demonstrated in the following case illustration by Jackson & Birchwood (2006).

> `J was a 21 year old African Caribbean man who developed psychosis following a period of withdrawal, depression and anxiety. J had had a difficult childhood. His father had died of a drugs overdose when he was 14, leaving J and his younger brother to be brought up by their mother. J found it difficult to talk about his father's death, and generally coped with premorbid aversive life events and traumas by keeping quiet and avoiding any conversation about them. He was a naturally socially anxious and shy child and this eventually extended into early adulthood... Following the emergence of his psychotic symptoms (including voices, thought broadcast and paranoia) and a period of non-adherence to medication, J began to deteriorate, and he was eventually admitted to a psychiatric hospital…he was treated with anti-psychotic medication, and after just less than four weeks was discharged. … Initially, he refused to discuss anything to do with his psychosis… and after a few months, having made a good symptomatic recovery… he started to experience flashbacks and intrusive thoughts and images related to his admission' (Jackson & Birchwood, 2006: 135)

From this case, it is clear that J's disposition of psychosis is highly complicated with a mixture of an unhappy childhood in terms child neglect, child abuse, and death of his father. Following this was a pre-morbid period in which J was entirely withdrawn, depressive, and anxious, properly being fully occupied with the recall of unhappy and traumatic past memories such as being abused or neglected by his parents. J became self absorbed and finally ended up with a psychotic breakdown with voices, thought broadcast and paranoia. The admission of J to a mental hospital did not reduce his mental instability. Instead, it was a traumatic experience. It further intensified his hallucinations and delusions. Initially, J refused to share anything and his condition was fair. Later, an empathic nurse approached him and gained his trust allowing J to share and release his unhappy traumatic experiences. It stabilized his mental state and J had a better recovery.

Trauma and Psychosis: Co morbidity

Romme and Escher summarized related studies on trauma and psychosis and listed them in Table 5:

Table 5. Studies for Trauma and Psychosis (Romme & Escher, 2006: 165)

Author and Studies	N	Nature of Population	Frequency of trauma
Muser et al. (1998)	275	Serious mental illness (schizophrenia and manic depressive)	98%
Drayer and Legeland (1999)	135	Psychiatric hospital patients	95%
Jacobson and Richardson (1987)	100	Psychiatric Hospital (29% psychotic)	87%
Goodman et al. (1995)	99	Homeless women (59% schizophrenic)	97%
Muenzenmaier et al. (1993)	78	Outpatients women (57% schizophrenic)	74%
Davies-Netzley et al. (1996)	105	Homeless women (47% schizophrenic)	77%
Craine et al. (1988)	105	Inpatients state hospital (41% schizophrenic)	51%
Carmen et al. (1984)	122	Psychiatric Hospital (18% psychotic)	53%
Romme and Escher (1996)	50	Voice hearers (36% schizophrenic)	77%

Similarly, Strauss (et al. 2009) reviewed related studies and concluded that co-morbidity between post-traumatic stress disorder and schizophrenia is around 19% to 66%. Based on this review, they described that positive, negative and first rank symptoms in schizophrenia are all influenced by the occurrence of post-traumatic stress disorder (PTSD). Psychotic positive symptoms for people with co-morbid PTSD and schizophrenia have more frequent violent thoughts, behaviors, and feelings as well as heightened paranoia, and greater severity of delusions and hallucinations. Regarding psychotic first rank symptoms, people with co-morbid schizophrenia and PTSD had more negative beliefs about themselves and others, which may mediate the relationship between trauma and paranoia. Also, their re-experiencing symptoms may mediate the link between trauma and paranoia and hallucination. For psychotic negative symptoms, the presence of PTSD in schizophrenia was associated with increased secondary negative symptoms, with deficit syndrome and primary negative symptoms associated with lower rates of current life diagnosis of PTSD. Rome and Escher (2006) interviewed 48 persons hearing voices (hallucination), and the relationship of their voices to their history of traumatic experiences (emotional neglect, physical abuse, sexual abuse) are shown in Table 6:

Table 6. Comparison of three groups of voice hearers relating to trauma (Rome & Escher, 2006: 169)

Related interpersonal traumas	People with Schizophrenia N= 18	People with Dissociative Disorder (N=13)	Non-patients (N= 15)
Emotional Neglect	12 (67%)	13 (87%)	10 (67%)
Physical Abuse	11 (61%)	10 (67%)	7 (47%)
Sexual Abuse	3 (17%)	8 (57%)	5 (33%)
No Abuse	3 (17%)	2 (14%)	4 (27%)

From the above table, it is clear that voices (hallucination) are closely related to the interpersonal traumas experienced by the individual. Rome and Escher (2006) further articulated both psychiatric patients and non-patients experience traumatic events in the same ways as these experiences were highly threatening to their survival in the following ways:

1. physically threatening to them with a possible fatal result or being seriously hurt
2. socially threatening as it threatened the continuity of one's expectations of the future such as losing one's beloved object
3. emotionally threatening as there were overwhelming emotional confrontation such as the death of one father who has abused him/her (Rome & Escher, 2006: 169)

All these threatening effects deepen the destructive effects of the traumatic experiences to a degree that, despite traumatic events being over and done with; related memories were still vivid and powerful. The individual `felt' that they were still occurring in forms of related voices of related parties within the traumatic events. For example, a sex abuse survivor may always hear the voice of abusers cursing or threatening them for sexual intercourse. These types of intrusive thoughts and voices may appear in forms of continuous paranoia and/or flash backs that greatly disturb the individuals' daily life to a degree that they may come to a conclusion that all people around him/her know his/her sexual abuse history and teasing around him/her.

Internal Process from Trauma to Psychosis

There is growing literature showing that psychosis is a prolonged result of post-traumatic stress disorder (PTSD). Jankowski (et al., 2006) summed up the process from PTSD to psychosis in the following way:

> 'The basic thesis is that the psychosis itself, characterized by perceptual disturbances, frightening delusions, feelings of persecution, and other threats to the self, may be sufficiently terrifying to qualify as `traumatic events' according to criterion A of DSM IV. This concept represents a modification of the traditional PTSD paradigm, which implies the traumatic stressor is an external event. (Jankowski et al., 2006: 88)

Regarding the process from PTSD to psychosis, there are quite a number of studies describing the details of this process. Most of them are within a cognitive behavioral orientation. Fowler (et al., 2006) tried to speculate the pathway from trauma to psychosis within four cognitive routes.

1. Direct associations between intrusive memories of traumatic or stressful experiences and delusions and hallucinations.
2. Indirect association between trauma and persecutory delusions and hallucinations mediated by negative evaluation of self and others (the schema route)
3. Indirect association between trauma and hallucination mediated by negative and self-critical rumination concerning the relationship between the individual hearing the voices and the voice identity.
4. Speculations about potential catastrophic interactions between trauma processes and information processing abnormalities, which characterize psychosis, which may magnify vulnerability to psychosis.
(Fowler et al., 2006: 100)

1. Direct associations between intrusive memories and persecutory hallucinations

The first cognitive route is the direct association between intrusive memories of traumatic or stressful experiences and delusions and hallucinations. There is consistent evidence that traumatic history can increase the risk of psychosis, and the severity of hallucinations being associated with the degree of hurt and harm in sexual abuse (Bebbington et al., 2004; Fowler et al., 2006). Morrison (2001) affirmed that normal intrusive memories in the form of images and voices in the state of anxiety, and other neurotic disorders in response to external threat, in intensive and frequent ways, could be gradually transformed into delusions and hallucinations. Fowler's (1977) study showed that there were four cases with a direct connection between traumatic events, such as being raped and bullied, and experiences of hallucinations. In these four cases, clients all harbored related auditory hallucinations of hearing voices in the form of critical comments and threats from abusers. There seemed to be a meaningful and direct connection between the past trauma and current symptoms of auditory hallucinations. Fowler (et al., 2006) illustrated this sort of direct connection in the following case.

> `Alice was a 35-year-old woman with a diagnosis of schizophrenia. She was severely thought disordered and initially the therapist had some problems in making sense of her difficulties... an experience she had every day when going off to sleep. Alice complained of hearing threatening voices coming from the loft. When she was going to sleep, she also had feelings of being sexually interfered with, which were accompanied by visions of the rapist. She believed strongly that her father lived in the lofts and was coming down to abuse her at night. Alice believed these to be real and current experiences and was afraid to go to bed at night. The night time events appeared to be linked to past experiences of being sexually abused, both as an adult by past partners, and as a child by her father.' (Fowler et al., 2006: 102)

From this case, it was clear that Alice's hallucination was closely related to her actual abusive experiences. As she was previously sexually abused both by a stranger in her adulthood and by her father in her childhood, her traumatic fear was highly dissociative, fearful and confused. All these dissociated fearful experiences were first repressed in the process of traumatic experiences. However, all these traumatic memories rebounded intensively in forms of frequent conscious flash backs as well as unconscious distressing nightmares. Gradually, it transformed into prevailing paranoia in which her father might come to abuse her at night. In her flash back, traumatic memories became intrusive images, voices and feelings that greatly disturbed Alice's life as well as distorted her own perception of reality. It also shattered Alice's self-integrity and cohesiveness to a state she was self-fragmented in having schizophrenia.

2. Indirect association between trauma and persecutory hallucination with negative view on self and others

Regarding indirect linkage between trauma and persecutory delusions and hallucinations, related studies showed that it is mediated by negative evaluation of self and others within a schema route. Recent studies (Fowler et al. 1997; Barrowclough et al. 2003; Teasdale and Barnard, 1993) showed that persecutory ideas and hallucinations are related to negative views of self and related negative emotions. They appear in a form of a vicious cycle. The more negative one's self esteem and emotions are, the more one becomes vulnerable to external negative comments, and the easier are all these negative emotions and lack of self-appreciation turned into persecutory hallucinations. That means, the combination of anxiety and negative self-evaluation may directly relate to psychotic experiences, especially paranoia, with a persistence of delusional ideas (Fowler et al. 2006: 110).

Persecutory hallucination and delusion can also relate to a negative view of others in which individuals assume others imposed harm, hurt, oppression, and criticism on them. All these negative views of others are normally accompanied with negative emotions, such as intensive anger and hate towards others, which is commonly observed in individuals with paranoia (Flower et al., 2006; Gilbert, 1992).

In many ways, the negative views of self and the negative views on others can come together within the experiences and recall of traumatic experiences. Fowler (et al., 2006) believed that the occurrence of persecutory delusions and hallucinations is not the only defensive response to negative self esteem (Bentall et al., 2001), but a catastrophic appraisal of social position of an extreme negative self and negative others. That means, both of them can be two sides of the same coin, reinforcing or compensating one another. The sense of being weak and inadequate can make one become highly vulnerable to others' comment. If all these negative comments from others are internalized, the individual becomes highly vulnerable to depressive self-harm and self-blame, However, a projection of anger by labeling others as threatening, critical and oppressive can lessen the internalization of others' negative comments and cover up individual senses of weakness and inadequacy. Unfortunately, the covering up of the individual's senses of inadequacy and weaknesses, and over-projection on others, make one detach from reality and become trapped within a dilemma of negative self-evaluation and anger with others. However, all of these are intolerable. They also become a vicious cycle; the more vulnerable one becomes, the more threatening and persecutory others are, and the more detached and oppressive the external reality becomes. It finally turns into a catastrophically negative and unrealistic appraisal of oneself and others in the form of persecutory or paranoid delusions and hallucinations in psychosis. Flower's (et al., 2006) study concluded the following:

> `The combined pattern of extreme self and other evaluations was associated with a history of humiliating trauma (bullying, assault, sexual abuse), and multiple regressions suggested that extreme self and other evaluations were the strongest mediator of the relationship between traumatic events and paranoia.... We have found clear evidence to suggest that extreme negative evaluation of self and others are more likely to be present among people with psychosis who have been exposed to either ongoing social adversity or specific social humiliation such as rape or bullying. The way in which past traumatic and stressful experiences may be linked to paranoia may then be via the mediating or negative self and others evaluations. This can occur as a result of adaptation and social learning in a similar manner that was suggested by psychological theorists of PTSD' (Fowler et al. 2006: 111)

That means traumatic experiences and recall are correlated with a negative evaluation of the self and others as well as negative emotions such as anger, depression, feelings of being threatened, which contribute to the onset of psychosis (Fowler et al. 2006; Dalglesih, 2004; Foa and Rothbaum, 1998). These four sets of factors relate to one another and can be shown in Figure 11.

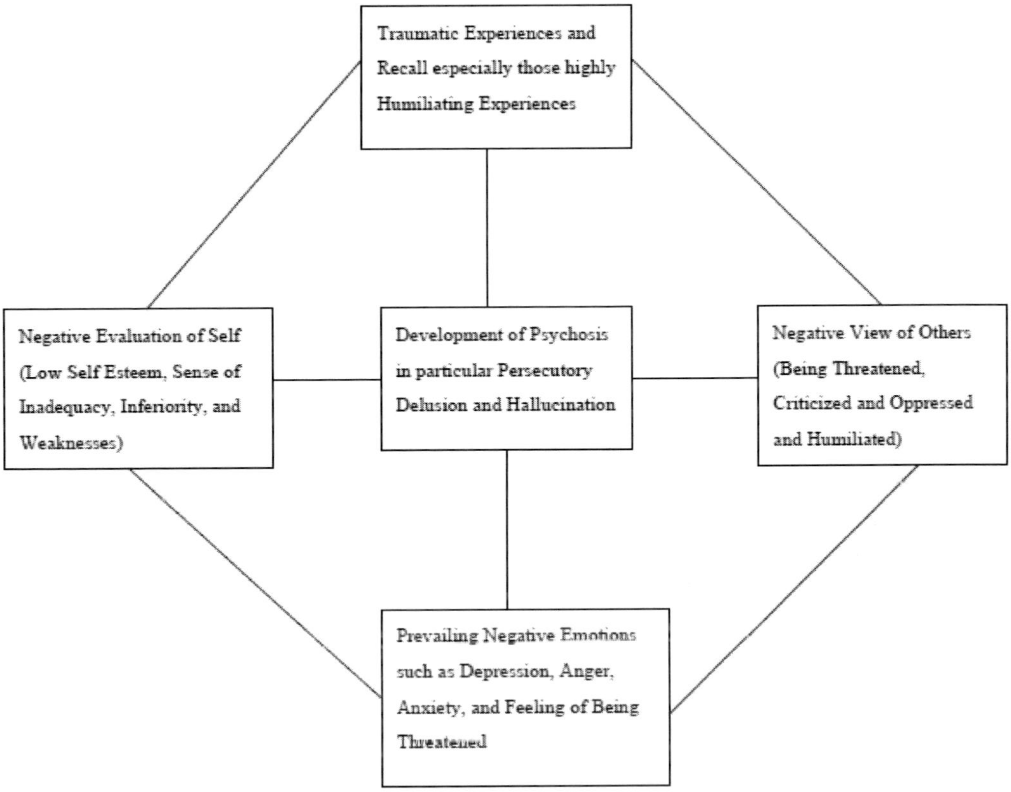

Figure 11. Negative Self and Others in Contributing Persecutory Delusion after Traumatic Experiences summarized from (Fowler et al., 2006).

3. *Indirect association between trauma and hallucination mediated by negative and self-critical rumination concerning the relationship between the individual hearing the voices and the voice identity.*

Many studies showed that hallucination can be regarded as a misattribution of one's own thoughts or internal dialogue because of self-monitoring and faulty interpretation of external stimuli (Bentall, 1990; Jonhs and McGuire, 1999) There is also evidence that auditory hallucinations are a sign of being humiliated and oppressed in the external environment in which the voice heard is closely related to the dominating and powerful persecutors within all these humiliating experiences (Birchwood and Chadwick 1997; Birchwood et al., 2000; Fowler et al. 2006). Vaughn and Fowler (2004) identified two appraisal processes in auditory hallucinations. The first one is that the related voices are highly dominating and close to the individual. The second one is that the individual is highly submissive to the voice heard. That means, in distressing auditory hallucination, which have been nurtured by traumatic experiences, individuals feel highly powerless to the overwhelming and prevailing powerful and oppressive abusers in their traumatic experiences. There seemed to be a spontaneous appraisal of subordination, humiliation, dominance, and oppression. It is a kind of self-dialogue and continuous rumination with the abusers' voices being vivid and real (Fowler et al., 2006). They described this in the following details.

> `People who have been traumatized and are vulnerable to having hallucinations might sometimes experience the product of such rumination as voices, i.e., their thinking or rumination about the interactions with their abuser occurring as voices rather than as ruminative thoughts or the experience of internal dialogue... The content of the voices does not directly reflect exactly what the voices said in the past. Often such voices criticize with respect to what the voice hearer is saying currently. In psychosis the abuser is often appraised as a figure who is current and real.' (Fowler et al., 2006: 113-4)

That means, the abusive and traumatic experiences are not only fixated or recalled after their occurrence. Instead, within the mind of the individuals, they are continuously developing and growing to a stage that the individual feels that the abuser is still real and powerful. The traumatic experiences, abuse, and humiliating experiences are also real and occur in different forms in everyday life. As all these prevail, the individual may complain that his/her persecutory delusions and hallucinations, with the voices of the abuser and oppressor continuously speaking in forms of teasing, blaming, criticizing and humiliating the individual. In response to these persecutory delusions and hallucinations, the individual involves in a form of self-dialogue. The self-dialogue can be either internalizing all these negative comments in forms of negative views of self and overwhelming senses of fear and inferiority, or trying place to hide, to avoid, or to deter all these running tracks of voices. The individual can also be involved in vigorous or irrational defense by curing, arguing, and blaming these voices. People around the individual, as they cannot hear or feel all these persecutory delusions and hallucinations, may think that the individual is 'crazy' or 'insane' by bizarre fear, gestures, and behaviors, angry voices, or yelling in the air.

A close look at the cognitive routes proposed by Fowler et al. (2006) can form a conclusion that can be a further combination and intensive form of the first, second and third cognitive routes. Within these routes, the individual's negative views of self and negative views of others are directly correlated with traumatic experiences in formulating the contents of persecutory delusions and hallucinations. It is also a direct maximization and generalization of the abusive and traumatic experiences by the abusers and oppressors in which they not only occur within traumatic experiences but are everywhere, every occasion, every situation, and every moment. The traumatic experiences become parts of everyday life in which the individual can escape nowhere.

4. *Speculations about potential catastrophic interactions between trauma processes and information processing abnormalities, which characterize psychosis, may magnify vulnerability to psychosis.*

In this cognitive route, severe negative views of self and others may finally distort the individual's normal information processing, in which cognitive processing with internal origins, such as images and thoughts are regarded as external origins in terms of hallucinations and delusions (Kapur, 2003; Hemsley, 1994). That means their negative views of self and others are further provoked and nurtured by spontaneous fear and continuous occurrence, and recall of traumatic experiences to a state that their cognitive process are greatly distorted. They have impairment in inputting new and spontaneous information from external reality. Instead, all these tend to be greatly distorted by prevailing negative emotions and recall of memories of traumatic experiences. This is a vicious circle in which the more negative emotion and recall of memories of traumatic experiences occur, the higher will be the deficit of reception and interpretation of new and spontaneous information from external reality. Fowler (et al., 2006) described this vicious circle as the following:

> 'That is an interaction between information processing abnormalities and normal processes associated with emotional reaction to stress and trauma, which may from the catastrophic change be observed as acute psychotic states. Such a catastrophic abnormality may distort and exaggerate the experience of the products of emotional processing, and extreme emotion may exaggerate information processing abnormalities. The idea that psychosis exaggerates emotional response deserves further investigation but is consistent with longitudinal observation of the build-up of emotions in combination with unusual symptoms in psychotic relapse, and with observations that include the occurrence of rare and unusual symptoms of emotional disturbance.' (Fowler et al., 2006: 114)

In short, the individual's sense of reality, appraisal of related stimuli, events, objects, and events in the reality is hindered by negative emotions and negative traumatic memories to a degree that the perception and response of external reality is distorted, alienated, and self constructed in forms of psychotic delusion and hallucinations. Hemsely (1994) asserted that information process models of PTSD and psychosis are similar in a way that both have intrusive thoughts that hinder the incoming information from reality. That means the distortion and problems of information processing can be manifested in several ways:

1. Regarding past traumatic experiences as current ones. Senses of anxiety, fear, and being threaten in PTSD from traumatic experiences are still felt as real and spontaneous by the individual. (Ehlers and Clark, 2000)
2. Problems in placing moment-to-moment experiences within appropriate context (Fowler et al., 2006). Individuals are either totally occupied by the recall of traumatic experiences or the present situations are still too traumatic and stressful that the individual tries to avoid or isolate them.
3. Individual fails to construct a coherent whole in shifting from past memories and new information input from related contexts.
   (Squire, 1992)

Along a similar line of thinking, Romme and Escher's (2006) concluded that there are seven paths in turning traumatic experiences into onset of psychosis. They are listed as follows:

1. The dissociative pathway
2. Turning the suffered powerlessness and aggression towards oneself
3. The abolition of all emotions or becoming like a robot
4. A flight reaction from the existing problems into a fantasy solution
5. Trying to fulfill impossible expectations
6. Denial or transforming what has happened
7. To surrender to a higher power
   (Romme & Escher, 2006: 171-173).

All these seven pathways can be gradually described as follows:

1. The dissociative pathway

In this pathway, the individual tries to dissociate him/herself from the traumatic experiences and recall. Romme and Escher's (2006) described this pathway as follows:

> `One of the dissociative pathways is to create a substitute. Another is the realization of partial splits. For example, during a trauma of sexual abuse, the person is emotionally and physically setting herself/himself apart, and looks from a distance at what is going on. Alternatively, another person may take his/her place. This other person may become a voice that reminds the listener what has happened. Most of this dissociation fails and the memory becomes intrusive with anxiety provoking images. (Romme and Escher, 2006: 172)

That means, after the traumatic experiences, especially those highly humiliating ones, there should be at least two tracks of voices (hallucination). Along Romme and Escher (2006) thinking, the writer formulates the process from dissociation to the onset of psychosis. First, there are two main types of voices (hallucinations). One represents the traumatic contents and details of the experiences (A). One represents the clients' own evaluations and reminders of the trauma (B). These two types of voices can be further split into the following:

A: Voices representing contents and details of the traumatic experiences
A1: One voice representing the abuser
A2: One voice representing the clients as a victim

B: Voices representing the individual's own evaluations and reminders of the trauma
B1: One voice representing the negative blaming and adverse consequences of the traumatic experience.
B2: One voice representing the client's needs to be supported, cared for, and protected by others

As a holistic person, in normal psychic functioning, A and B should be correlated together. In dissociation, A is separated from B (primary dissociation), A1 is separated from A2 (secondary dissociation), or B1 is separated from B2 (secondary dissociation). The dissociation pattern in both levels can be quite confusing and irregular. In developing from dissociation into psychosis, there may be several stages.

In stage 1, the individual only hears one track of voice at one time consistently, A1, A2, B1, or B2. The choice of any voice is determined by which parts of the traumatic experiences need to be dissociated, and which part needs to be recalled into memories. For example, the occurrence of A1 means that there is a recall of the abuser, but a dissociation of the individual (A2), adverse consequence (B1), and demanded support (B2) within the traumatic experiences.

In stage 2, the individual may hear the voice of A1, at the other time, s/he may hear A2 or vice versa. Similarly, s/he may hear B1 at one time and B2 or another time or vice versa. In hearing one kind of voice, the individual is not able to relate to another type of voice. That means the individual dissociation mechanism is less stable than in stage 1, in which the individual shifts from one type to another type of voice. In doing so, s/he may use one type to cope with another type of voice. For example, while s/he hears the voice of the abuser for a period of time his/her sense of anger, fear, and helplessness gradually increases to an intolerable degree that s/he needs to shift to another voice symbolizing the pain and sufferings of the victims (A2). Similar lines of shifting may happen between B1 and B2. The shifting of one voice to another voice implies instability of the mental state and increased dissociation mechanism, which tends to nurture a vigorous unstable self-splitting process.

In stage 3, the shifting from one voice to another voice can become more and more quickly to an extent, the individual feels that s/he does not only hear one track of voice but several tracks of voices one after another. As the time between one voice (hallucination) is so close to another one, the individual simply interprets this as they occur together. There may be several mixtures among these four tracks of voices. There can be two tracks of voices mixing together (A1A2, B1B2, A1B1, A1B2, B1A2 and B2A2). There can be three tracks of voices mixing together (A1A2B1, A1A2B2, B1B2A1, B1B2A2). There can be four tracks of voices mixing together (A1A2B1B2). Comparing voices in stage 1, stage 2, the voices occurring together in stage 3 are highly disturbing to the individual. At that moment, the individual is already on a stage of psychotic onset in which s/he feels highly confused, alienated from the reality, and is absorbed in all these voices (hallucinations).

In stage 4, these voices not only occur one after another and together but they are related to one another. That means, the voices can argue with one another. For example, A1 (the voice representing the abuser) can argue with A2 (the voice representing the client himself/herself in a form of a victim). Similarly, B1 (the voice representing the evaluation of adverse consequence of trauma on the individual) can argue with B2 (the supportive and caring others urged by the individual in facing the traumatic experiences). As these voices are arguing with one another, it makes the individual feel more confused and massive. It also implies a full manifestation of first rank symptoms in which the individual's ego boundary is highly diffused and the sense of reality is also severely disturbed to an extent that s/he may need immediate psychotic treatment or hospitalization to minimize the risk of potential harm to oneself and others.

2. Turning the suffered powerlessness and aggression towards oneself (Aggression turns inwards)

This proposition is described in psychodynamic approach in which the individual turns others' oppression inwards and turns into self-aggression. Romme and Escher (2006) described this in details:

> `physical abuse and intense verbal aggression over a longer period, we observed, can often result in an abolition of emotion of aggression. People don't feel those emotions any more or mix them up with other emotion. When this is combined with a negative self-image and guilt feelings, psychosis develops when the defense is attacked by circumstances... Aggression turns into negative hallucinations or delusions combined with anxiety provoking intrusive images, and then guilt, which results in suicidal ideation (Romme and Escher, 2006: 172)

Romme and Escher's (2006) idea, described above, is quite similar to Fowler et al. (2006) stance in which the individual's negative emotions and negative self image come together making externalized negative emotions turn inwards and become prevailing auditory hallucinations in psychosis. Romme and Escher's (2006) description can be further elaborated into the following stages of development:

a. Physical abuse and intense verbal aggression for a long period of time in which related feelings of anger, helplessness, and fear in this abuse repeatedly occur at an intolerable level.
b. To cope with all these prolonged negative feelings and continuous traumatic experiences, one needs to distance himself/herself from all these negative feelings by internalizing and absorbing them.
c. In absorbing and internalizing these negative feelings, the individual mixes them with negative self images and a sense of guilt (Instead of the attributing the abuse and aggression to the fault of abusers, the individual begins to regard them as a part of his/her own faults that deserve the abuse. That is always the schema of the abuser and aggressor in justifying the continuous abuse and aggression.)
d. The self defense as well as self-image and boundaries are gradually eroded by these internalized senses of guilt and other negative feelings of helplessness, fear, and aggression aroused by continuous abuse and aggression by others.
e. There is a formation of paranoid hallucinations or delusions combined with anxiety provoking intrusive images, and then guilt, which results in suicidal ideation

3. The abolition of all emotions or becoming like a robot (Depressive pathway)

In this path, the individual may turn from depressive reaction towards the traumatic loss of a loved one and gradually become delusive in hearing the voices (hallucination of the lost but loved one). These voices may finally turn into a full growth of schizophrenia.

> `Individuals after being rejected in love, after suicide of a loved one, or confrontation of unresolved issues of sexual identity.... When the compensation fails, the lost lover might start speaking as a voice, or a compensatory delusion might develop. When the person is not able to interpret the experience... coping with these experiences is more difficult. Secondary reaction can mimic a full picture of schizophrenia. (Romme and Escher, 2006: 173)

The loss and depressive path to form psychosis as described by Romme and Escher (2006) can be further elaborated in the following stages of development.

a. Loss of a loved one
b. Compensation by focusing on sports, exercises and meaningful activities
c. Failure of the compensatory mechanism
d. Development of voices of the loved one (assuming that the loved one is delusively present)
e. Inability to interpret these voices as a signal of existing emotional problems
f. Sense of confusion of reality
g. Full growth in psychosis with a poor and diffused sense of reality and self-identity.

4. A flight reaction from the existing problems into a fantasy solution

In this pathway, as the traumatic experiences are continuously threatening, the individual is involved in a flight and fight reaction. S/he tried to avoid facing the traumatic experiences and external threats. However, the traumatic threat is still there. Thus, the individual can only escape the external threat by involvement in fantasy in terms of constructing his/her own hallucination. It is a kind of delusional fantasy. In doing so, the individual's sense of reality, space, and time changes accordingly. Below is the example described by Romme and Escher (2006).

> `one women's marital relationship was near divorce at the time her mother died. She also had difficulties at work because she worked at the same office as her husband. When it became clear that divorce could not be prevented, she heard the voice of her mother telling her that she should take an airplane to Iswahan, because she would find a new husband there.' (Romme and Escher, 2006: 173)

From this case, it is clear that the following stages of development, from stressful and traumatic experiences to auditory hallucinations, can be found in the client (A).

a. Highly stressful and traumatic experiences (A's divorce, death of mother)
b. The traumatic experiences cannot be avoided and continued (A was still working with the husband in the same office)
c. Involvement in a fight and flight mechanism in facing the traumatic threat (A's divorce. It could not be avoided but A emotionally and unconsciously wanted to avoid facing all these)
d. As in the reality, avoiding the traumatic threat is impossible (A's husband was still in the same office), individual had to strive for delusive escape (taking air plane to Iswahan) as well as delusive support by others (her deceased mother).
e. The absorption in delusive escape, support, and fantasy become a habitual way for the individual to face the continuously oppressive reality (A heard the voice of her mother telling her that she should take an airplane to Iswahan, because she would find a new husband there).

5. Trying to fulfill impossible expectations (the manic depressive pathway)

In this pathway, the individual first experiences a manic depressive episode before the onset of persecutory hallucination (Romme & Escher, 2006). Gradually, the manic episode becomes uncontrollable to an extent that it finally comes up with a psychotic breakdown. The following example may serve a way to illustrate this pathway. Related parties' consensus to use their stories for academic purpose is sought. For the sake of confidentiality, their personal information and identity are properly disguised.

> `P was a client suffering from schizo-affective disorder. His father died when he was only ten years old. His mother married his stepfather who was an alcoholic and abused his mother and P regularly. P was accustomed to protecting his mother by taking the abuse and fighting back towards his father. Later his stepmother was caught by the police because of drug trafficking, and finally died in prison. When P was twenty years old, his mother died because of lung cancer. P suffered a lot from severe depression and later recovered under the care and concern of his intimate girlfriend who was a caring nurse

working in the hospital where her mother died. They planned to marry at first but P's girlfriend intended to study in London. Their marriage was thus postponed. Unfortunately, his girlfriend was terribly sick in the period of her study and was cared by her schoolmate, who was a medical practitioner in London. Later, they fell in love and married. P was totally shocked by their marriage and his depressive episode prevailed for a few days. Then he was troubled by an intensive manic episode saying that he had super power to convince the wife to return to Hong Kong. He firmly believed that their marriage was an unhappy one and his girlfriend did it involuntarily under the abuse and threat of an evil British medical practitioner. One month later, his manic episode turned into a psychotic breakdown. He harbored continuous voices (auditory hallucination) saying that many Chinese women in London, including his girlfriend, were crying for help. They urged P to save them). P even went to the airport armed with a sharp knife and wanted to take a flight to London. He yelled at the airport that he had to save all abused women in London. He was thus finally caught by the police and was sent to a mental hospital. He was thus hospitalized and diagnosed as suffering from schizoaffective disorder with a prevailing paranoid delusion.'

In line of Romme and Escher (2006) and Bock's (2000) orientation, P's development of prevailing hallucination can be formulated in the following stages:

a. Continuous suffering and hardship in life including childhood, adolescence, and adulthood. (P's father died in his childhood. He was continuously abused by his stepfather in childhood and adolescence. His stepfather and mother died in his adolescence and youth. His girlfriend left him in adulthood.)
b. Depressive mood was easily provoked by spontaneous loss of significant others in life (P lost his father, stepfather, mother, and girlfriend, which made him become highly vulnerable to depression.)
c. To survive within hardship and difficulties in life, individuals were accustomed to lifting their depressive mood by mild manic episodes in the form of intensive self struggle, tough fighting back to opponents, over-sensitive responses to external criticism, and formulation of omnipotent ideas and belief (P was accustomed to defending his mother from his step-father's abuse, fighting with his step-father.)
d. Individuals come to a point that the continuous loss of significant others were far beyond their limits of resilience and coping. (The loss of the love of his girlfriend was intolerable to P.)
e. Individuals' habitual coping by manic episodes and intensive self-struggles can no longer cope with the prevailing depressive mood caused by this traumatic loss and accumulated effects of previous losses (P lost the love of his girl friend plus the accumulated loss of his mother, his father, as well as his stepfather all made him feel highly uncomfortable and intolerable. All these were far beyond the coping and resilience limits of P. His manic episode and intensive self struggle could no longer cope with that sort of accumulated and traumatic loss.)
f. Individual's manic episode and intensive self struggle was gradually transformed into grandiose delusions and hallucinations with voices telling the individual that s/he was really omnipotent and could accomplish an impossible mission (P thought that he was omnipotent and could save his girl friend and other Chinese females who were abused by evil British males).

6. Denial or transforming what has happened

This is a process of denial in which the individual cannot accept what has happened. This can be one of the following:

a. Being rejected in a loving relationship (Romme & Escher, 2006)
b. Struggling in an unacceptable sexual identity (Romme & Escher, 2006)
c. Being abused/abandoned by a beloved object/person

All of these unacceptable events are highly painful and intolerable for the individual to cope with; self-isolation and projection of critical voices from the outer world that explain, continue, or argue with the individual. Gradually, these sorts of voices change to auditory hallucinations and delusions of schizophrenia. Romme and Escher (2006) did not explain, in detail, how this process actually happens. In clinical practice, the writer discovers that the process of denial of abusive and humiliating experiences is associated with the dissociative path. Within the intense dissociation mechanism, the individual easily denies, suppresses, and represses their unacceptable experiences and relationship. In doing so, the individual's normal ego functioning and sense of reality are also repressed and suppressed. That means, the more the individual is dissociated from all these traumatic memories and experiences, the more s/he is vulnerable to related triggers and the less s/he can repress and suppress with all these unpleasant experiences. As a consequence, all these repressed memories and experiences easily rebound. As the sense of reality is so weak, and ego functioning is so inadequate, the re-bounce and triggering of these traumatic experiences may disturb the individual's consciousness in forms of uncontrollable delusions and hallucinations. All these delusions and hallucinations can represent the individual's experiences of being rejected, abandoned, and uncared for by others. It also represents the highly inferior and ambivalent feelings of the individual in all these traumatic experiences.

7. To surrender to a higher power (The spiritual path)

To cope with abusive and traumatic experiences, individuals may regard voices (auditory hallucination) as a symbol and sign from a supernatural power. It can be both positive and negative. In a positive sense, individuals can regard these voices as advice from a supernatural god helping individuals to deal with difficulties and hardship. In clinical practice, once individuals have already resolved these difficulties and hardship, all these auditory hallucinations would thus vanish (Romme & Escher, 2006). In a negative sense, they can be regarded by individuals as evil spiritual forces, such as being possessed by demons and evil spirits in bringing them bad luck, including traumas and abuses. All these spiritual attributions can gradually distort and lessen one's sense of reality. Romme and Escher (2006) did not go further to describe the process of how such spiritual attributions finally become psychotic hallucinations and the onset of schizophrenia.

The writer, in his clinical practice, had encountered the following case in which the individual attributed her bad luck and traumas to the possession of an evil spirit. Related parties agreed to use their stories for academic purposes. For academic purposes, their personal information and identity were properly disguised.

> `F was a female Chinese with mental retardation. She had suffered from paranoid schizophrenia for ten years. She was born in a family in rural China. Initially, she was a

> normal and happy baby and her parents loved her deeply. She also had an older brother and a younger sister. F's parents worked very hard to support a hand-to-mouth lifestyle. Unfortunately, when F was ten, a high fever nearly took her life. She recovered but with a deficiency in her brain function with a mild grade of mental retardation. Her mother also died because of a lung infection seven years later. F's father could hardly accept the loss of his wife and became an alcoholic. He could no longer support the whole family financially and psychologically. He thus abandoned F on a vacation trip to Hong Kong. From that time onwards, F was institutionalized in a children's home run by a social welfare agency. F was deeply shocked by the loss of her mother and the traumatic abandonment by her father; she became highly inert and withdrawn. She was highly sensitive to strangers and unfamiliar social environment, including the new institutional life, for two years. The social workers in this social welfare agency were far too busy to take care of her. One day, F ran away and intended to return to her own home in rural China. In fact, she did not know where to go and she finally lost her way. She slept in the park and was dreadfully lonely, fearful, and sad. At that time, she was even approached by a drunken old man who intended to rape her. Fortunately, she was saved by a passing policeman, and was escorted back to her children's home. From that time onwards, F harbored a strong auditory hallucination and persecutory delusion that all her bad luck in life were caused by a male evil spirit. F said this evil spirit was cunning, seductive, and evil. F insisted that the voices of the evil spirit were always at her ear telling her that she was a seductive and beautiful woman and wanted to have sex with her. Also he said he tried every means to get rid of F's relatives as they all opposed her having sex with him. He first killed her mother. Her father abandoned her to avoid the whole family being killed by the evil spirit. She had to sacrifice herself in order to save the life of her whole family. Gradually, F's auditory hallucination became more and more frequent. Finally, one day, in the children's home, she cried desperately saying the evil spirit came over and took her way. She began to tear off her clothes saying that she needed to have sex with the evil spirit so that she could save her whole family. Related workers in the children's home took her to a mental hospital and she was diagnosed as suffering from paranoid schizophrenia.

From this case, it was clear that F's auditory hallucination was an attribution to a supernatural force that caused all the misfortunes in her life, including her severe fever in childhood that caused her mental retardation, the death of her mother, her abandonment by her father, and the sexual harassment by the drunken man in the park. Within this evil spirit, all these misfortunes became meaningful. The death of her mother, the abandonment by her father, and sexual harassment were all arranged by this evil spirit to have sex with her. That means, within the spontaneous voices of the evil spirit, F was no longer a woman with mental retardation that was looked down upon by others, or being abandoned by her family members. Instead, she was an attractive young lady that attracted the evil spirit who tried every means to possess her. She also needed to sacrifice herself to save her family members.

Implications to Mental Health Recovery to Clients with Schizophrenia

The above-mentioned perspectives in describing traumas and psychosis can be summed into the following:

1. A breakdown of the ego system in facing traumatic experiences (breaking down of beliefs, ways of life, mental structures, defense, goodness of objects, and protective function of the psychosocial environment and perception of reality) (Garland, 1998).

2. Three coping mechanisms (self-splitting, identification of lost objects, and dissociation of body and mind) occur together and interact with one another after the occurrence of the trauma. However, if the identification and/or dissociation process fails, the self-splitting mechanism prevails and leads to schizophrenia.
3. The failure of dissociation leads to the onset of schizophrenia. It is an autistic referential process with a gradual decrease of consciousness on the environment due to avoidance of being triggered by a wide range of objects; restricted daily life because of over-involvement in maintaining the deteriorating dissociation dynamism; as well as a deep interference of the remaining parts of the self-system in maintaining normal ego functioning (Sullivan, 1956)
4. There is plenty of research evidence showing that there is a high co-morbidity of psychosis in relation to child abuse, victimization experience, post-traumatic stress disorder, internal processes from traumatic memories, emotions and the negative self (Larkin & Morrison, 2006)
5. There are seven paths in turning traumatic experiences into the onset of psychosis (the dissociative pathway; turning the suffered powerlessness and aggression towards oneself, the abolition of all emotions or becoming like a robot, a flight reaction from the existing problems into a fantasy solution, trying to fulfill impossible expectations, denial or transforming what has happened, and to surrender to a higher power) (Romme & Escher, 2006: 171-173).
6. The loss of a beloved one can also lead to the onset of schizophrenia when the compensatory mechanism fails. It consists of several stages (loss of a loved one, compensation by focusing on sports, exercise and meaningful activities, failure of the compensatory mechanism, development of delusive voices of the loved one, inability to interpret these voices as a signal of existing emotional problems, sense of confusion of reality, and full growth in psychosis with a poor and diffused sense of reality and self identity.) (Romme & Escher, 2006).
7. Cognitively speaking, there are four ways in which traumatic experiences can lead to psychosis (direct associations between intrusive memories of traumatic or stressful experiences and delusions and hallucinations, indirect association between trauma and persecutory delusions and hallucinations mediated by negative evaluation of self and others (the schema route), indirect association between trauma and hallucinations mediated by negative and self-critical ruminations concerning the relationship between the listener and the voice identity, and speculations about potential catastrophic interactions between trauma processes and information processing abnormalities, which characterize psychosis that magnifies vulnerability to psychosis. (Fowler et al., 2006: 100)

Putting these together, it is clear that traumatic experiences have a prevailing breaking and splitting effect on the individual. The splitting effects can be counteracted by the identification of lost objects or depressive paths or/and dissociation paths that similarly occur during the traumatic process. There are several pathways leading to the onset of psychosis. They are described as follows:

1. The individual, in his/her developmental process, fails to develop a cohesive self-system. That means s/he is vulnerable to the traumatic process. Even a mild or short-

term trauma may have enough power to break the client's self-system leading to the onset of psychosis.

2. The trauma is spontaneous and repetitive (*such as continuous sex abuse or physical abuse by significant others*), when the individual can cope with one incident of trauma with residual breaking, losing and dissociative effects on the self-system, another traumatic incident come in. As a consequence, the self system becomes more and more vulnerable. The accumulated breaking effects finally come to a point that leads to a self-splitting result of schizophrenia.
3. The trauma is too severe and intensive (*such as serious traffic accidents, horrible disasters, warfare and severe criminal offense*), which is entirely out of the resilience and tolerance level of the client. That means the individual cannot cope with the trauma either by dissociative or identification mechanism. It simply breaks the individual's self-system, and sense of reality leading to the onset of schizophrenia.
4. The individual first uses the dissociation mechanism to cope with the trauma. For various reasons (*It can be overloading of the dissociation mechanism because of many other unpleasant events. It can be that the related social context is full of triggers so that the dissociation mechanism fails. It can also be that the individual is too self and socially isolated so it weakens his/her dissociative mechanism*) the dissociation mechanism fails and finally leads to the onset of schizophrenia.
5. The individual first uses the identification mechanism to cope with the trauma. For various reasons (*It can be the individual being too attached and enmeshed with the lost object. It can also be the failure of the compensatory mechanism. It can also be further losses after the traumatic loss of a beloved object. For example, the loss of one's wife in a car accident can also lead to losses of employment and investment because of depressive moods and alcoholic addictions.*), this identification mechanism fails. Finally, the identified and split ego parts turn into psychotic delusion and hallucinations.
6. The individual uses both identification and dissociation mechanisms to cope with the trauma. For various reasons (*It can be that this traumatic incident triggers recall or re-bounce of many former memories. It can also be the individual is rapidly shifting around various mechanisms in coping with the traumatic experience. It can be the individual does not have good use of this coping mechanism*), these two coping mechanisms fail. Finally, the breaking and splitting of the self-system prevails with a result of onset of schizophrenia.

All these have important implications to mental health recovery for clients with schizophrenia. It can be summarized as follows:

1. Related professionals and caregivers should understand and accept that the content and manifestation of clients' delusions and hallucinations are closely related to their memories of traumatic experiences.
2. It is important to provide a secure, supportive, and caring social environment for clients with schizophrenia so that they are free from further traumatization, which certainly worsens their psychotic confusion. In many cases, there are further traumatizations through inappropriate institutionalization, control, over-dosage of psychiatric medications, isolation, and labeling induced by harmful treatment and

intervention. All these should be avoided in related parties for the recovery of clients with schizophrenia.

3. Since clients have suffered from former traumatic experiences before the onset of schizophrenia, related parties should allow clients to be free from related objects, persons, and issues that can trigger rebounding traumatic experiences. That means, clients should also be free from former oppressive environments such as engulfing parents, dehumanized colleagues, abusive and bullying peers as well as oppressive significant others. In doing so, related professionals should ensure that related service context be a highly supportive, caring, nurturing, and humanistic environment for clients with schizophrenia.
4. As clients' delusions and hallucinations are a symbolic expression of clients' traumatic experiences, related professionals should help clients ventilate their unfulfilled needs, release their suppressed negative emotions, and heal their hurt and harm underlying traumatic experiences. All these should be done in a gradual, prolonged and natural process within clients' normal and integrated daily activities and interaction.
5. The psychotic break is partially because of the vulnerability of the self-system even before the traumatic incidents. Thus, to have a full mental health recovery, it is crucial that related professionals should facilitate clients to strengthen their self-system through constructive activities and development of their potentials. In other words, their sense of uniqueness, sense of consistency, sense of agency, sense of coherence, sense of integrity, and sense of substantiality should be fully developed for a good and complete mental health recovery.

Conclusion

In conclusion, this chapter attempts to discuss various approaches in describing the psychosocial causes of schizophrenia in terms of oppressive environment, self-destructive power, and ontological insecurity as well as parent-child psychodynamics in the formation of schizophrenia.

The discussion starts with social construction of mental illness, including schizophrenia, in terms of language, discourse, social exclusion, and labeling. Within Foucault's line of thinking, individuals with schizophrenia are powerless. They have to construct their own truth and right. However, all the self-constructed truths and rights are only delusive, and unacceptable to the powerful. Nevertheless, the dominance, oppression, and humiliation of actual reality are overwhelming and inescapable for the powerless. Thus, within the delusive reality, individuals build up their own power and right to dominate others. That means, within the delusive reality, they are powerful. The self-constructed delusive reality is labeled by professional knowledge in terms of schizophrenia. Medical professionals are trained to exercise diagnostic labeling, medical treatments, institutionalized detention, and social exclusion of the powerless with delusive empowerment in delusive reality.

In terms of self-constructed power, Glass (1995), based on Freud's articulation affirmed that delusions and hallucinations are self-destructive psychotic regression. Within this sort of regression, there is a prevailing manifestation of one's inherent instinct of aggression and self-destruction with a severe impairment of one's ego functioning. This self-destructive power is unconscious, continuous, and highly powerful to a degree that psychotic time is a withdrawal from reality on one hand and transcendence of external time and power on the other hand.

Within the existential and phenomenological perspective, ontological security is actualized in terms of sense of uniqueness, sense of agency, sense of substantiality, sense of consistency, sense of cohesiveness, and sense of integrity within an interpersonal mutual support network. However, within a continuous oppressive social environment, the individual suffers from ontological insecurity by engulfment, implosion, and petrification. Engulfment is created by intrusive, controlling, and manipulative others. Engulfment by other tends to suffocate senses of uniqueness and consistency with a result of diffusion of self-identity and self-boundary. Implosion is nurtured by crushing reality. Implosion is a denial and deprivation of one's senses of agency and cohesiveness with a result of being absorbed in continuous confusion and uncontrollability in reaching an external environment. Petrification is created by spontaneous neglect, exclusion, and isolation. Petrification and depersonalization is a denial and deprivation of one's sense of substantiality and integrity with a result of being traumatized by oppressive others, dissociation and isolation from the related environment. Gradually, self-fragmentation occurs as the individual intends to protect his/her own inner self. Instead of being engulfed, imploded, and petrified by others, the individual engages in a process of self-engulfment, implosion, and petrification. All these lead to psychotic self-fragmentation.

Within a psychodynamic perspective, Arieti (1974) affirmed that schizophrenia is developed from a spontaneous hostile, disengaged, and critical parent-child relationship. The pre-psychotic development of childhood has the following process:

1. highly critical or highly disengaged mother
2. intolerable external reality and painful inner world
3. poor permanent and internalized negative maternal image
4. negative image of self and others
5. poor I-Thou relationship
6. the negative and vicious circular response of the mother and father
7. negative self image, body image, gender identity and early defense system

As a result, pre-psychotic development tends to nurture two types of personality, schizoid and stormy personality. Within these two types of personalities, the individual child and early adolescent develop extensive detachment and rebellion from parents, unavoidable stressful involvement in competitive life and self-injury, poor conceptual thinking, and self-image as well as psychosexual conflict. In adolescence and early adulthood, the individual could face a pre-psychotic panic in which the individual develops extreme fear and panic towards distressing others. Finally, in the period of psychosis, individuals turn to intensive fear and panic.

Many studies also show that there is a close relationship between trauma and the onset of psychosis. Psychodynamic approaches articulated that the occurrence of trauma, in fact, stirs up all unresolved emotional and developmental complexes in life. There are three major groups of concepts in describing how an individual's self-system can be fractured by the traumatic experiences. The first group is the description of the break down of the ego system in traumatic experiences and recall (Individual's weak and fragile ego system is gradually or abruptly broken down by traumatic experiences and related recall (Garland, 1991). The second group of studies is the failure of dissociation mechanism (dissociation of traumatic experiences protects the individual from traumatic recall and allows the individual to absorb the negative impact of the traumatic experience gradually. However, the failure of the dissociation mechanism implies an overwhelming negative impact on the individual. The loss of the protective mechanism leads to a final fracture of the individual's self-system (Sullivan, 1956). The third group of studies is spontaneous evidence and co-morbidity between traumatic experiences (child abuse, bullying, victimization) and psychosis (Morrison et al., 2006). There are numerous studies in this decade showing that trauma is one the major psychosocial causes leading to psychosis in which positive symptoms, negative symptoms, and first rank symptoms are closely related to process, details, contents of traumatic experiences, individual experiences in abuse, victimization, bullying, and disasters, in particular those happening in childhood and adolescence.

Putting various described perspectives together, it is obvious that the psychosocial cause of schizophrenia is closely related to an oppressive environment in which individuals are spontaneously engulfed, imploded, and petrified by oppressive and powerful others, in particular those significant ones. The powerful ones use their overwhelming power to construct the truth, right and reality. They dominate and circulate the powerless to an extent that the powerless ones cannot exercise their power, their rights and even cannot engage in their own reality. The only way they can do this is to construct their own power and reality in their delusions and hallucinations. In doing so, the individual's self-constructed power is highly destructive to an extent that it fractures the integrity, cohesiveness, uniqueness, consistence, and substantiality, as well as agency of the self-system of the individual. It also ruins his/her sense of reality, self-boundary, and self-identity. As a consequence, the individual self system is gradually split and fragmented. In many ways, the powerful oppressive ones can be the parents of the individuals. Comparing other oppressive others, parental oppression can be the most powerful and destructive to the individual, in particular in infancy, childhood and adolescence in which his/her self-system in undergoing a construction process. Facing a highly critical parent, the individual child's self identity, image, and boundary are severely threatened by parental criticism. S/he also feels dreadfully lonely in facing parental detachment and disengagement. Gradually, the individual child develops a negative image and attitude towards oneself and others and a poor I and thou relationship, which can breed a pre-psychotic personality in late childhood and early adolescence. Finally, the pre-psychotic personality will turn into first onset of psychosis under continuously oppressive psychosocial environment. Within related recent studies on trauma and psychosis, it is clear that this sort of highly critical and disengaged parents can be abusive, imposing trauma on their children even if they do not abuse them. Their severe criticism and disengagement towards children may mean that they may ignore, neglect, or even blame their children for inviting others' traumas and abuse. In some cases, their severe criticism can also be intensive enough to become traumatic experiences for the children. In many ways, all these traumatic experiences, as well as continuous abuse, criticism, and neglect by parents are depowering mechanism for the individuals. The development of hallucinations and delusions can be interpreted as an intermingling of spontaneous rebound of these depowering traumatic experiences, as well as a self-induced but delusive empowerment process for the individual with schizophrenia in facing the oppressive reality. The relationship among Foucault's delusive reality of truth, right, and power, Glass's regressive but destructive power of delusions and hallucination, Laing's ontological insecurity, and Arieti's developmental process from highly critical and detached parents, as well as traumatic experiences in persons with schizophrenia can be briefly summarized in Figure 12.

External oppressive environment in terms of prevailing domination from the powerful groups: 1. The powerful ones construct the reality, truth and right and exercise their power in social network and related institution 2. The powerless have to submit and internalize reality, truth and right constructed by the dominating powerful. Their own reality, truth and rights are thus oppressed	**Development of psychosis in terms of construction of their own delusive reality of truth, right and power of the powerless group** 1. The powerless have to construct their own rights, power and truth.. Within this, one's sense of consciousness, time, space, body and self image are empowered. The powerful exclude and label the powerless as unacceptable and psychotic. It s hould be punished and depowered 2. The more the exclusion and labeling, the more the powerless need this delusive reality to survive and more powerless, detached and psychotic they become. This is highly destructive to the individual. It shatters his/her integrity, cohesiveness and senses of time, space and reality.
External oppressive environment in terms of Ontological Security: 1. Individual's senses of uniqueness and consistency are engulfed by others 2. Individual's senses of agency and cohesiveness are imploded by others 3. Individual senses of substantiality and integrity are petrified by others	**Development of psychosis in terms of formation of divided self** 1. Gradual loss of sense of self (uniqueness, consistency, agency, cohesiveness, imploded, substantiality and integrity) by engulfing, imploding and petrifiying others 2. Development of delusive senses of self and denial the senses of self in actual reality. Delusive sense of self is strengthened by self engulfment, self implosion and self petrification. 3. Delusive senses of uniqueness and consistency becomes psychotic first rank symptoms, delusive senses of agency and cohesiveness turns into positive symptoms, and delusive senses of substantiality and integrity is replaced by negative symptoms
External oppressive environment in terms of highly critical and/or detached parents: 1. Internalized negative parental image and self image 2. Poor I-thou relationship 3. Development of pre-psychotic personality in terms of stormy and schizoid personality 4. Vulnerable self system and psychosexual conflicts 5. Pre-psychotic panic and onset of psychosis.	**Development of psychosis in terms of construction of self construction of paranoia and grandiosity and self fragmentation:** 1. Growing detachment from distressing others and development of poor self system 2. Failure of dissociation mechanism with overwhelming fear and threats from distressing others and oversensitivity to others' rejection, exclusion, criticism and humiliation. 3. Over-whelming fear gradually develops into active hallucination and delusion by self construction of delusive paranoia and grandiosity. Oversensitivity to others' rejection and fragile self system finally leads to self fragmentation, self regression and self confusion.
External oppressive environment in terms of traumas and abuse: 1. Breaking down of ego system in traumatic experiences and recall 2. Failure of dissociation mechanism that protect the individual from negative effect of trauma 3. High co-morbidity between abuse, trauma and psychosis 4. Relationship of psychotic positive, negative and first rank symptoms to experiences and related scheme in traumas and abuse	**Development of psychosis in terms of transformation of abusive and traumatic recall into oppressive delusions and hallucinations and self fragmentaion** 1. Ego system is far too fragile and vulnerable to further stress and difficulties, it is finally split and fractured 2. Dissociation failure induces tremendous symbolization and fantasy to face continuous and intensive triggering from external reality with a result of severe ego disturbance and development of delusion and hallucination 3. Abusers and related persons in traumatic experiences can gradually develop into a intensive negative cognitive schema of self and others. Memories (voices and images) of abusive experiences

Figure 12. Psychosocial Causes and Multi-dimensional Perspectives of Power, Oppression, and Development of Psychosis.

From the above figure, it is clear that an oppressive psychosocial environment tends to be a breeding ground for the development of psychosis. Different perspectives simply imply different ways in the formulation of psychosis. Glass and Foucault's view implies that external domination from overwhelming powerful figures in all directions is internalized by the individual. Since the individual cannot assert his/her own rights, truth, and power in the reality, s/he can only assert it within his/her own delusions and hallucination. In Laing's view, the formation of psychosis comes from the sense of ontological insecurity because of external engulfment, implosion and petrification by oppressive others. They engulf, implode, and petrify the individual to an extent that the individual's sense of self and existence (senses of agency, cohesiveness, uniqueness, consistency, integrity and substantiality) are denied and suffocated. It finally leads to the formation of psychotic symptoms in which the individual is self-engulfed, imploded, and petrified in their own positive and negative psychotic symptoms. Similarly, within Arieti's line of thinking, the oppressive others are the individual's highly critical and/or detached parents in which the individual gradually develops a poor self image as well as a poor sense of others. Under this influence, individuals usually develop poor I-Thou relationships with others. It further nurtures his/her pre-psychotic personality in the form of stormy and schizoid personality patterns in which s/he is highly sensitive to others' comments and criticisms, and intensively detaches from actual reality. It finally creates a psychotic episode and a mental breakdown into an onset of schizophrenia.

Oppression can also occur in a form of traumatic experiences, particularly abusive experiences. Firstly, traumatic experiences can have intensive effect of breaking down individual's ego system especially in spontaneous traumatic recall. The ego system becomes highly fragile and vulnerable to further stress and frustration. Together with these are unresolved inner conflicts that surface because of the breaking effects of the trauma. All these finally become intolerable to the individual and s/he develops psychotic symptoms. Secondly, traumas can also lead to failure of the dissociation mechanism. It induces tremendous symbolization and fantasy to face continuous and intensive triggering from external reality, with a result of severe ego disturbance, and development of delusion and hallucination. Thirdly, many studies showed that there is a high co-morbidity between abuse, trauma and psychosis. There is also a strong correlation between psychotic positive, negative, and first rank symptoms, and related experiences and schema in traumas and abuse. Abusers and related persons in traumatic experiences can gradually develop into an intensive negative cognitive schema of self and others. Memories (voices and images) of abusive experiences can finally develop into related hallucinations and delusions in schizophrenia. All these clearly show that schizophrenia is actually nurtured by a continuously oppressive psychosocial environment in which the individual self-system is entirely fractured by external oppressive power. In the next chapter, the author described the process of self-fragmentation in schizophrenia. In other words, mental health recovery for clients with schizophrenia should be done within a highly supportive, caring and humanistic social environment. In most cases, clients with schizophrenia have long been humiliated and even abused within a highly oppressive social environment and are accustomed to detaching from oppressive reality. They may lose their trust of others. They may still appear as inert, passive and withdrawn even in facing supportive others. Related parties and professionals should be very patient and enduring in waiting for the gradual response of clients with schizophrenia. In fact, clients with schizophrenia earnestly yearn for love, caring, acceptance and support from significant others. It is crucial that related parties, particularly professionals, provide persistent caring and support, which can finally pull clients with schizophrenia out of their introverted delusions and hallucinations back to the substantial and caring reality. Only by doing that can clients with schizophrenia have a holistic and multi-dimensional mental health recovery.

References

Arieti, S. (1974). *Interpretation of Schizophrenia (2nd edition)*: Completely Revised and Expanded, London: Crosby Lockwood Staples.

Barrowclough, C., Tarrier, N., Humprhrey, L., Ward, J., Gregg, L., & Andrews, B. (2003). Self esteem in schizophrenia: Relationships between self evaluation, family attitudes and symptomology, *Journal of Abnormal Psychology*, 112,93 - 99.

Bebbington, P., Bhugra, D., Brugha, T., Singleton, N., Farrell, M., Jenkin, R. et al. (2004). Psychosis, victimization and childhood disadvantage: Evidence from the second British National Survey of Psychiatric Morbidity. *British Journal of Psychiatry*, 185: 220-226.

Beck, J. and van der Kolk, B (1987). Reports of childhood incest and current behavior of chronically hospitalized psychotic women. *American Journal of Psychiatry,* 1444, 1474-1476.

Bemporad, J. R. (1967). Perceptual disorders in schizophrenia. *American Journal of Psychiatry*, 123: 971-975.

Bentall, R. P. (1990). The illusion of reality: A review and integration of psychological research on hallucination, *Psychological Bulletin*, 107, 82-85.

Bentall, R. P., Corcoran, R., Howard, R., Blackwood, R., and Kinderman, P. (2001). Persecutory delusions: A review and theoretical integration. *Clinical Psychology Review*, 21, 1143-1192.

Bentall, R. P., Kinderman, P., & Kansey, S. (1994). The self, attributional processes and abnormal beliefs: Towards a model of persecutory delusion. *Behaviour Research and Therapy*, 32:331-341

Birchowood, M. J. (2003). Pathways to emotional dyfunctioning in first episode psychosis. *British Jorunal of Psychiatry,* 182: 373-375.

Birchwood, M. and Chadwick, P. G.. I. (2003). Omnipotence of voices: Testing the validity of a cognitive model. *Psychological Medicine,* 27: 1345-1353.

Birchwood, M., Meaden, A., Trower, P., Gilbert, P. and Piastow, J. (2000). The power and omnipotent of voices: Subordination and entrapment by voice and significant others. *Psychological Medicine,* 30: 649-656.

Carmen, E., Rickers, P. P., and Mills, T. (1984). Victims of violence and psychiatric illness, *American Journal of Psychiatry*, 141: 378-383.

Craine, L. S., Henson, C. E., Colliver, J. A., and MacLean, D. G. (1988). Prevalence of a history of sexual abuse among female psychiatric patients in a state of hospital system, *Hospital and Community Psychiatry,* 39:300-304.

Davies-Netzley, S. Hurlburt, M. S., and Hough, R. (1996). Childhood abuse as a persecutor to homelessness women with severe mental illness. *Violence and Victims*, 11, 129-142.

Drayer, N., and Langeland, M. A. (1999). Childhood trauma and perceived parental dyfunction in the etiology of dissociative symptoms in psychiatric inpatients. *American Journal of Psychiatry,* 156, 379-385.

Ehlers, A., and Clark, D. M. (2000). A cognitive model of post-traumatic stress disorder, *Behavior Research and Therapy*, 38, 319-345.

Ellenson, G. (1985). Detecting a history of incest. *Social Casework*, November, 525-532.

Ensink, B. (1992). *Confusing Realities*, Amsterdam: Vu University

Famularo, R., Kinscherff, R., and Fenton, T. (1992). Psychiatric diagnoses of maltreated children: Preliminary findings. *Journal of the American Academy of Children Adolescent Psychiatry,* 31, 863-867.

Foucault, M. (1965). *Madness and Civilization*, Translated R. Howard, New York: Routledge.

Foucault, M. (1976). *Power/ Knowledge: Selected Interviews and Other Writings 1972-1977* C. Colin (Edited) New York: Harvester Press.

Foucault, M. (1980). *Power/ Knowledge: Interview and Lecture by Michael Foucault*, New York: Pantheon Books.

Foucault, M. (1982). The subject and power, in J. Scott (Edited) *Power,* Vol. 1., London: Routledge.

Foucault, M. (2006). *History of Madness*, New York: Routledge.

Foucault, M., (2002). *Power,* (translated by R. Hurley) London: Allen Lane.

Fowler, D. (1997). Direct and indirect links between the content of psychotic symptoms and past traumatic experience: Evidence from therapists reports from the London-East Anlia study of cognitive behavior therapy for psychosis. *Paper presented at the British Association of Behavioral and Cognitive Psychotherapy Annual Conference*, Southport, Italy.

Fowler, D. Freeman, D., and Steel, C. et al. (2006) The catastrophic interaction hypothesis: How do stress, trauma, emotion in W. Larkin, W. & A. P. Morrison, (Edited) *Trauma and Psychosis: New Directions for Theory and Therapy. pp. 101-124..* London: Routlege.

Freud, A. (1967). *The Ego and the Mechanisms of Defense*, New York: International Universities Press

Freud. S., (1924/1983). Neurosis and Psychosis' in *Sigmund Freud: on Psychopathology,* Penguin Books.

Garland, C. (1998). `Thinking about trauma', in C. Garland (Edited) *Understanding Trauma: A Psychoanalytical Approach,* pp: 9-31, London: Duckworth.

Gilbert, P. (1992). *Depression: The Evolution of Powerlessness.* Hove: Erilbaum

Glass, J. M. (1995). *Psychosis and Power: Threats to Democracy in the Self and the Group*, London: Cornell University Press.

Goodman, L. A., Dutton, M. A., and Harris, M. (1995). Physical and sexual assault prevalence among episodically homeless: women with serous mental illness. *American Journal of Orthopsychiatry,* 65, 468-478.

Heins, T., Gray, A., and Tennant, M. (1990). Persisting hallucinations following childhood sexual abuse. *Australian and New Zealand Journal of Psychiatry*, 24, 561-565.

Hemsely, D. R. (1994). A cognitive model for schizophrenia and its neural basis, *Acta Psychiatric Scandinavia*, 90, 80-86.

Hemsley, D. R. and Stell, C. (2004). A cognitive model for schizophrenia and its neural basis. *Acta Psychiatric Scandinavin*, 90, 80-86.

Holowka, D., King, S., Saheb, D., Pukall, M., and Brunet, A. (2003). Childhood abuse and dissociative syptoms in adult schizophrenia. *Schizophrenia Research*, 60, 87-90.

Honig, A., Romme, M., Ensink, B. Escher, S. Pennings, M., and de Vries, M. (1998). Auditory hallucinations: A comparison between patients and non-patients. *Journal of Nervous and Mental Disease*, 186, 646-651.

Jackson C., Birchwood, M. (2006). Trauma and first episode psychosis. in W. Lakin & A. P. Morrision (Edited) *Trauma and Psychosis: New Directions for Theory and Therapy. pp.127-147.* New London: Routledge.

Jankowski, M. K. Muser, K.T., and Rosenberg, S. D. (2006). Psychosis with comorbid PTSD, in W. Larkin, W. & A. P. Morrison, (Edited) *Trauma and Psychosis: New Directions for Theory and Therapy. pp. 75-100.* London: Routlege.

Laing R.D., (1960). *The Divided Self*, London: Tavistock Publication.

Laing, R. D. & Estersen, A. (1970). *Sanity, Madness and the Family.* (2nd Edition) London: Tavistock Publications.

Larkin, W. & Morrision, A. P. (2006). (Edited) *Trauma and Psychosis: New Directions for Theory and Therapy*, London: Routlege.

Lipschitz, D. Winegar, R., Hartnick, E., Foote, B., and Southwick, S. (1999). PTSD in hospitalized adolescents: Diagnostic comorbidity and clinical correlates. *Journal of the American Academcy of Child and Adolescent Psychiatry*, 38, 385-392.

Morrison, S. P. (2001). The interpretation of intrusion in psychosis: An integrative cognitive approach to psychotic symptom, *Behavioral and Cognitive Psychotherapy*, 29, 257-276.

Muenzenmaier, K., Meyer, I., Strauening, E. and Ferber, J. (1993). Childhood abuse and neglect among women outpatients with chronic mental illness, *Hospital and Community Psychiatry,* 44, 666-670.

Muser, K. T., Goodman, L. B., Trumbetta, S. L., Rosenberg, S. D., Osher, F. C., Vidaver, R. et al. (1998). Trauma and posttraumatic stress disorder in severe mental illness, *Journal of Consulting and Clinical Psychiatry,* 66, 493-499.

Read, J. Agar, K., Argyle, N. and Aderhold, V. (2003). Sexual and physical abuse during childhood and adulthood as predictors of hallucinations, delusions, and thought disorder. *Psychological and Psychotherapy: Theory, Research and Practice*, 76,1-22.

Read, J. Rudegeair, T., & Farrelly, S. (2006). The relationship between child abuse and psychotic public opinion, evidence, pathways and implication', W. Lakin & A. P. Morrision, A. P. (2006). (Edited) *Trauma and Psychosis: New Directions for Theory and Therapy*, pp. 26-45, London: Routlege.

Read, J., and Argyle, N. (1999). Hallucination, delusions and thought disorders among adult psychiatric inpatients with a history of child abuse. *Psychiatric Services*, 50, 1467-1472.

Romme M.A.J., & Escher A.D. (1989). `Hearing voices' *Schizophrenia Bulletin*, 22: 209-210.

Romme, M. A. J. & Escher, S. D. M. (1996). Empowering people who hear voices. In G. Haddock and P. Slade (edited) *Cognitive Behavioral Intervention with Psychotic Disorder,* (pp. 137-151), London: Routledge.

Romme, M. A. J. & Escher, S. D. M. (2006). Trauma and hearing voices' W. Lakin & A. P. Morrision (Edited) *Trauma and Psychosis: New Directions for Theory and Therapy. pp.162-191..* New London: Routledge.

Sansonnet-Hayden, H., Haley, G., Marriage, K., and Fine, S. (1987) Sexual abuse and psychopathology in hospitalized adolescents. *Journal of the American Academy of Child and Adolescent Psychiatry,* 150, 1037-1042.

Squire, L. (1992). Memory and the hippocampus: A synthesis from finding with rats, monkeys and human, *Psychological Review*, 99, 195-231.

Strauss, G. P., Duke, L.A. Ross, S. A. & Allen, D.N. (2009). Post-traumatic stress disorder and negative symptoms of schizophrenia. *Schizophrenia Bulletin*, 35(4): 1093- 1123.

Strauss, J. S. (1989). Subjective experience of schizophrenia: toward a new dynamic psychiatry II. *Schizophrenia Bulletin*, 15, 179-187.

Strauss, J. S., Hafez, H., Lieberman, P. & Harding, C. M. (1985). The course of psychiatric disorder III: Longitudinal principles. *American Journal of Psychiatry*, 142(3): 289-296.

Sullivan. H. J. (1954). *Clinical Studies in Psychiatry*, New York: W.W. Norton & Company.

Teasdale, J. and Barnard, R. (1993). *Affect, Cognition and Change: Remodeling Depressive Thought.* Hillsdale, New Jersey, Erlbaum.

United States Department of Health and Health Sciences (2004). *National Consensus Statement on Mental Health Recovery,* Washington, DC: United States Department of Health and Health Sciences.

Vaughan, S., and Fowler, D. G. (2004). The distress experienced by voice bearer is associated with the perceived relationship between voice bearer and the voice, *British Journal of General Psychology*, 43, 143-153.

Yip, K.S. (2014). *Emotionality and Mental Illness: A Multi-Dimensional Model*, New York: Nova Science.

Chapter 3

A Conceptual Review of Self-Fragmentation and Self-Integration Dilemma in Schizophrenia: Implication to Mental Health Recovery

Introduction

In the previous chapter, various psychosocial causes of schizophrenia were discussed. Within the highly oppressive psychosocial environment, the development of schizophrenia can be understood and interpreted as a process of self-splitting and fragmentation. While self-splitting implies that the self system is divided into two separated but loosely related parts, self-fragmentation means that the split self system can be further fractured into many confused but related components. It is a form of deep confusion and severe disorganization in which ego functioning, social functioning, sense of reality, and the self-system are deeply hindered or even impaired by the self-fragmentation. The fragmented self, in response to the prevailing and unavoidable oppressive social environment, goes astray with highly creative delusive paranoia, grandiosity; self-constructed reality as well as high detachment and inertness, or even lifelessness in normal functioning and representation. Each fragmented part or component may represent one part or picture of delusive reality in response to the threatening and ontologically insecure external environment. In this chapter, the writer attempts to describe this process of self-splitting and self-fragmentation in detail. The process of self-fragmentation, similar to the psychosocial causes of schizophrenia, is mentioned in many schools of thoughts. The most representative ones are mentioned in the following section. Their implications to mental health recovery for persons with schizophrenia are also discussed.

Conceptualization of Self-Fragmentation and Splitting in Schizophrenia

Frosch's Self-Splitting and Self-Fragmentation

Part Self and Part Object Splitting in Schizophrenia

All the above-mentioned subjective experiences of persons with schizophrenia in positive symptoms, negative symptoms, and first rank symptoms represent a self-fragmentation for persons with schizophrenia. It is a process of breaking the integrated self systems into unrelated or conflicting parts with a confusing and destructive effect on the individual's self image, self-boundary and ego functioning. Frosch (1983) had a good description about the self-fragmentation process in psychosis.

> `I view fragmentation as a very primitive stage in psychotic development, proceeding even to formation of part-self and part-object images. It is a precursor to splitting. Splitting comes into play at a high level of psychotic development although it still occurs at a stage where the part-self and part-object images have not been integrated and synthesized.' (Frosch, 1983: 221)

Frosch (1983) affirmed that schizophrenia is a part self and part object splitting. That means that both the self-system and perception of others fails to integrate into two interactive and cohesive systems.

Self-Fragmentation and Psychotic Features

Frosch (1983) affirmed that self-fragmentation is the crucial feature in schizophrenia in which self and object can be fragmented into parts. It accounts for the bizarre delusions or body image distortions.

> `I have referred to a psychotic character who felt that his head was not securely fastened to his neck, and grew his beard quite long so that it might help to keep his body intact. Such splitting may also be resorted to at times to preserve the object. *One patient, for instance, was able to split me into various parts so that she could destroy some of these parts and still preserve me and herself. It was easier to express her anger at me by directing it against one part. If she killed only that part, I could go on living.* It would be terrible if she destroys me, yet she had to express her hatred' (Frosch, 1983: 221)

According to Frosch's articulation, self-fragmentation is a form or an end of self-splitting in which the individual self system continuously splits into parts. Apart from splitting of the self-system, the individual also split external objects into parts. Paradoxically, that sort of splitting with a result of fragmentation is also a mechanism for preservation of self-system as well as others. Both the self and external objects can split into parts. These parts can be good and bad, past or present, external or internal, major or minor; or favorable and not favorable. The individual can express his/her anger towards the part of self or part of others that s/he dislikes most without being totally destroying or rejecting his/her own self system or his/her beloved object. However, once the splitting mechanism moves on, the individual's mental state will move into a state of confusion. The confusion and ambiguity may exist in several forms:

a. A confusion and ambiguity of reality and fantasy
b. A confusion and ambiguity of internal and external world
c. A confusion and ambiguity of what one's needs and what is actually available in the environment
d. A confusion and ambiguity of one's own self identity
e. A confusion and ambiguity of presence of external objects

All the ambiguity and confusion will further speed up the process of self-splitting with a result of ongoing and severe self-fragmentation.

Implications to Mental Health Recovery

Frosch's (1983) idea clearly shows that self-fragmentation of the self-system or perception of others mainly serves two functions.

1. To split and fracture the self-system into good and bad parts.
2. To split the fracture perception of others (object/images of objects) into good and bad parts
3. To destroy bad parts of self-system delusively to preserve the self-system subjectively.
4. To destroy bad parts of object/object images delusively to make objects/object images be non-threatening to the self system subjectively.

In doing so, s/he actually takes the cost of being ambiguous and confused in his/her senses of reality, self-identity and the presence of external objects. This is a highly paradoxical and dynamic process. On one hand, the individual fractures his/her self-system and perception of others to preserve himself/herself as well as the perception of the external. On the other hand, that sort of fragmentation leads to further confusion and ambiguity, which leads to a mentally suicidal destruction of aliveness of one's self-system and external reality. Behind all these, as mentioned in the previous chapter, the individual exists within a highly oppressive and painful but unavoidable psychosocial and physical environment in which minimal survival of the self-system and perception of reality is being deeply threatened. All these have strong implications to mental health recovery for clients with schizophrenia.

1. Availability, stability, and regularity of a highly supportive and acceptable psychosocial and physical environment.
2. Within this environment, there should be stable supportive others (good others).
3. All these supportive others should be highly acceptable, supportive, and caring to clients' fractured self-system and perception of others.
4. A prolonged acceptance, support, and interaction with these supportive others enable the individual to believe and perceive there are substantial and integrated good objects/object images in the actual reality. It also brings him/her a strong sense of ontological security.
5. Gradually, the individual can reduce his/her self-fragmentation process and rebuild a normal cohesive self-system with an actual and realistic perception of external objects in the actual reality.

Laing's Self-Splitting and Fragmentation in Divided Self

Self-Splitting in Schizoid Position

Laing (1960) in his masterpiece `Divided Self', affirmed that self-splitting is an inherent mechanism in facing a threatening environment.

> `The splitting is not simply a temporary reaction to a specific situation of great danger, which is reversible when the danger is past. It is, on the contrary, a basic orientation to life, and if it is followed back through their lives one usually finds that they seem…. the normal individual, in a situation all can see to be threatening to his being and to offer no real sense of escape, develops a schizoid state in trying to get outside it, if not physically, *at least mentally; he becomes a mental observer, who looks on, detached and impassive, at what his body is doing or what is being done to his body*. If this is so in the normal, it is at least possible to suppose that the individual whose abiding mode of being in the world is of this split nature is living in what to him, if not to us, is a world that threatens his being from all sides, and form which does not exist. (Laing, 1960: 79)

Laing affirmed that self-splitting in schizoid position has the following nature:

1. It is an inherent mechanism for individuals in facing external threat and dangers
2. It is an intense threat to one's being and existence
3. The threatening situation cannot be escaped or avoided. There is no exit.
4. Self splitting can occur mentally and/or physically
5. In the self-splitting, the individual becomes a mental observer, observing what has been done or is being done to his/her body.

The Dilemma in Self-Splitting

> `The self then seeks, by being unembodied, to transcend the world and hence to be safe. But a self is liable to develop feelings that it is outside all experiences and activity. *It becomes a vacuum. Everything is there, outside; nothing is here, inside. Moreover, the constant dread of all that is there, of being overwhelmed, is potentiated rather than mitigated by the need to keep the world at bay.* Yet, the self may at the same time long, more than anything, for participation in the world. Thus, its greatest longing is felt as its greatest weakness and giving in to this weakness is its greatest dread, since in participation the individual fears that his vacuum will be obliterated, that he will engulf or otherwise lose his identity….' (Laing, 1960: 80)

Laing (1960) affirmed that once the self undergoes a process of self-splitting, the self is trapped within a dilemma. On the one hand, it feels safe as it is being detached from the external world. On the other hand, the loss of contact from the outside makes it feel dreadful and becomes a vacuum. It has a strong urge to participate in the outside world. As a result, the individual's self-system is trapped between an approach and avoidance to the outside world. This dilemma tends to speed up the self-splitting process.

Primary and Secondary Splitting

Laing (1960) describes two basic type of splitting in persons with schizophrenia. The first type is primary splitting in which the self-system, because of ontological insecurity, split into two parts, the inner self, and the unembodied self. An embodied self embraces a two-way interaction (substantial real perception and meaningful action) with others. A split self-system with split inner self and an unembodied self fails to have a substantial and real interaction with others. Instead, the unembodied self engages in an unreal perception with others and responds with futile, meaningless, and purposeless action towards others. *The split inner self is totally separated from the external world with a dreadful loneliness and emptiness in itself. The approach and avoidance to the ontologically insecure external reality pushes the individual to have secondary self-splitting, into a true and false self.*

> `Anything may be concealed from others, but nothing must be hidden from himself. In this, the self attempts to become a relationship, which relates itself to the exclusion of everything and anything. We have here the seed of secondary splitting with the self. The individual's being having become cleft into a true and false self, and the true and false selves lose their realness as already indicated, but also they both in turn break into sub-systems within themselves. Thus, in the relationship that the self has with itself, one finds a second duality developing whereby the inner self splits to have a sadomasochistic relationship with itself. (Laing, 1960: 83)

In the secondary splitting, the inner self, without contact of the external reality is forced to relate itself to itself. That means, the inner self itself become a system in which it can further split into an inner false self and an inner true self. The secondary splitting allows the inner true self to reject, to expel, and to condemn the inner false self to further exclude possible threats from the environment. In doing so, the individual starts to lose his/her own integrated identity before self-splitting.

Molar and Molecular Self Splitting

Laing (1960), from an existential and phenomenological perspective, asserted that after the process of psychosis, self-splitting occurs vigorously resulting in a lifeless embodied self. It becomes an unembodied false self as a cocoon of the individual's inner self because of stress and oppression from the external environment. Further splitting will go on with a final consequence of self-fragmentation. Laing (1960) addressed this splitting as molar and molecular splits.

> `Janet has differentiated dissociation or splitting into molar splits and molecular splits. The hysterical split personality is a molar split. The schizophrenia consists of molecular splitting. In Julie's case, there seemed to be both. The overall unity of her being had being broken up into several partial assemblies or partial systems (quasi-autonomous complexes, inner objects), each of which had its own little stereotyped personality (molar splitting). In addition, any actual sequence of behavior was fragmented in a much more minute manner (molecular splitting). Even the integrity of words, for instance, would be disrupted (Laing, 1960: 196).

According to Laing (1960), there are two types of self-splitting in clients with schizophrenia. The first type is molar splitting in which the individual's personality may be split (changed) into different parts in which each part becomes a partial system having their own uniqueness and characteristics. Very often, a person with active delusions may proclaim that in his/her mind there is an angel and a devil. S/he can clearly present the fighting and argument between the angel and devil. In some case, the individual even develops a shifting identity that s/he is an angel at some time and is a devil at another time. The angel and devil represents different internal object that have its own identity, characteristics, uniqueness, and special functioning and meaning to the individual and his/her related environment. The second type of splitting is molecular splitting in which the individual's behaviors, thoughts, attitudes, and talking are fragmented and unrelated fragments.

Partial Self System as Separated Units

> `The fact that her being was not assemblies in an allover manner, but was split into various partial assemblies or systems, allows us to understand various functions, which presuppose the achievement of personal unity or at least a high degree of personal unity could not be present in her, as indeed they were not.
>
> A personal unit is a pre-requisite of reflective awareness that is the ability to be aware of one's own self-acting, relatively unselfconsciously, or with a simple primary no-reflective awareness. (Laing, 1960:197)

In the self-splitting, each split part is actually a unique partial system with its own reflective awareness, focus, boundaries, autonomy, its own interpretation and interaction with another partial system.

> In Julie, each partial system could be aware of objects, but a system might not beware of the processes going on in another system, which was split off from it. For example, if, in talking to me, one system was speaking, there seems to be on overall unity within her whereby `she' as a unified person could be aware of what this system was saying or doing.
>
> In so far as reflective awareness was absent, `memory', for which reflective awareness would seem to be a pre-requisite, was very patchy. All her life seemed to be contemporaneous. The absence of a total experience of being as a whole meant that she lacked the unified experience on which to base a clear idea of the boundary of her being. Thus, Federn's term, ego boundary, is unsatisfactory. One needs another term for the total of which the ego is a part. Rather, each system seemed to have a boundary of its own. That is to say, to the awareness that characterized one system, another system was liable to appear outside itself......
>
> Each partial system seemed to have its own focus or center of awareness; it had its own very limited memory schemata and limited ways of structuring percepts; its own quasi-autonomous drives or component drives; its own tendency to preserve its autonomy, and special dangers which threatened its autonomy. (Laing, 1960: 197-198).

In other words, within Laing's articulation, self-splitting is an ongoing process in which the self-system undergoes self-division into various partial systems. Each partial system tends to serve a special function for coping with demands and frustrations, both internally and externally. The more these partial systems are split, the more fragmented the individual becomes and the more the individual's wholeness and uniqueness is lost. Instead, s/he turns into a bundle of highly diversified but connected fragmented partial systems in which each of them has its own focus, awareness, function and boundaries. All these partial systems in interaction, interpretation and sometimes, conflicting to one another, imply a fragmentation as well as confusion of one's own holistic ego functioning, boundaries as well as ability to interact with external reality.

Partial Self-System and Confusion of Self-Identity and Boundary

> `She would refer to these diverse aspects as `he' or `she' or address them as `you'. That is, instead of having a reflective awareness of those aspects of herself, `she' would perceive the operation of a partial system as though it was not of `her', but belonging outside. She would be hallucinating.
>
> Together with the tendency to perceive aspects of her own being as not-her, was the failure to discriminate between what `objectivity' was not her and what was her. This is simply the other aspect of the lack of an overall ontological boundary. She might for instance feel that rain on her cheek was her tears.....a tendency to become what one perceives...(Laing, 1960: 198)

After the formulation of various partial systems of the self, the individual with schizophrenia will have the following psychotic transformation:

1. Shifting the reflective awareness of those aspects of him/herself to a detached observation to partial systems of self as an external being
2. Encountering difficulties and problems in discriminating between what `objectivity' is not oneself, and what is oneself.
3. Regarding external objects as one's symbolic identity or merging one's identity with external objects.

After the fragmentation of the cohesive self-system into various partial systems of the self, the individual loses his/her ability to have a clear self boundary as well as cohesive and substantial feelings of being in his/her fragmented self system. In a way, external objects can easily intrude into one's own self-system, including one's self-identity and feeling of being. Similarly, individual objects, as well as one's own emotion, thoughts, as well as identity can easily merge with any object/s in the external environment. That means, parts or partial systems of self can easily unite with external objects with a result of a highly confusing shifting of self-identity or a feeling of being one object then another object, from one situation to another situation, and from one symbol to another symbol. In other words, the more the self-system is fractured into various partial systems, and the more severe the molecular splitting is, the more confused and detached the individual becomes. As his/her self-system is severely fractured, any split part can easily merge with external objects making the individual feel highly insecure, confused, and fearful.

> All perception seems to threaten mergence and all sense of being perceived by other threatened her similarity. This meant that she was living in a world of constant persecution and felt herself to be doing to others what she dreaded as happening to her. Almost every act of perception appeared to involve a confusion of self with no self. The ground was prepared for this confusion by the fact that, since a large aspect of her person was partially outside herself, it was easy to confuse those split off aspects of her being with other people... To love was therefore very dangerous. To like = to be like = to be the same as... . She is thinking thoughts a, b, c. I express closely similar thoughts a1, b1, c1. Therefore, I have stolen her thoughts' (Laing, 1960: 198-199).

Dilemma of Self-Splitting versus Self-Cohesion

In other words, the individual with schizophrenia involves a highly confusing process, which regards his/her partial self-system as an external object and regards external object as his/her self. In doing so, s/he actually engages within a dilemma of *self-splitting versus self cohesion*. Within a fractured and fragmented self-system and a diffused self-boundary, the individual has an intense fear of losing his/her self-identity and generates an intensive urge to restore it by merging with any available external object. However, the merging of the external object with the partial self-system brings along further splitting and fragmentation of the self-system into more conflicting and disconnected partial systems. As the dilemma proceeds, the fragmented partial system enters life more and more. In many cases, each partial self-system may represent one voice (hallucination), one identity (delusion) and one sort of thought insertion and thought broadcasting. The conflicts between the fragmented partial self-systems may also imply argument between commenting voices (hallucination) or fighting between two delusive figures and identities. In this process, the individual is deeply trapped by prevailing fear and confusion.

Implications to Mental Health Recovery

Laing's (1960) description on self-fragmentation can be summed up in the following points:

1. Self splitting starts because of unavoidable external threat that is highly intolerable and inescapable to the individual
2. The individual undergoes self-splitting to mentally withdraw from the oppressive environment. That means, s/he sacrifices the external layer of the self system to preserve the whole self system
3. The splitting includes two processes, the primary process, and the secondary process. In the primary process, the self-system is split into the inner self and unembodied self. When the primary process cannot cope with the external threat, the secondary splitting process moves on. It is a splitting of the inner self into the true self and false self. Clinically speaking, there can be tertiary splitting process, in which the true self can further split into the inner true self and inner false self.
4. Within the primary and secondary splitting process, there are two types of splitting, molar, and molecular splitting. Molar splitting is a splitting of personality, self-identity, and structure. For example, one split part as an angel and another part as a devil. Molecular splitting is a confusion of behaviors, attitudes and cognition, emotions in each split part.
5. All split parts in the self-system are unique with its own unique partial system. Every part has its own reflective awareness, focus, boundaries, autonomy, with its own interpretation and interaction with another partial system.
6. Together with the self-splitting process is also a self-cohesion process. Both self-splitting versus self-cohesion occurs together in which the external split parts (such as the unembodied self, the false self and inner false self) connects with the oppressive reality so that the inner split parts (such as embodied self, true self and inner true self) can be preserved and survive within the oppressive reality.

All these have important implications to mental health recovery for clients with schizophrenia that can be listed as follows:

1. The greater and the more serious the individual's self-system is split, the more confused the individual's mental state is confused.
2. Related professionals need to accept and understand that clients' delusions and hallucinations is actual a split part of self-system. In other words, their contents, forms, details, and manifestation can be fully interpreted within clients' own background, personality and experiences as well as unfulfilled needs and aspiration.
3. Clients' delusive self-identity and diffused ego boundary can be understood by its unique structure and identity within one partial split self-system or confused interaction within several split partial self systems.
4. A full mental health recovery should be founded on a highly accepting and caring social environment in which the individual's inner true self, true self and embodied self can be fully extended and developed. In other words, the self-cohesion process can be done within an actual reality rather than within a delusive identity and grandiose delusions and hallucinations.
5. The recovery process should be a reverse process of the self-splitting to self-cohesion process including the following stages:
   a. From very severe splitting (inner true self, inner false self, false self, and unembodied self) to severe splitting (true self, false self and unembodied self)
   b. From severe splitting (true self, false self and unembodied self) to moderate splitting (inner self and unembodied self)
   c. From moderate splitting (inner self and unembodied self) to mild splitting (inner self and occasionally/temporarily unembodied self)
   d. From mild splitting (inner self and occasionally/temporarily unembodied self) to slight and normal adaptive self adjustment (inner self and social self)
6. Regularizing and normalizing the self-cohesion within different social contexts and social environment.

Arieti's Fragmentation of Perception of the Whole

Problems in Perceiving the Wholeness of Objects

Arieti (1974) based on Bemporad (1967)'s experiments described that for persons with schizophrenia, most of them have problems in perceiving the wholeness of objects in their related environment. It is a fragmentation of perception.

> `Many years ago, I noticed the fragmentation of a whole in the drawing of very regressive patients.......For instance, when she wants to draw a profile, she could not finish it. Parts of the profile were disconnected; furthermore, some of these parts were repeated several times, conferring a confusing appearance to the whole drawing. Some patient reported to me that during the acute episode they were aware that they were losing perception of wholes and were making conscious of efforts to reconstruct these wholes, but the attempts were only partially successful. At times, the parts that replaced the missing ones were not appropriate, and distorted the wholes resulted. (Arieti, 1974:280)

Within Arieti's description, individuals with schizophrenia focus only on the parts of the external object. However, the relations of the parts as wells the profile of the whole object is repeatedly missing. Interestingly, even though they are conscious about losing their perception of the whole, and try all effort to reconstruct these wholes, their attempts are unsuccessful with only inappropriate replacement of parts or distortion of whole. That means, there is a splitting or unreachable gap between what the individual perceives, and what the individual can attain or do with objects in the external reality. The individual's ability in getting the wholeness of objects in the external environment is dissociated, suppressed, or even repressed. It may indicate the concurrence of Laing's (1960) idea that individuals with schizophrenia suffer from prolonged ontological insecurity from oppression in the external environment in terms of engulfment, implosion, and petrification. They try all means to detach themselves from the external reality. In doing so, the individual's perception of wholeness in the related environment are also fragmented and split. That sort of fragmentation and splitting may facilitate the individual to detach from the related oppressive environment.

Part and Whole Perception in Different Stages of Schizophrenia

Arieti (1974) further described the Bemporad (1967) experiment as follows:

> Bemporad (1967) did experiments with four groups of patients by using four pseudo-isochromatic plates for testing color perception…Three cards showed a number made up of different sized dots against a field of dots of contrasting colors. The fourth card was unambiguous, showing a clearly defined number against a field of contrasting color.
>
> The acute schizophrenia group showed almost exclusive fragmentation of perception with response to the part rather than the whole percepts. This fragmentation occasionally persisted to the fourth card, which did not lend itself to partial perception. The chronic and recovered schizophrenia groups correctly identified a great number of whole percepts than the acute group, but the majority also fragmented the card data. These groups also show more than twice as many incorrect whole responses as the acute group.
>
> Bemporad concluded that in many schizophrenic patients, there is an autonomous fragmentation of perceptual wholes followed by an instantaneous reintegration according to the primary process, rather than the secondary process (Arieti, 1974: 280-281)

Bemporad's (1967) experiment clearly showed that different stages of the schizophrenic process might have different impacts of perception of the external environment. The acute groups tend to have fragmentation of perception with response to the part rather than the whole. The chronic and recovered schizophrenia groups identified a great number of whole percepts than the acute group, but majority also fragmented the card data. They also showed more than twice as many incorrect whole responses as the acute group. That means, in the acute state, where positive symptoms such as hallucinations and delusions prevail, individuals tend to ignore the whole and focus on parts of related objects in the external environment. In doing so, they have an active interaction or may be over sensitive to any stimuli in the external environment. However, the focus on the part and detachment from the whole also implies that they may have less chance to fragment the whole external object. In chronic and recovery states, in which negative symptoms always outweigh positive symptoms. Individuals are less sensitive to the external stimuli as their positive symptoms are subsideded by the negative symptoms. Thus, they focus on the whole, rather than the part. They tend to be less detached from the external environment. Thus, they can perceive the wholeness of external objects more frequently than the acute group. That means, they have a higher frequency in fragmenting the whole.

Implications to Mental Health Recovery

Arieti's (1974) articulation of clients' perception of part and whole can be concluded as follows:

1. For normal persons without psychosis, they tend to have a good balance perception of whole as well as perception of part. That means, they can have a refined perception of parts when they need to focus on parts (for example, in concentrated reading of a book, people focus their attention on the book and their attention on other objects and people in the environment may be detached). They can perceive the whole when they need to do so (for example, during a meeting, we need to note the interaction of various members as well as the entire atmosphere of the whole meeting).
2. For people with schizophrenia, in their pathological developmental process, their perception of the whole is gradually affected and weakened. As the environmental process is highly oppressive, the individual tries to detach their attention from the whole (abusive and oppressive others) to those parts where they feel better and secure. For example, in a formal meeting in which the individual feel inferior or oppressed by the others, to make him/her feel better, s/he may try to focus his/her attention on some secure minor details or activities. S/he may engage and concentrate on drawing cartoons in a page of minutes of the meeting. The drawing must be small and with refined details to make him concentrate. The more the individual concentrates on the drawing, the more comfortable s/he feels by detaching himself/herself from the unpleasant meeting.
3. As the psychotic symptoms become more and more severe, the individual is more and more detached from the actual reality. In that sense, his/her perception of the whole deteriorates more and more and his/her perception and attention on the delusive parts become stronger and stronger.
4. In the acute state of schizophrenia, the individual's perception of parts, particularly delusive parts, become much stronger than their perception of whole in the actual oppressive reality.
5. As time goes by, in the chronic state, as negative symptoms prevail in clients with schizophrenia, both his/her attention and perception on parts and whole deteriorate accordingly. In a very chronic state, the individual is inert, passive, withdrawn, and highly institutionalized. His/her perceptions on the environment may be institutionalized, inert, and fixated. His/her perceptions of details on parts may decrease accordingly as his/her psychic energy in concentration and attention deteriorates accordingly.

All these have strong implications to the mental health recovery of clients with schizophrenia. The following intervention strategies may be considered in the mental health recovery of clients with schizophrenia.

1. Related professionals should provide a highly supportive, caring, and empathic social environment for the recovery for clients with schizophrenia.
2. Within this supportive and caring environment, related professionals should first help clients to focus on their supportive parts such as symbolic objects, related persons and contexts that can trigger clients' good past memories.
3. Gradually, related professionals should guide clients to shift their attention to other supportive parts within a non-threatening and caring actual reality.
4. Related professionals should help clients express their unfulfilled needs, aspirations, and positive emotions in relation to all these attentive parts within a supportive actual reality.
5. Smoothly and naturally, clients with schizophrenia should be able to re-engage in meaningful activities and interaction with related objects, issues and people within an actual reality in daily life. Their perception of the whole and parts in various social contexts can thus become flexible and effective.

Burnham's Dividedness as a Consequence of Faulty Integration

Dividedness As the Main Features of Schizophrenia

In terms of the need-fear dilemma, Burnham (1969) described dividedness in individuals with schizophrenia as the main features of schizophrenia.

> `Dividedness is a pathognomonic feature of schizophrenia; witness the literal meaning of the word and the many similar terms which have been employed, including splitting, dissociation, segregation, segmentalization, and sejunction' (Burnham et al. 1969: 23)

Burham (etal. 1969) affirmed that dividedness exists in several forms:

1. splitting
2. dissociation
3. segregation
4. segmentalization
5. sejunction

Schizophrenia is regarded as a regressive breakdown of ego and an undoing of differentiation acquired through a primitive mental process. That means, the individual is in a process of self-disintegration, which is a process of de-differentiation. That means the individual fails to differentiate he/she and the external environment; internal objects and external objects; his/her own feelings and others' feelings; as well as his/her perceptions and others' perception.

The Process of De-differentiation and Object Addiction

The process of de-differentiation implies that the individual fails to maintain his/her own self-boundary, self-image and self-identity in terms having his/her own feelings, internal objects, and perceptions without influence by others.

> `In this process, which also involves disintegration, affects, assume the form of engulfing, uncontrollable, intense floods of feeling, instead of their normal form as modulated signals, which alert and guide the person to adaptive action……
>
> Dividedness and faulty integration go hand in hand with defective reality constructs, which fail to assimilate significant areas of experience. The range of experience that a person can assimilate into his reality construct depends, in considerable part, upon what he has been taught is or is not acceptable for inclusion in his definition of self and others…
>
> Because he is poorly differentiated and integrated; he lacks reliable internal structure and an autonomous control system. Accordingly, he has an inordinate need for external structure and control. He requires others to provide the organization and regulation, which he is unable to provide for himself. It involves no stretch of the imagination to say that his very psychological existence depends upon his maintaining contact with objects, as individuals or as part of a social structure...the schizophrenic person is an object addict.' (Burnham et al. 1969: 28)

Regarding the process of de-differentiation, apart from a prevailing oppressive environment, Burnham (1969) affirmed that it originates from a weak and poor internal structure, and an autonomous control system. That means, s/he has a poor internal and external self-structure. S/he fails to provide his/her own stable internal and external structure. S/he exerts a very strong urge to depend on others' relationships, perceptions, attitudes, as well as feelings for psychological existence.

The Fear of Disturbing Other and Fear of being Abandoned

In doing so, the individual becomes very vulnerable to other's comments, criticisms, or negative feelings. S/he is highly dangerous for others' abandonment. S/he can constantly be fearful of distrusting others and demand constant proof of the object's constant togetherness. In many ways, his/her perceptions of abandonment are originated from his/her internal instability. S/he may even attempt to deny this need and fear of separation.

> `The excessiveness of his needs for objects also makes them inordinately dangerous and fearsome since they can destroy him through abandonment. Hence, he fears and distrusts them. He may attempt to alleviate the threat of abandonment by repeated pleas or demands for proof of the object's constancy. Such pleas are insatiable because much of the inconstancy of his perception of objects stems from his inner instability. Another defensive tactic, also of limited value, is the attempt to deny his needs and his fear of separation. (Burnham et al. 1969: 28)

From Fear and Dependence of Object to Breakage

> `The schizophrenic person's fear of objects stems not only from their power to frustrate his need for them but also from their enormous power to influence him. They can make or break him. Because he is so lacking in separation and autonomy, he is particularly fearful of *domination, enslavement, or engulfment*. In addition, the influence of object is threatened to dissolve his tenuous self/oneself boundaries and even to collapse his entire structure of self. (Burnham et al. 1969: 28)

In other words, the process of self-fragmentation of individuals with schizophrenia consists of the following stages:

1. fragile internal structure and lack of power to differentiate oneself from others in feeling, thinking, decisions and perception.
2. a strong need to depend on an external object
3. prevailing fear of separation of an external object
4. external object is highly influential to the individual
5. the external object can either make or break the individual
6. the individual is thus sensitive, vulnerable and breakable to others' domination, enslavement, or engulfment.
7. individual's self-boundary and structure can be easily fractured and dissolved by all these external domination, enslavement and engulfment.

Self-Fragmentation and Impacts on Ego, Id and Superego

Within the process of self-fragmentation, the individual's internal structure is highly vulnerable to external influences just like being a ship within a rough sea. Individuals can flow with any external waves. The fragmentation and splitting process may proceed differently to various sectors of the individual. At one time, the individual's superego may become highly affected. At the other time, the individual's id and ego are influenced.

Influence on the Ego System

> `Influence in the ego sector may not be threatening at all, at least for a time. The object may be experienced as a friendly, reliable mentor and regulator. Dramatic clinical improvement of a schizophrenic patient may attend an object's functioning as an auxiliary ego. However, such an arrangement has distinct limitations. For one thing, it may lead to excessive dependence and severe anxiety whenever the patient is separated from the object. (Burnham et al. 1969: 28)

Within the fragile internal structure, the object is experienced as a friendly and reliable regulator. The external object is highly influential to an extent it becomes the individual's auxiliary ego. That means, the individual's ego system cannot be completed with the linkage of this auxiliary system (external object). If this auxiliary system is lost, the individual may come to a stage of severe anxiety.

> `In addition, the continuous presence of the auxiliary ego is difficult, if not impossible, to maintain. Eventually a heavy backlog of mutual anger may accrue from the patient's resentment of the dependent position and the auxiliary ego's resentment of continuous 24-hour duty. Accordingly, such relationships are basically unstable and liable to eventual disruption.' (29)

As auxiliary ego (the external object) is not always available, the individual may turn his/her attachment and dependence to being angry at his/her dependent position. That means, s/he is kept within a dilemma. On one hand, s/he is highly dependent on external objects (auxiliary ego). On the other hand, s/he is angry at his/her own dependence. The situation is particular complicated if the auxiliary ego is unavailable.

Influence on the Superego

Self-fragmentation not only has an impact on the ego but also on the superego and id. As the self-control system declines because of self-fragmentation, the individual's superego turns into a primitive state. Its rigid arbitrary rule is being shaped by an external authority rather than one's own internal autonomous judgment.

> `We noted earlier that the schizophrenic person's control system consists of a primitive superego based on rigid arbitrary rules, closely derived from external authorities rather than from his autonomous judgment. Consequently, objects easily influence his superego system, usually in one of two ways, through severity or leniency. Each type of influence may evoke object fear and inner instability. When the influence of the superego is severe, the object is experienced as a dreaded purveyor of threat, condemnation, restriction, and punishment. Primitive flight or fight defenses are employed to ward off the intrusive authority of the object. Obviously, any relationship in which the object attains this meaning becomes strained and liable to disruption. However, the person with unreliable inner control may also welcome harsh influence, since it affords him relief from guilt and minimizes his fear of losing control of his impulses. Schizophrenic patients often seek punishment and may beg to be sent to a judge in the hope of receiving a sentence of imprisonment or execution. (29-30)

That means, within the influence of primitive superego, the individual loses his/her own autonomous moral judgment. Instead, s/he is spontaneously shaped by judgment and criticism from an external authority. Gradually, these criticisms and judgments, no matter how mild they are, become highly threatening to the individual. They may be regarded as severe condemnation, oppression, restriction, and punishment imposed by external objects. Thus, a flight or fight response will be employed to ward off all these threats. Nevertheless, the meaning and relationship with the external object may minimize all avoidance mechanisms. Instead, the individual with schizophrenia will be overwhelmed by severe guilt. S/he may seek self-punishment to release this sense of severe guilt. In other words, his/her primitive harsh but externally influenced superego tends to oppress his/her own ego in terms of condemnation and oppression.

The sense of guilt and his/her dependence of external objects make the individual avoid shifting his/her superego to become a lenient superego. His/her harsh superego implies a sense of self-control. The lenient superego means a loss of self-control, at the same time a loss of a sense of agency. It tends to be the only way to ensure that the individual's unwanted impulses can be under proper control. Also, a lenient superego may also imply a sense of disloyalty and mistrust to the highly critical external object.

> 'one might assume that the schizophrenic person would welcome a lenient influence on his typically harsh, restrictive and arbitrary control system, but this assumption fails to take into account the fact that his superego, though harsh, constitutes his major means of self control. Hence, a lenient influence, especially if sudden and massive, may threaten him with total loss of control. Removal of old controls without the opportunity for adequate development of new, flexible controls is likely to result in chaotic impulse discharge ... the schizophrenic person's deep-rooted belief that loosening of superego structures, though yearned for, constitutes traitorous disloyalty and usurpation of authority.' (Burnham et al. 1969:30)

The shifting from a harsh superego to a more flexible and lenient superego may also trigger the sense of guilt of self-condemnation and self-mortification of the individual.

> `In fact, he may regard moving towards modifying his superego as tantamount to destroying the original external authority. Accordingly, any move toward replacing the internalized original authority by a more reasonable and flexible authority is likely to trigger reparation measures, such as severe self-condemnation and self-mortification. A state of panic with fear of imminent world collapse may be precipitated.' (Burnham et al. 1969:30)

According to Burnham (1969), a harsh superego, in line with the weak ego structure and strong dependence of the individual, is a compensation for the fear of losing the attachment of the external object. That means, the harsh superego, by fueling the sense of guilt, enables the individual to ensure that that the highly authoritative external object can tolerate his/her dependence. However, the individual also pays the price of taking a risk of being shattered by the harsh superego.

Influence on the Id

Together with the influence on the superego and ego is also the id being influenced by the powerful external object.

> `The schizophrenic person's id system is also highly susceptible to influence. An approach toward interpersonal intimacy mobilizes frightening and potentially unmanageable impulses, while upsetting tenuous internal balances. When this occurs, the object is viewed as dangerous. Part of the danger is the mobilization of primitive urges to obtain unlimited, unconditional, and magical oral supplied from the object. In their extreme form, these urges are felt as literal cravings to devour or merge with the object. The arousal of these and other primitive id impulses causes great discomfort in both the schizophrenic person and his/her objects. The usual result is mutual withdrawal and disruption of relationships. (Burnham et al. 1969: 31)

As the individual's internal structure of ego is weak and highly dependent on the intimacy with the external object, the individual actually relies on the external object to fulfill his/her unmanageable primitive impulses. S/he is addicted to merging with the external object to satisfy his/her prevailing impulses. When this occurs, both the external object and the individual will be in state of intense anxiety and discomfort. To decrease this sense of discomfort and cool the overwhelming desires, the individual and his/her external object may consciously or unconsciously avoid and withdraw from one another.

The Need and Fear Dilemma in Schizophrenia

When all these are put together, the individual will be in a state of need and fear or approach and avoidance dilemma. Within the process of self-disintegration and de-differentiation, the individual seriously needs the external object. S/he is highly attached to the external object. However, the more s/he is attached or dependent on the external object, the more s/he feels uncomfortable and anxious. This sort of fear and need dilemma exerts a strong influence on ego, superego, and id of the individual.

First, the individual needs the external object as an auxiliary ego to complete his/her integrity in ego functioning. Secondly, the superego of the individual becomes primitive, harsh, condemning and highly criticizing. However, the individual welcomes this, as it is the only way to ensure that s/he can depend on the external object as long as s/he can be self-humiliated, condemned, and oppressed. S/he does not prefer a lenient superego as it may risk losing the care of the autocratic object. Thirdly, the closer the individual gets to the external object, the more his/her primitive impulses and desires are aroused and prevail. As a consequence, s/he risks losing his/her total control of overwhelming desires and primitive impulses. Thus, s/he may try his best to avoid getting close to his/her autocratic external object.

This need and fear dilemma of self-fragmentation in persons with schizophrenia can be represented by Figure 1.

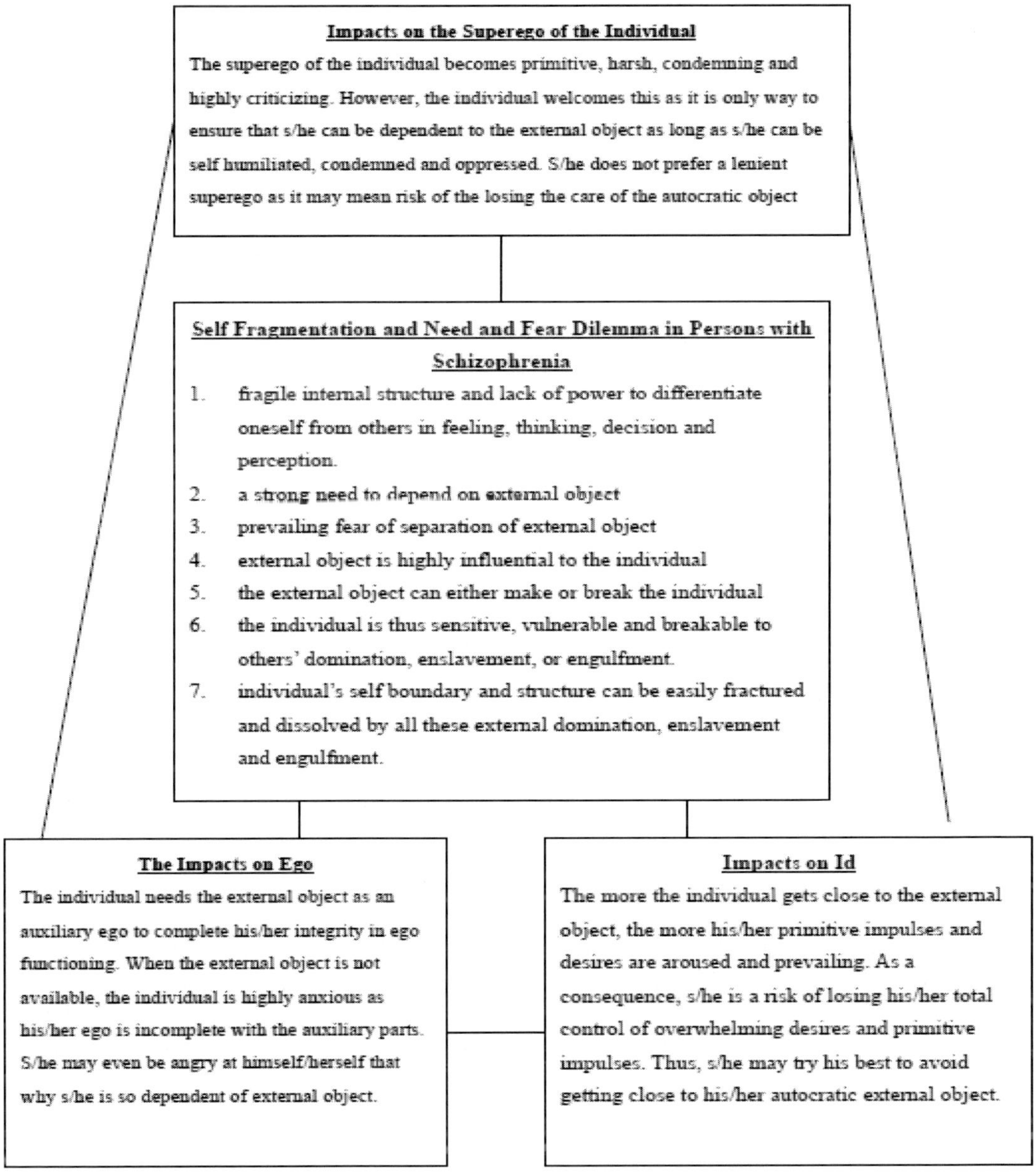

Figure 1. Self-Fragmentation and Need and Fear Dilemmas Described by Burnham (1969).

As mentioned above, the individual is highly dependent on the external object for ego integrity and functioning. However, the harsh superego and highly sensitive id make the individual become highly anxious and uncomfortable in encounters with the external object. Thus, the individual may also develop intense fear towards the objects. The fear may take many forms in persons with schizophrenia.

> `The fear of object influence takes various forms. The patient may directly voice fear that the object will dominate, control or enslave him and thereby deprive him of this separateness, independence, and identity. He may dread being literally swallowed up and devoured, or may refer to concerns that proximity to the object will contaminate, poison or otherwise infect him with bad stuff. Complaints of non-personified influencing agents such as electricity, mysterious rays, or machines are frequent. In whatever form, his fear of influence reflects his sensed lack of autonomy and corresponding need, fear of heteronomy. As we have indicated, the patient not only dreads what the object may do to him, but also what he may do to the object. He especially fears that the primitive, incorporated form and intensity of this object need will destroy the object.' (Burnham et al. 1969: 31)

The fear of the external object takes several forms. The first is that the individual fears that the external object dominates, controls, and enslaves him/her so that his/her autonomy, separateness, independence, and identity are threatened. The second is that fear of the external object, when getting close to the individual, will do something bad to him/her, such as infecting, poisoning or inserting some bad thing on him/her. The third is that external non-personified objects, such as electricity, rays, or machines, as well as other visible or invisible moving objects, may be able to control one's thoughts and thinking.

Implications to Mental Health Recovery for Clients with Schizophrenia

It is clear Burnham (et al., 1969) provided another important aspect to describe the fragmentation process in schizophrenia. While Frosch (1983) emphasized the splitting of self-system and others into good and bad parts, Laing (1960) stressed the splitting of the unembodied self, inner self, false self, inner true self, and inner false self. All these come to a highly oppressive environment in which the individual has no way to avoid or to empower him/her in facing the oppression. However, both Forsch (1983) and Laing (1960) did not explain why the individual needs to get close to the oppressive others. In that sense, Burnham (et al., 1969) affirmed that the individual cannot separate himself from the oppressive others. Instead, s/he needs the oppressive others to construct his own self-system. In that sense, he internalizes the negative comment from the oppressive other/s, which is highly painful and intolerable. In other words, he enters within a need and a fear dilemma. It is the need and fear dilemma that speeds up the process of self-fragmentation in schizophrenia. According to Burnham (et al., 1969) the process of self-fragmentation consists in the following stages:

1. fragile internal structure and lack of power to differentiate oneself from others in feeling, thinking, decisions and perceptions.
2. a strong need to depend on external objects
3. prevailing fear of separation of external object
4. external object is highly influential to the individual
5. the external object can either make or break the individual
6. the individual is thus sensitive, vulnerable and breakable to others' domination, enslavement, or engulfment.

7. individual's self boundary and structure can be easily fractured and dissolved by all the external domination, enslavement and engulfment.

The need-fear dynamics have a strong impact on ego, id, and superego.

Impacts on the Superego of the Individual

The superego of the individual becomes primitive, harsh, condemning and highly criticizing. However, the individual welcomes this since it is the only way to ensure that s/he can be dependent on the external object as long as s/he can be self-humiliated, condemned, and oppressed. S/he does not prefer a lenient superego as it may risk losing the care of the autocratic object.

The Impacts on Ego

The individual needs the external object as an auxiliary ego to complete his/her integrity in ego functioning. When the external object is not available, the individual is highly anxious, as his/her ego is incomplete with the auxiliary parts. S/he may even be angry at himself/herself, which is why s/he is so dependent on the external object.

Impacts on Id

The more the individual gets close to the external object, the more his/her primitive impulses and desires are aroused and prevailing. As a consequence, s/he risks losing his/her total control of overwhelming desires and primitive impulses. Thus, s/he may try his/her best to avoid getting close to his/her autocratic external object.

There are three types of fear towards external objects:

1. The fear that the external object dominates, controls, and enslaves him/her so that his/her autonomy, separateness, independence, and identity are threatened.
2. The fear that the external object, when getting close to the individual, will do something bad to him/her such as infecting, poisoning, or inserting something bad onto him/her.
3. The fear that external and non-personified objects, such as electricity, rays, machines, as well as other visible or invisible moving objects, enable the control of one's thoughts and thinking.

All these have a strong implication on mental health recovery for persons with schizophrenia. That means, mental health recovery for patients with schizophrenia should imply a proper resolution of their need and fear dilemmas. The need and fear dilemma in clients with schizophrenia may be resolved by the following intervention strategies;

1. Related professionals should be fully beware that beneath the need and fear dilemma, clients with schizophrenia may appear as detached and inert to other on one hand, but have an intense need to attach and to get closer to other, on the other hand. That means, despite the reluctance, inert, withdrawal and passivity of clients with schizophrenia, related professionals should still insist on getting close to them to help

them get away from their pathological absorption in their delusions and hallucinations.

2. Similarly, many clients with schizophrenia harbor prevailing paranoid delusions and hallucinations. Their paranoid delusions and hallucinations can also be understood in terms of clients need and fear dilemmas. To alleviate their paranoid delusions and hallucinations, it is crucial that related professionals provide a highly secure, caring, and supportive social environment free from control, domination, and oppression.
3. Clients with schizophrenia indeed have strong attachment needs to their significant others. At the same time, their significant others may also be highly oppressive and even abusive. Thus, it is important for related professionals to facilitate clients to be away from oppressive significant others, on one hand, and to fulfill their attachment needs in order to substitute good others, on the other hand. This can be done by having empathetic professional workers, as well as supportive and caring clients, in various social service contexts.
4. Related professionals should facilitate clients with schizophrenia to establish a stable interpersonal relationship as well as stable and positive self-image and self-identity. By doing so, clients' need and fear dilemma can thus be gradually resolved.

Bion's Projective Identification, Fragmented Ego, and Objects into Whole

Projective Identification and Schizophrenic Splitting

Definition of Projective Identification

Bion (1984), based on Melanie Klein's concepts of schizoid position and depressive position, extended Klein's concept of projective identification to describe the process of splitting both the individual's ego and external object. He described projective identification as follows:

> `Projective identification is a splitting off by the patient of a part of his personality into the object where it becomes installed, sometimes as a persecutor, leaving the psyche from which it has been split off correspondingly impoverished.' (Bion, 1984: 37)

Internal and External Factors of Schizophrenic Splitting

Bion (1984) affirmed that schizophrenic splitting is merely due to a pathological interaction between environment and personality in which the individual projects his/her split identity on the external object. It originates from an oppressive environment as well as a problematic personality. Regarding problematic personality there are four aspects, destructive impulses, hatred of internal reality, dread of imminent annihilation, as well as premature formation of objective relation.

> `Schizophrenic disturbance (splitting) springs from an interaction between 1) the environment and 2) the personality. In this paper, I ignore the environment and focus attention on four essential features of the schizophrenic personality.
>
> First is a preponderance of destructive impulses so great that even the impulses to love and be suffused by them turn into sadism.

> Second is a hatred of reality, as Freud pointed out, which extends to all aspects of the psyche that allow awareness of it.
>
> Third, derived from these two, is an unremitting dread of imminent annihilation.
>
> Fourth is a precipitate and premature formation of object relations, foremost amongst which is the transference, whose thinness is in marked contrast to the tenacity with which it is maintained. The pre-maturity, thinness, and tenacity are pathognomic and are alike derived from the dread of annihilation by the death instinct.
>
> The schizophrenic is pre-occupied with the conflict, never finally resolved, between destructiveness, on the one hand, and sadism on the other.' (Bion, 1984: 37)

According to Bion (1984), schizophrenia should be ego splitting primarily due to interaction between the problematic environment and the personality. That means the related environment may be highly oppressive. At the same time, the individual is also vulnerable to an adverse environment. As the developmental process moves on, the interaction of the oppressive environment and vulnerable personality may become a vicious cycle making the individual more and more vulnerable to adversity, hardship and oppression to a degree that results in schizophrenic splitting and fragmentation. Bion (1984) articulated four aspects of a vulnerable personality. The first aspect is an overwhelmingly destructive impulse, which makes an individual turn love into hate in facing others. This may due to fact that the individual is continuously oppressed for such a long period of time that his/her anger or impulse to destroy is accumulated but not released as time goes on. The second aspect is a hatred of internal reality. That means, the individual, in facing spontaneous oppression without an appropriate chance to fight back or resist it, not only harbors anger towards external objects, but also hates himself/herself because s/he cannot fight back or escape from it effectively. The continuous scene of being oppressed is also dreadfully traumatic to the individual. As a consequence, s/he may feel deep hatred of his/her internal reality, which is highly confused and full of senses of helplessness, worthlessness, and anger. The third aspect is an unremitting dread of imminent annihilation. Being fueled by an overwhelmingly destructive impulse and hated internal reality, the individual does harbor a strong urge to diminish the external object. However, this urge of taking revenge is strictly inhibited by the weak ego and his/her own feelings of hatred towards the individual's own internal reality. Instead, s/he harbors an unrealistic wish that external objects can save him/her from the highly oppressive environment. His/her own incomplete ego also requires a strong external object to identify and strengthen with. However, as s/he gets close to the external object, s/he also projects his/her destructive impulse and unremitting dread of imminent annihilation onto the external object. Thus, s/he is constantly kept within a dilemma of premature transference and identification with the external object, as well as projecting destructive and dreadful identification onto the external object.

Projective Identification in Terms of Counter-transference towards the Analyst

Bion (1984) affirmed that all these internal features in schizophrenic splitting could be represented by the strong projective identification on the external object. The projective identification is thus not only an intensive but premature identification with the external object but also a projection of his/her prevailing destructive impulses as well as dreadful hatred of internal reality of the external object.

> `To sum up, ignoring the effect of the external environment, the schizophrenic personality depends on the existence in the patient of four features:
> a conflict that is never decided between life and death instincts;
> a preponderance of destructive impulses
> hatred of existential and internal reality
> a tenuous and tenacious object relationship.
> This peculiar endowment makes it certain that the schizophrenic patient's progression through the paranoid schizoid and depressive positions is markedly different from that of the non-psychotic personality. This difference hinges on the fact that this combination of characteristics leads to a massive resort to projective identification.' (Bion, 1984: 38)

That sort of projective identification is clearly shown when clients with schizophrenia interact with their therapists.

> `The relationship with the analyst is premature, precipitate, and intensely dependent. When the patient broadens it under pressure of his life or death instincts two concurrent streams of phenomena becomes manifest: First, projective identification, with the analyst as an object, becomes overactive with the resulting painful confusional states...Second, mental and other activities, which are the dominant impulse, be it life instinct or death instinct, striving to express itself, are at once subjected to mutilation by the temporarily subordinated impulse. Driven by the wish to escape the confusional states and being harassed by the mutilations, the patient strives to restore the restricted relationship; the transference is again invested with its characteristic featurelessness. Whether the patient walks straight past me into the consulting room as if scarcely aware of my presence, or whether he/she displays an effusive, mirthless, bonhomie, the restricted relationship is unmistakable. Restriction and expansion alternate throughout the analysis.' (Bion, 1984: 38)

As Bion (1984) described, the therapist/analyst is always regarded by the client with schizophrenia as an important external object in which s/he casts his/her projective identification. S/he is the target of receiving the client's dominating but unresolved impulse to destruction. S/he is also the object to be identified for the client's weak and fragile ego. The client's life and death instinct manifests towards the analyst. S/he may appear as fearing or being of the analyst's presence. On the contrary, s/he can also be highly exciting, happy, and adhesive to the analyst. That sort of conflict, according to Bion (1984), is already the foundation of self-splitting in persons with schizophrenia.

Projective Identification and Psychotic Splitting

Bion (1984) affirmed projective identification, involved in schizoid and depressive positions, which were mentioned by Klein, are common among individuals in the developmental process from infancy to adolescence. Thus, there should be a distinction between psychotic and non-psychotic splitting.

> `Projective identification of conscious awareness and the associated inchoation of verbal thought is the central factor in the differentiation of the psychotic from the non-psychotic personality. I believe it takes place at the outset of the patient life. These sadistic attacks on the ego and on the foundations of inchoate verbal thoughts, and the projective identification of the fragments, make certain that from this point on there is an

> ever-widening divergence between the psychotic and non-psychotic parts of the personality until at last the guild is felt to be unbridgeable.' (Bion, 1984: 39)

From Bion's description, psychotic splitting originates from projective identification, and consists of the following:

1. sadistic attack on the ego
2. projective identification of the fragments
3. immature development of verbal thought
4. unbridgeable sense of guilt

For non-psychotic projective identification, the individual is able to introject good others and turn the schizoid position into a depressive position in which s/he integrates his/her whole expelled ego particles back into the ego system through awareness of his/her own shortfalls and weaknesses. Together with this is a sense of resolvable guilt leading the person gradually into maturity. However, for psychotic project identification, the individual is unable to move to a depressive position. Instead, s/he is over-whelmed by an unreachable sense of guilt in which s/he rather continuously expels the ego particles outside. The ego system becomes more and more split, leaving the individual ego system with fractured ego particles, which are difficult to introject back.

From Splitting to Fragmentation

Schizophrenic splitting is an on-going process with final consequences of fragmented parts of the ego system in which the individual's ego functioning and ability is impaired. S/he is being trapped in his state of mind of confusion and inability to perceive the external reality.

> `In so far as the destruction is successful, the patient experiences a failure in his capacity for perception.... The patient feels imprisoned in the state of mind he has achieved and is unable to escape from it because he feels he lacks the apparatus of awareness of reality, which is both the key to escape and the freedom, itself, to which he would escape. The sense of imprisonment is intensified by the menacing presence of the expelled fragments within whose planetary movements he is contained....In the patient's fantasy the expelled particles of the ego lead to an independent and uncontrolled existence outside the personality, but either containing or contained by external objects, where they exercise their functions as if the ordeal to which they have been subjected has served only to increase their number and to provoke their hostility to the psyche that ejected them. In consequence, the patient feels himself to be surrounded by bizarre objects. (Bion, 1984: 40)

In the ego splitting process, by means of projective identification, part of the individual's ego was projected outward and identified with external objects. Expelling particles of the ego outside imply that the ego system loses its own components with a result of losing part of its own ego functioning. Thus, the individual's ability to face reality, to be aware of his/her own limits, the perception of external objects as well as the ability to be independent and free from external constraints, are all subsided by the expelling of parts of the ego system. The merging of expelled ego particles and the external object allow the individual to have a clear target to which his/her prevailing hostility and sadism can be directed. His/her dreadful internal reality can also be projected outward making the individual feel much better within his/her constructed fantasy.

Consequence of Psychotic Splitting and Projective Identification

As a consequence of the psychotic splitting because of spontaneous pathological projective identification, the individual results in self-fragmentation, in which the individual's ego system is fragmented into particles. These expelled particles merge with external objects. Thus, the individual sense of reality is deeply disturbed. Finally, in interacting with others, both the ego and external objects are also split.

Nature of Fragmented Particles

> `Each particle is felt to consist of a real external object which is encapsulated into a piece of personality that has engulfed it. The character of this complete particle will partly depend on the character of the real object, says a gramophone, and partly on the character of the personality that engulfs it. If the piece of the personality is concerned with sight, the gramophone when played is felt to be watching the patient. If with hearing, then the gramophone when played is felt to be listening to the patient. The object, angered at being engulfed, swells up, so to speak, and suffuses and controls the piece of personality that engulfs it; to an extent, the particle is felt to have become a thing. Since these particles are used by the patient as if they were prototypes of ideas - later to becomes words, they are the actual thing they name, and so too the confusion that arises because of what the patient equates, but does not symbolize.' (Bion, 1984: 41)

In the process of psychotic projective identification, the expelled ego particles consist of certain natures of the real external object as well as the individual's ego system. The merging of part of the ego system and part of the external object make the individual become highly ambivalent. The individual may personalize the external object as an engulfment to him/her, making him/her feel that s/he is being swallowed, eaten up or inserted by the external object. At the same time, the individual may also feel that within that sort of engulfment, being swallowed and eaten up, the part of ego that merges with the external object turns into a thing, or becomes dead. Thus, projective identification is where the individual projects part of his/her ego by identifying with external objects resulting in a merging of expelled ego and external object. On the one hand, the expelled ego is lost, becomes dead, or is rejected by the individual. On the other hand, the individual, because of the merging of external object, feels that s/he is being eaten up or engulfed by the external object. That means the individual is trapped within *a dilemma of splitting and cohesion*. In terms of splitting, the individual split his/her ego system into particles in which certain particles of ego are expelled outside. In terms of cohesion and merging, the individual merges expelled ego particles with external objects. The merging and splitting of ego particles and external objects continues and manifests in first rank symptoms of schizophrenia.

Diffused Sense of Reality

As the ego fragmentation and merging with external objects move, individuals begin to lose their sense of reality.

> `The patient now moves, not in a world of dreams, but in a world of objects, which are ordinarily the furniture of dreams. These objects, primitive yet complex, partake of

> qualities which in the non-psychotic are peculiar to matter, anal objects, sense, ideas, superego, and the remaining qualities of personality. One result is that the patient strives to use real objects as ideas and is baffled when they obey the law of natural science and not those of mental functioning.
>
> Associated with projective identification is the psychotic personality's inability to introject. (Bion, 1984: 42)

The individual, after ego fragmentation, fails to embrace a clear sense of reality and self-boundary between himself/herself and the external objects. Instead, s/he projects part of him/herself into the external objects. S/he may proclaim that external objects are extensions of his/her own superego, body, ideas, and sense. At the same time, external objects can also intrude into his/her own body, mind, and ideas. Within this process, most things s/he encounters in the immediate reality are not real and substantial. Instead, s/he seems to live within a dream in which everything, including himself/herself tends to be flexible, changeable, and merging with one another. However, s/he needs to use actual real objects for normal daily communication and activities. In doing so, s/he is deeply puzzled by the merging of external objects and his/her ego particles. That means s/he is trapped within *dilemmas of substantial reality and a delusive dream* in his/her own sense of existence in the related environment. On the one hand, s/he engages in a dream with everything flexible, changeable, and merging with one another. On the other hand, s/he needs to seek his/her own functioning, roles, and meaning with substantiality of unchangeable external objects.

Projective Identification and Splitting of Ego and External Object

Bion (1984) in his article `Notes on the Theory of Schizophrenia' affirmed that the individual with schizophrenia, in the process of self-splitting, also embraces a tendency to split his/her objects. On the one hand, s/he identifies the external object. On the other hand, s/he projects his/her self-splitting experiences towards the object. Bion (1984) articulated that sort of projective identification in terms his own transaction with his patients in which they tried to split him as an analyst.'

> `As this moment I want to consider only his use of it (language) as a mode of action in the service either of splitting the object or its projective identification. It will be noted that this is but one aspect of schizophrenic object relation in which he is either splitting or getting in and out of his object.
>
> The first of these uses is in the service of projective identification. In this, the patient uses words as things or as split-off parts of himself in which he pushes forcibly into the analysis. Typical of the consequences of this behavior is the experience of a patient who felt he got inside me at the beginning of each session and had to be extricated at the end of it.
>
> Language is again employed as a mode of action for the splitting of his object. This obtrudes when the analyst becomes identified with internal persecutors, but it is employed at other times too. Here are two examples of this use of language; The patient comes in the room, shakes me warmly by the hand, and looking piercingly into my says, "I think the sessions are not for a long while but stop me every going out" I know from previous experience that this patient has a grievance that the sessions are too few and they interfere with his free time. He intended to split me by making me give two opposite interpretations at once… . My second example has wide implications; the patient speaks in a drowsy manner calculated to put the analyst to sleep. At the same time, he stimulates

> the analyst's curiosity. The intention is again to split the analyst, who is not allowed to sleep and is not allowed to keep awake. (Bion, 1984)

Both examples, illustrated by Bion (1984), showed that individuals with schizophrenia, in the process of ego splitting also try to split his/her external objects. The first example might represent the client that projected his *approach and avoidance dilemma* towards the analyst. That means, on one hand, he wanted to gain more attention from the analyst. On the other hand, once being rejected, he tried to demonstrate strong rejection towards the analyst. S/he might also be caught within a complex of love and hate towards him/her as well as towards others. On one hand, s/he may hate or be pitiful with him/her. On the other hand, s/he may hate himself/herself, thinking that s/he is not lovable. Thus, in the process of projective identification, s/he may project all these love and hate dilemmas towards the external object - the analyst. The second example might illustrate the individual's own sense of ambivalence towards his/her sense of being or existence. On one hand, s/he may want to disguise himself/herself from the oppressive reality (in a sleeping state). On the other hand, s/he manifests a need to be discovered, attended, and appreciated by others (a state of being). That sort of disguise and manifestation dilemma has been projected and identified to the external object (analyst). It is also a kind of dissociation and re-association dilemma. On the one hand, the individual intends to dissociate from the oppressive reality. On the other hand, s/he keeps himself/herself awake to be attentive to get others' acceptance and appreciation. That sort of dissociation and re-association dilemma also projects on the client's external object (analyst) making the analyst feels highly dissociated but is unable to detach from the client as s/he continues to pull the analyst back into consciousness.

Splitting and Failure of Symbolization

Bion (1984) articulated that for clients with schizophrenia, severe splitting of the ego system decreases his/her ability to use symbolization in interpreting external objects.

> `The severe splitting in the schizophrenic makes it difficult for him to achieve the use of symbols and subsequently of substantives and verbs. It is necessary to demonstrate these difficulties to him as they arise, of this we shall shortly give an example. The capacity to form symbols is dependent on:
>
> 1. the ability to grasp whole objects
> 2. the abandonment of the paranoid schizoid position with its attendance splitting
> 3. the bringing together of splits and the ushering in of the depressive position.
>
> (Bion, 1984: 26)

The individual with schizophrenia, because of his splitting of the ego system, his/her ability to symbolize incoming objects becomes slim. In fact, it is entirely a means to interact with the external environment in terms of symbols and verbs. The ability to symbolize external objects, according to Bion, depends on three inter-related abilities. The first one is the ability to grasp the whole object. That is the overall impression of the external object, especially the familiar one. For example, in normal situations, the individual knows his/her mother as a whole from his/her mother's past, present, and future impressions, or memories. That sort of understanding also encompasses his/her relationship with the individual as well as his/her mother relationship with the other family member. Even though his/her mother is harsh to him/her at this time, his/her ability to grasp the whole object enables him/her to understand that his/her mother is actually good and kind to him because of prolonged good and kind experiences with his/her mother. However, in the case of schizophrenia, the individual may focus on the current situation and interpret that his/her good mother has changed into a bad mother. Or s/he has two mothers, one is good and one is bad. Either of these 'two mothers', or both of them, is unreal and delusive.

The ability to grasp the whole object may also imply the meaning of the whole sentence or underlying message in a dialogue. In normal daily interactions with others, individuals should be accustomed to putting various short unrelated sentences or words into meaning, according to various social cultural contexts, norms or related impressions or memories formed in contacting and relating to others. For example, within formal occasions, such as in a formal meeting, everyone should speak in a polite way and presumes the ability to hold every word or sentence spoken by everyone in a cohesive way. Nevertheless, in case of a person's schizophrenia, or while one is highly furious with another one, even in a formal meeting, the individual may pick on a unrelated word or a sentence spoken by others as doing something very harmful or threatening to him/her that s/he needs to fight back. It appears as a kind of exaggerating feedback to the related psychosocial environment (Strauss et al., 1985)

It can also be the meaning of a series of behaviors or actions performed by others. It can be the meaning of a set of phenomena/events performed by various parties around a similar focus. Every day, the individual needs to grasp all these meanings in order to respond spontaneously to the external environment. Nevertheless, in the process of self-splitting, both the individual's ego system and the external object are split. The individual's attention will thus focus his/her attention on the split parts or the conflicting situations among the split parts. S/he fails to grasp a normalized meaning of the whole object.

The second ability and third ability happens together in the process of symbolization. Based on Melaine Klein's idea, Bion (1984) affirmed that symbolization is based on the ability to abandon the paranoid schizoid position in self-splitting so that the individual can use the depressive position to glue the split parts together and avoid further damage. When the individual encounters a significant other that is going to leave him/her alone and is no longer a lovable object, the individual may undergo a splitting process where both him/her, as well as the external object, will split into good and bad parts. S/he projects his/her anger towards the external object. On the one hand, s/he perceives external objects as bad and evil, and needs to attack. In doing so, s/he actually projects his/her bad self and identifies it with the bad part of others. The splitting then continues with an inclination of a schizophrenic nature. At that moment, if s/he is able to symbolize the incoming message clearly, s/he is able to integrate further symbolized messages from past memories or the current environment, the significant other's leaving or threatening is only temporary or part of the message. Thus, s/he is able to abandon the paranoid schizoid position and turns into a depressive position that attributes the leaving of and turning back of his/her significant others part of his/her own faults. That means, s/he needs to improve himself/herself so that s/he can win the intimacy, acceptance, and caring of his/her significant others.

The individual loses his/her ability to symbolize incoming messages and fixates his/her thinking and feeling in the schizoid position. Within this position, verbal thoughts are also affected. Individuals fail to integrate and actively synthesize incoming message from external objects. Thus, the recognition of the internal persecutor and the loss of the good object cannot be compensated by returning to the depressive position. In other words, s/he cannot resolve his/her inner psychic reality by symbolizing messages from external objects in related social environment.

> `Since the verbal thought depends on the ability to integrate, it is not surprising to find that its emergence is intimately associated with the depressive position, which, as Melaine Klein has pointed out, is phase of active synthesis and integration. Verbal thought sharpens the awareness of the psychic reality and therefore of the depression, which is linked with destruction and loss of good objects. The presence of internal persecutors, as another aspect of psychic reality, is similarly unconsciously more recognized. The patient feels the association between the depressive position and verbal thought is one of cause and effect - itself a belief based on his capacity to integrate - and this adds one more to the many causes of his hatred, already well in evidence, of analysis, which is after all a treatment which employs verbal thought in the solution of mental problems (Bion, 1984:26).

In the primitive schizoid position, the individual fails to symbolize the new incoming message as different from those projected by his/her bad self. S/he simply regards most external objects s/he encounters as bad others and persecutors. Similar fear and paranoia can also transfer to the therapist/analyst. The projective identification of the analyst as a bad self/bad others overwhelm the individual and consequently decrease his/her willingness to use his verbal ability as a means of symbolizing incoming messages.

> `The patient at this stage becomes frightened of the analyst, even though he may concede that he feels better, but, and this is where the kernel of our problem lies, he shows every sign of being anxious to have nothing whatsoever to do with his embryonic capacity for verbal thought. That is felt to be better left to the analyst; or, as I think it is more correct to say, the analyst is felt to be better able than he to harbor it within himself without disaster. The patient seems, despite all the work I had done, to have reverted to the use of language that I have described as characteristic of the schizophrenic before analysis. He has greater verbal capacity but prefers to employ it as he did when it was slight.' (Bion, 1984:27)

The Urge of Whole in Dream

Bion (1984) tended to take another stand on ego fragmentation of persons with schizophrenia. Instead of describing the process of ego fragmentation, he pointed out the urge of the individual with schizophrenia to have a cohesive whole object, helping him/her to glue his/her fragmented or split ego. This urge of integration of both ego and object reflects clearly in one's dream.

> `The peculiarity of the dream to the psychotic is not its irrationality, incoherence, and fragmentation, but its revelation of objects, which are felt by the patient to be whole objects and therefore fit and proper reason for the powerful feelings of guilt and depression, which Melanie Klein has associated with the onset of the depressive position. (Bion, 1984:80)

Unresolved Dilemmas in Fragmentation of Ego and Object

> `Their presence is felt to be evidence that real and valued objects have been destroyed. The immediate oscillation to fragmentation, however, does not, as I have shown in my account of the stream association with a running commentary on the

patient's feelings, afford any true relief, because it merely substitutes persecutory anxiety for the dreaded depression.......a patient who brings fragments together to make a whole object can be so disturbed by the cohesion of the fragments that an immediate explosive fragmentation follows. I supported his findings in my paper `Some Notes on the Theory of Schizophrenia' ......The danger here lies in the possibility of suicide, on the one hand, or on the other, a return to the paranoid schizoid position. (Bion, 1984:80)

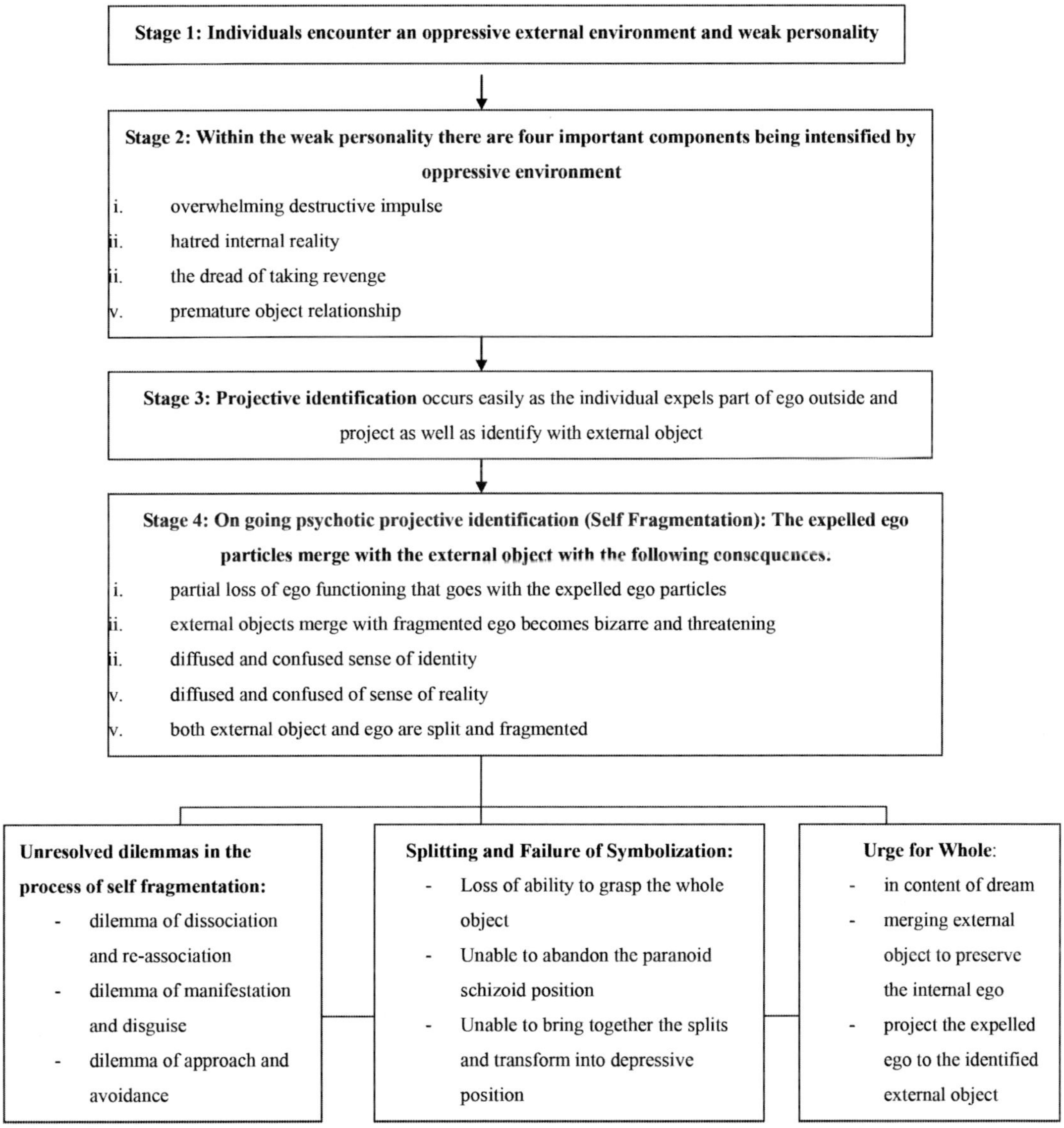

Figure 2. From Projective Identification to Self Fragmentation described by Bion (1984).

Bion (1984) affirmed that the urge for a whole object appears in dreams for individuals with schizophrenia. The individual constructs a holistic object in his/her dream but in reality, his/her object has been destroyed. It represents several dilemmas. *The first dilemma is splitting and integration.* In reality, the individual is undergoing a process of splitting into fragmented ego. In dream, the individual tries to integrate his/her ego by constructing an object as a whole. *The second dilemma is concealment and visibility.* On one hand, the individual with schizophrenia tries to conceal his/her urge for integration and existence in dream with a projection to a whole object. On the other hand, s/he tries to visualize his/her guilt feeling by splitting up his/her own ego as well as his/her object by manifesting related paranoia and ruling commenting hallucinations on himself/herself. *Thirdly, s/he also keeps within a dilemma of destruction and preservation.* As the valued and real object is destructed, his/her ego is also undergoing a threat of vanishing by continuous splitting. Thus, s/he has to glue his/her split ego by bringing the fragments together and reconstructing a whole object.

Thorough Ego Fragmentation and Problems in Reparation

Nevertheless, the more s/he brings the fragments together, the more intolerable and guilty s/he becomes. Following this is an immediate and further fragmentation to the object and ego.

> `It seems as if the patient, regressing from the depressive position, turns with increased hatred and anxiety against the fragments that have shown their power to coalesce and splits with great thoroughness; as a result we have a danger of a fragmentation so minute that reparation of the ego becomes impossible and the prospects of the patient become correspondingly hopeless. (Bion, 1984: 80)

Bion followed Melanie Klein's orientation of the depressive position and the schizoid position in describing the ego fragmentation. He affirmed ego fragmentation is actually a regression from the depressive position to the primitive schizoid position in which the individual diverts his anxiety and hatred towards the fragmented objects and ego with a result of further fragmentation happening on the ego and objects. Finally, the fragmentation will be so thorough that reparation of the ego may become impossible whereas the individual may be hopeless to recover from fragmentation.

Implications to Mental Health Recovery for Clients with Schizophrenia

The process of self-splitting from projective identification to fragmentation, described by Bion (1984), can be summarized into five stages. In the first stage, the individual faces an oppressive external environment as well as a weak personality. Bion (1984) tends to focus on the weak personality. In the second stage, the oppressive environment tends to intensify the weak personality of the individual with four important components including overwhelming destructive impulse, hatred of internal reality, the dread of taking revenge, and premature object relationship. In stage three, within these four forces, the individual frequently involves in projective identification. S/he tends to expel the bad part of his ego outside and merge with the external object. In normal projective identification, the individual is able to turn/transform his/her schizoid and paranoid position into a depressive position in which s/he is able to integrate back the expelled ego parts by introjection of good parts of the external object. However, in stage four, in psychotic projective identification, the prevailing oppressive environment makes the individual unable to transform his paranoid schizoid position back to a depressive position. Instead, more and more expelled ego particles merge with related external objects with the following consequences. Firstly, there is a continuous partial loss of ego functioning, which goes with the expelled ego particle. Secondly, as more and more ego particles merge with external objects, the ego feels highly threatening and bizarre toward external objects. Thirdly, the individual's identity becomes more and more diffused. Fourthly, this is also a diffused sense of reality. Finally, both the individual's ego and the external object are also split. That means, the individual's self-fragmentation goes on. Together with these are three unresolved dilemmas in the process of self-fragmentation. The first is the dilemma of dissociation and re-association in which the individual tries to dissociate him/her from reality and ego. At the same time, s/he also tries to re-associate himself/herself with the related environments and external objects. The second dilemma is the manifestation and disguise or visibility and concealment. On the one hand, s/he wants to disguise himself/herself from external oppressive environment. On the other hand, the expelled ego projects outside and merges with the external object. The individual manifests himself/herself by merging with external objects. The third one is the dilemmas of approach and avoidance. The individual wants to approach the other to build a transitional object relation. Once this relation is built, the psychotic identification mechanism prevails making the individual project the dreaded internal reality into the external object. The individual projects all his/her inner anger, and sense of revenge into the external object. To avoid further provoking of this intolerable anguish and anger, the individual avoids further contact with the external object. Finally, in the process of painful ego fragmentation, the individual harbors an intensive urge for the whole. The urge of whole is especially reflected in the content of dream. It also reflects in the spontaneous merging of the external object to preserve the internal ego. Furthermore, the project of unwanted ego particles into the external object also implies the deep but distorted wish or death instinct; that once the bad or unpleasant part of the ego is extinguished, the ego can be purified and survive.

All these have strong implications to mental health recovery of clients with schizophrenia. In fact, it is important for them to stop their psychotic projective identification. Related intervention strategies can be described as follows:

1. Related professionals should be fully alert of clients' dilemmas in psychotic projective identification. They are dissociation and re-association; approach and avoidance; as well as visibility and concealment. That means they should be enduring and persistent in believing that clients with schizophrenia, despite being detached from reality, confused in the mind, bizarre in their behaviors and/or inert and passive, within their mind, still urge for togetherness, integrate with reality, as well as associate with objects, issues and persons with the reality. In other words, related professionals should try their best to arrange supportive and caring objects, issues, and persons so that clients with schizophrenia can identify with good external objects without expelling parts of their ego system.
2. Related professionals should help clients with schizophrenia to connect with the supportive reality in terms of gradual, smooth, and natural activities and interaction with supportive objects, issues, and persons in the reality. All these should be done within a normalized daily life and integrated community context so that clients with schizophrenia can gradually develop a constructive and healthy sense of reality.
3. With a good restoration of a healthy and normal sense of reality, clients with schizophrenia should be facilitated to ventilate and air out their hated internal reality, overwhelming destructive impulse, the dread of taking revenge, and premature

objective relationship in their continuous encounter/attachment with oppressive significant others in their previous life. By doing so, they do not represent all these inner unconscious complexes symbolically through manifestation of delusions and hallucinations.

4. Clients with schizophrenia need to strengthen and rebuild their self-system in terms of self-identity, self-image, as well as self-boundary. Only by doing so, can they have a better resilience system in facing further challenges in the actual reality and environment. All these can be done by developing clients' strengths, potential and talents with regular and empathic appreciation by their significant others.
5. It is crucial that clients with schizophrenia, in the recovery process, after the restoration of a healthy self system within a supportive and caring environment, are able to learn and become accustomed to using normal projective identification in facing oppressive others in actual reality. This can be done by facilitating them to have good support from supportive significant others in facing difficulties and frustration in life, if their significant others are still highly oppressive.

Dynamic Forces in Psychotic Self-Fragmentation

For persons with schizophrenia, self-fragmentation is not merely a pathological process with the development of positive, negative, and first rank symptoms. It is also a coping mechanism in facing the highly oppressive, exclusive, and rejecting but unavoidable external reality. According to the above-mentioned literature review, within the self-fragmentation and self-integration dilemmas, there are three types of dynamic forces that can be identified. They are listed as followed

1. Self-splitting versus self cohesion
2. Self-concealment versus self visibility
3. Self-destruction versus self preservation

Within a deficit and pathological orientation, it is clear that individuals, within the process of development of schizophrenia, continuously split their self-systems into parts, isolate and exclude themselves from oppressive reality by concealment within a self constructed delusive reality, and destruct their own ego functioning and social functioning within actual reality. Within a coping and strengths-based perspective, it is clear that the individual, facing the prevailing and unavoidable oppressive environment, tends to split his/her self system to maintain self-cohesion; to destruct his/her self-system to ensure his self-preservation; and to conceal his/her identity in order to attain a kind of self-visibility within others' existence. All these self-cohesion, self-preservation, and self-visibility are inherent inner psychic forces originated from the ontological needs and drive of senses of uniqueness, consistency, agency, cohesion, integrity, and substantiality. The self-fragmentation, as mentioned by Burnham (1969), can exist in various forms such as:

1. Splitting (the self system is divided into two or more parts)
2. Dissociation (part of the self system is suppressed and even repressed)

3. Segregation (part of the self system is being separated from other part/s)
4. Segmentalization (each of the separated parts in the self system is isolated from one another)
5. Sejunction (disjoining cohesive parts of the self system)

From all these various forms of self-dividedness, it is clear that there are several inherent forces within the self-system. The first one is the concealing force (part of the self-system is suppressed and even repressed). The second one is the destructing force (part of the self-system is being separated and disjoined from others). The third force is splitting forces (the self system is split and segmented). Within a deficit orientation, these three forces can be regarded as highly negative causing various pathological symptoms in schizophrenia. However, within a coping and strengths based orientation, all these three forces are highly defensive and protective for the self-system from the prevailing but avoidable and highly oppressive social environment. The concealing force enables the individual to protect other parts of the self-system by hiding from the oppressive others. The destructive force enables oppressive others to know that individual's self-system is destroyed and they cannot destroy it anymore. Hence, it preserves other concealed but living parts of the self-system. The splitting force separates the visible but destroyed parts of the self-system from other parts of the self-system so that the self-system can maintain a certain degree of cohesion. In other words, the self-splitting versus self-cohesion, the self-concealment versus self-visibility, the self-destruction versus the self-preservation forces simply occur together. Self-splitting, concealment, and self-destruction are originated or targeted on self-cohesion, self-visibility, and self preservation. The inherent forces of self-cohesion, self-visibility, and self-preservation, in fact, are manifested and actualized within a highly oppressive and destructive social environment. In line of Freud, the self-splitting, destruction, and concealment forces originating from the individual's death and aggression instincts turn inwards, and exclude, destruct, and repress the part of the self-system that is directly being depowered, humiliated, and depersonalized by oppressive others in actual reality so as to preserve, to glue up, and to actualize the rest of the self-system within a highly symbolized delusive reality.

Along Bion's (1984) thinking, who adapted the schizoid and depression position mentioned by Klein (1935, 1946), these three sorts of dilemmas are originated from the projective identification in which part of individual's ego is projected outward and identified with the external object. The expelling of particles of ego outside implies that the ego system loses its own components with a result of losing part of its own ego functioning including:

1. ability to face reality,
2. to beware of his/her own limits,
3. the perception of external objects, and
4. the ability to be independent and free from external constraints

Also, the merging of expelled ego particles and the external object make the individual have a clear target at which his/her prevailing hostility and sadism can be directed. His/her dreadful internal reality can also be projected outward making the individual feel much better within his/her constructed fantasy. Bion (1984) also affirmed that the urge of a whole object always appears in dreams for individuals with schizophrenia. In other words, the individual constructs a holistic object in his/her dream but in reality, his/her object has been destroyed. It also represents the above-mentioned three dynamic forces. The first dynamic force is splitting versus cohesion. In reality, the individual is undergoing a process of splitting into a fragmented ego. In dream, the individual tries to integrate his/her ego by constructing an object as a whole. The second dynamic force is concealment versus visibility. On one hand, the individual with schizophrenia tries to conceal his/her urge for integration and existence in dream with a projection to a whole object. On the other hand, s/he tries to visualize his/her guilt feelings in splitting up his/her own ego as well as his/her object by manifesting related paranoia and ruling commenting hallucinations on himself/herself. S/he also keeps within a dynamic force of destruction versus preservation. As the valued and real object is destructed, his/her ego is also undergoing a threat of vanishing by continuous splitting. Thus, s/he has to glue his/her split ego by bringing the fragments together and reconstructing a whole object. Sullivan (1956) affirmed that in individuals with schizophrenia, the occurrence of delusions and hallucinations originate from the failure of the dissociation mechanism, leading to a loss of control of content consciousness in which those fantasies, in forms of delusive images, voices, and cognitives occurring only in the sub-conscious and unconscious state of mind in dreams, comes into conscious level and turns into delusive reality in psychosis. That means the three dynamic forces, self-splitting versus self-cohesion, self-concealment versus self-visibility, as well as self-destruction versus self-preservation, originate from the following components:

1. Prevailing and overwhelming oppressive environment imposes unavoidable and inescapable oppression in terms of engulfment, implosion, and depersonalization (Laing, 1960) to the individual.
2. To face and cope with this oppressive environment, the individual needs to undergo a process of self-fragmentation by splitting out, visualizing and destructing the part that being engulfed, imploded, and depersonalized by oppressive others. In doing so, the individual can maintain the cohesion, to conceal and preserve the remaining parts of the self-system that have not been engulfed, imploded, or depersonalized by others. In doing so, related dilemmas, self-splitting versus self-cohesion, self-concealment versus self-visibility and self-destruction versus self-preservation occurs.
3. Within the process of fragmentation, projective identification is an important mechanism in facilitating related dilemmas in self-fragmentation and self. Based on Klein's schizoid and depressive positions, the individual's self-system can be divided into 'good' and 'bad self'. Object (others) in the external environment can be divided into 'good' and 'bad' others. Within a highly oppressive environment, there is a continuous occurrence of 'bad others' and the prolonged absence of 'good others'. The 'bad other' abuses the individual and labels him as bad and rejecting. In doing so, the individual tends to internalize this oppression in which his 'bad self' develops drastically, which is intolerable for the individual. As the individual cannot display his/her anger, or fight back and avoid the negative comments of the oppressors, projective identification becomes his/her mechanism for survival. In this mechanism, individuals try to split his/her 'bad self' and project it outwards. Then, this projected and split unwanted 'bad self' is identified and united with the external objects.

In fact, projective identification is a strong splitting force. Identification is a force in which the individual tries to identify with external objects to build up his/her own self-organization. It is an internalizing force pulling external objects inward and become part of the self-organization. In a normal and healthy developmental process, if the external object is a good and significant other, like a kind and empathic mother, a nurturing and appreciating father, the identification process enables the individual to build up a good self-organization with good self-boundary, identity and ego function. Kohut (1985) articulates this process of identification of good others as a presence of an idealized parental image in which the individual is able to have idealizing and mirroring transference in identifying and internalizing an omnipotent self object. However, if there is a lack of idealized parental image (good self object/good other), the individual may lack good material to build up his/her own self-organization, the self-organization of the individual cannot be fully actualized and built. In that case, an individual may have a poor or diffused self-organization in which his/her self-identity, self-boundary, and ego functioning is poor, inadequate and even diffused and harbors an intensive urge to identify with others.

Projection means that one tries to attribute to others one's own unpleasant thoughts, feelings, and impulses (Freud, 1967). For example, a man who tries to hide his sexual urges because of the appearance of an attractive and sexy woman may defend women that are seductive and immoral. Instead of admitting and criticizing his unpleasant thoughts and impulses, this man projects these to the faults of others. A white-collar worker who wants to steal belongings from his/her company may attribute these immoral deeds to the faults of colleagues who put their belongings everywhere. In doing so, the individual pushes out his/her desires, unhealthy thoughts, and negative emotions outwards to resolve the conflict between morality and desires, personal limitations and expectations, as well as environmental demands and internal anxiety. Once, related conflicts and inconsistencies are resolved, the mechanism of projection and pushing force ends with very slight impact on the integrity and cohesion of the self-system.

In projective identification, the pushing and pulling forces happen together. It creates a strong breaking and tearing impact on the individual's self-system. In her book *Psychoanalytic Diagnosis*, Nancy McWilliams points out that projective identification combines elements of projection (attributing one's own feelings, thoughts, and motives to others) and introjection (incorporating the feelings, motives, and thoughts of others). Projective identification, in a way, validates one's projection by making the projection real (McWilliams, 1994). 'In projective identification, parts of the self and internal objects are torn off and projected onto the external object, which then becomes possessed by, controlled, and identified with the projected parts' (Segal, 1973:27).

In other words, the pulling forces of identifying and relating external objects inwards, forming part of the individual's self-organization, occurs together with the pushing force that pushes part of an individual inner conflicts, unwanted desires and negative emotions outwards. These forces intermingle with one another and become an intensive breaking and tearing force in the individual's self-system.

4. The pushing and pulling force in projective identification is, in fact, a tearing and breaking (splitting) force that pushes part of the self that identifies with external objects outward. It is also a destructing force, diminishing the unwanted part of the self, which is labeled and oppressed by others. It is also a concealing force, in which the torn part is projected outwards. The identification with others is a force of cohesion in which the expelling of the unwanted 'bad self' can be an internal cohesion of the 'good self' from the oppression of the 'bad others'. It is also an external cohesion forces in which the individual 'bad self' is united with the 'bad others'. The identification with others is also a force of visibility in which the individual depends on others to see his/her unwanted desires, motives, and thinking. The identification with others is an also a force of preservation; with the projection of the bad self on others, s/he can successfully preserve the good self.
5. The destructive impacts of projective identification on the integrity and cohesion of the self-system can be in various forms and degrees, ranging from temporary self-breaking and tearing to highly confused self-breaking and tearing.

Implications to Mental Health Recovery of Clients with Schizophrenia

These three dynamic forces, self-concealment versus self-visibility, self-splitting versus self-cohesion, and self-destruction versus self-preservation are survival based on pulling and pushing forces in self-fragmentation. Within an oppressive reality, individuals need to visualize, to split and to destruct part of self-system to detach, to separate, and to diminish linkage with the oppressive others in the immediate social context. In doing so, individual's inner true self is preserved, cohesive, and concealed. As mentioned above, within a pathological perspective, the individual is self-destructive, concealed, and split. Within a strengths perspective, the individual is self-preserved, visualized, and cohesive. The self-splitting, concealment, and destruction mechanisms all happen within an oppressive reality. That means, within a supportive and caring reality, the individual does not need to conceal, split, and destruct part of his/her self-system. Instead, the self-preservation, cohesion, and visualization all happen within an actual reality. To achieve this, the following intervention strategies are suggested:

1. Related professionals should have a thorough and deep understanding of clients' unpleasant and traumatic experiences, as well as supportive significant others and oppressive significant others. Also, under what conditions, persons, objects and context is the individual accustomed to undergo psychotic projective identification, and activitation of the self-fragmentation and self-integration dilemmas.
2. Related professionals should help clients to be free from the adverse influences of their oppressive others (family members, colleagues, peers and highly autocratic and apathetic professionals) as well as highly institutionalized and controlled service context. In doing so, clients' self-splitting, self-concealment and self-destruction mechanisms can be minimized.
3. With a deep understanding of clients' experiences and significant others, related professionals should develop a caring, supportive and empathic environment for

clients with schizophrenia. It can be clients' supportive caregivers, caring and empathic professionals, as well as good clients' peers and colleagues.

4. With the support of good others (caregivers, professionals, peers and colleagues), clients with schizophrenia can manifest their inherent self-preservation, self-cohesion, and self-visualization within a healthy and supportive reality. In doing so, clients' positive and negative symptoms can thus be gradually alleviated.
5. Related professionals should facilitate clients to develop a cohesive and healthy self-system with positive self-image, self-identity and clear self-boundary through proper recognition and development of clients' strengths, talents and potentials with constant and deep recognition and appreciation from good and supportive others.

In terms of the degree of impacts of self-breaking and tearing, there can be four different stages.

Stage 1: Temporary Self-Breaking and Tearing

Stage one is temporary self-breaking and tearing because of the occasional use of projective identification to deal with anxiety in hardship and frustration in life. For example, a colleague needs to use this to deal with his supervisor's occasional critical comment on his/her job performance. On one hand, s/he needs to project his/her poor performance as a result of his/her supervisor's insufficient supervision. On the other hand, s/he also admits s/he is a bit stupid, naïve, and dependent that s/he misunderstands his/her supervisor's comment. The push and pull force makes him/her feel a bit of self-breaking and tearing as s/he cannot face both the critical comment from his/her supervisor and the idea that s/he is stupid and naïve. Fortunately, his/her supervisor is not always critical. Once, the critical comment goes away, the individual does not need to use the projective identification and his/her self-breaking ceases and s/he can regain his/her self-integrity and cohesion.

Stage 2: Partial Self-Breaking and Regular Use of Projective Identification

In stage two, there is a partial self-breaking and regular use of projective identification to certain areas and social cycles of the individual. The individual does not have a good and cohesive self-organization. His/her self-boundary, self-image, and self-identity is a bit inadequate and incompetent. In addition to that, at least one of his/her social circles, such as work, school, family or peers is continuously oppressive. Thus, in facing this oppressive social environment/s, s/he needs to regularly use projective identification in facing the oppressive others. His/her inadequate self-organization makes him/her need to identify with the oppressive other so that s/he can maintain proper ego functioning within this environment. On the other hand, s/he needs to project these internalized bad aspects out to protect his/her own self-image, boundary, and identity. Prolonged and regular use of projective identification causes the individual to become self-breaking, self-tearing, and segmented within this oppressive environment. However, as this oppressive environment is only one of the individual environmental contexts, his/her partially broken self-system can be glued together again in another supportive and caring environment.

Stage 3: A Full Self-Breaking and Tearing with Diffused Sense of Reality and Delusions

In stage three, there is a full self-breaking and tearing in which the individual has a highly diffused sense of reality with prevailing delusions and hallucinations. In this stage, the individual is not only facing one aspect of social context that is highly oppressive. Instead, most of his/her related social contexts such as family, peers, and work are oppressive, exclusive, and rejecting. Prolonged encounters and personal development within all these oppressive social contexts makes the individual's self-organization become highly fragile and diffused. S/he certainly has a poor and fragile self-identity, self-image, and diffused self-boundary. The frequent, overwhelming, and habitual use of projective identification fractures the individual's self-system. In every occasion, s/he is accustomed to project his/her false self, which is already being condemned, rejected, and excluded by oppressive others. In every social interaction, s/he is used to identify, introject, and internalize other's comment, especially those negative and critical ones. S/he eagerly seeks positive comment and appreciation so that his/her weak self-organization including self-boundary, self-identity, and ego functioning can be strengthened. However, the more s/he earnestly joins with others', the more s/he hates and rejects himself because of full introjection and internalization of others' negative comments. Gradually, the full-fledged and overwhelming projective identification may develop related psychotic symptoms. S/he may suffer from persecutory hallucinations and delusions since his/her prevailing identification mechanism makes him/her feel that everyone around is related to him/her. His/her projection mechanism projects his/her bad self in terms of an intensive sense of inferiority and self-hate making him/her feel that every person around is trying to criticize, reject, expel, or even harm and hurt him/her. The prevailing projective identification mechanism also makes the individual's ego functioning and self-organization become more and more fragile, weak, and vulnerable to external interference. The more parts of the individual self-system are being projected out, the weaker the remaining good inner-self becomes, and the more diffused is the self-boundary.

Stage 4: A Highly Confused Self-Breaking and Tearing with Highly Fragile Self-System

In stage 4, there is a highly confused self-breaking and tearing process happening with the vulnerable and highly fragile self-system. The individual's self-system is no longer functioning properly. It is broken not only into the good and bad self but also other fractured divisions such as the inner good self, outer good self, inner bad self, and outer bad self. Projective identification occurs out of the control of the individual and intermingles with other ego defense mechanisms such as regression, denial, and fantasy. These ego mechanisms move on automatically in every environment and context. Even if the social context is non-threatening and not oppressive, such as accepting and empathic professionals in the counseling process and supportive significant others, the projective identification still prevails. A person with schizophrenia still project his/her bad self onto others in a way, s/he firmly criticizes and concludes others are bad, intrusive and persecutory. In doing so, his/her delusive and grandiose identity is actualized to a state that s/he uses this to command and defend the projected bad others. For example, a client with schizophrenia, in seeing his/her psychiatrist may affirm that his/her psychiatrist is controlled by the demon or is the demon that comes to hurt him/her. At the same time, s/he may say that s/he does not fear the demon psychiatrist, as s/he is the angel sent by God to defeat all demons in the world. The highly split and torn components of self, inner good self, inner bad self, outer good self and outer bad self implies that there are changes in the delusive paranoia and grandiose identity. The individual, after proclaiming that s/he is the mighty angel, comes to this world to defeat the demon psychiatrist, as s/he sees a female psychiatric nurse drops in, then, s/he proclaims, s/he is now change to the mighty God, the female psychiatric nurse is actually the leader of the demon group. All these prevailing and active shifting, from one delusive identity to another, as well as from one paranoid delusion and hallucination to another, and the hallucinations are highly confused and disturbing not only to the individual himself/herself but also to others. The more frequent is the shifting, the more fragile, and vulnerable the individual's self-system becomes. The more vulnerable the self system is, the more frequent is the breaking and tearing, and the more confused and overwhelming the projective identification becomes.

In the coming session, based on the above-mentioned literature on self-fragmentation, the writer will mention each of these dilemmas in detail.

Self-Splitting versus Self Cohesion

Self-splitting versus self cohesion is the first dynamic force in the self-fragmentation and self-integration of the self-system in schizophrenia. Within a fractured and fragmented self system and a diffused self boundary, the individual has an intense sense of fear in losing his/her self identity and s/he generates an intensive urge to restore it by merging with any available external object. However, the merging of external objects with the partial self-system brings along further splitting and fragmentation of the self-system into more conflicting and disconnected partial systems. According to Laing (1960), each partial self-system wants to merge with external objects as an unclear and highly diffused self-boundary (self-cohesion by merging with external object) but further splitting in order to be alike (swallowed) by the external object. Within that sort of dilemma, the self-system is in a state of confusion. The more the individual fractures his/her self-system, the more diffused his/her self-boundary becomes, and the more it seeks to merge with the external object. However, the more it merges with external objects, the more fragmented the self-system is.

In the self-splitting versus self-cohesion dynamic forces, the individual needs external organization and regulation to attain a pseudo sense of self-cohesion. As what Burnham (et al., 1969) mentioned:

> `He requires others to provide the organization and regulation, which he is unable to provide for himself. It involves no stretch of the imagination to say that his very psychological existence depends upon his maintaining contact with objects, as individuals or as part of a social structure… the schizophrenic person is an object addict.' (Burnham et al. 1969: 28)

In other words, the self-splitting process not only occurs by internal forces of splitting, of segmenting and separating the part that has been humiliated, engulfed, imploded, and petrified by oppressive others; it also contains an external force of gluing this part with the external object, despite its being oppressive and humiliating. That means the self-system in self-splitting versus self-cohesion is very loose both in self-organization and self-boundary, in a way, it needs external organization, structure, and boundary to restructure its own organization and boundary of the split part.

This is a pull and push force that originates the self-splitting versus self-cohesion dynamic force. The individual pushes the parts of 'unembodied self' or the 'false self' out, and glues it up with the external object's self-organization, structure, and boundary. In doing so, the individual enables himself/herself to pull up the residual parts of his/her inner self so that s/he can remain cohesive and integrated inside without being oppressed and humiliated by others. The pull and push forces work together making the self-splitting versus self-cohesion dynamic force prevail.

Burnham (et al., 1969) affirmed that the push and pull force in this dilemma originates from the need and fear dilemma in schizophrenia. It is the need to be related to others, combined with the fear of being rejected and isolated by others. On one hand, the weak and poor self-organization pushes the individual to relate to others to depend on others' self-organization to complete his/her own self-organization. However, once the individual relates or interacts with others, the fear of being swallowed, indulged, and occupied by others prevails. The need and fear is originated from two sources. The first source is prolonged oppression and humiliation by others with a result of a fragile self-system as well as being highly sensitive to others' criticism and comment. The fragile self-system embraces poor self-organization and needs to depend on others to temporarily complete it. The sensitivity to criticism and experiences of humiliation can be attributed to the deep fear of being rejected and swallowed by others. The second source is prolonged abandonment and separation by significant others, making the individual feel highly anxious to attach and depend on the other. However, once s/he relates to another, the prevailing fear is that sooner or later, his/her significant other may leave and even abandon him/her. In both situations, the individual's self system is under-developed with poor self-organization and dependence as well as a strong urge to depend on others for survival. In both cases, the individual does not have any confidence or prior successful experiences so that s/he can relate to good others. The need and fear dilemma activates, continues, and worsen the self-splitting versus self-cohesion dynamic force. The individual becomes highly vulnerable to others' slightest comment, criticism, rejection, and isolation. All these external stresses, in extreme cases, no matter how enlightened they are, under the self-splitting versus self-cohesion dynamic force, can have a strong breaking effect on the self system of the individual. The individual needs to glue the split part together by relating to others. However, the more s/he relates to others, the easier s/he will be broken and split in his/her self-system by others. Finally, s/he will enter into a state of serious self-fragmentation process. Within this process from slight self-splitting to severe self-splitting, there are several stages of changes, which can be described as follows:

Stage 1: Temporary Self-Splitting versus Self-Cohesion to Significant Others Only

In this stage, the self-splitting versus self-cohesion is just temporary in a way; this dilemma only occurs occasionally during stress or unpleasant environments. Also, the need and fear dilemma merely focuses on client's significant others. S/he needs to attach to his/her significant others such as family members, close friends or peers, teachers in schools, and colleagues in work to compensate for his/her weak self-organization and ego functioning in facing stressful environments and oppression. However, s/he is also afraid of being controlled by these significant others. Nevertheless, all these significant others accept and tolerate these need and fear dilemmas. That means, the self-splitting versus self-cohesion dynamic force can function well to cope with stress and external oppression. Once stress and oppression ends, the individual can regain a normal ego and social functioning.

Stage 2: Partial Self Splitting versus Self Cohesion to Persons and Event in the Reality

In this stage, related external oppression and abuse is not only temporarily happening. They happen constantly and continuously within a certain scope of life or certain context of the individual. For example, there can be a constantly abusive family, work, or community, which the individual cannot avoid. However, within this context, individuals embrace an intense need and fear dilemma in which s/he needs to engage in a self-splitting versus self-cohesion dynamic force. For example, an individual needs to attach to an abusive father in a single parent family. As the only attachment figure, the individual, on the one hand, needs his/her father for attachment purposes. On the other hand, s/he harbors deep fear towards his/her abusive father. Because of continuous abuse in the developmental process, the individual is weak in developing a healthy and good self-organization; s/he needs to depend on his father's approval and acceptance. However, once s/he joins with his/her father, s/he is vulnerable to be abused and tortured. Thus, within the family context, s/he is engaging in a self-splitting versus self cohesion mechanism for survival and integrity of his/her self system. The individual can encounter a highly supportive and empathetic boss who supports, appreciates, and develops the individual's self-system; the individual does not need to engage in a self-splitting versus self-cohesion mechanism. Instead, s/he can develop a good self-system in his/her work context to compensate his/her difficulties in the family context. In that sense, the individual is only engaged in a partial self-splitting versus self-cohesion dynamic force in the reality.

Stage 3: Full Self-Splitting versus Self-Cohesion to Persons and Events in the Delusive but Organized Reality

In this stage, the individual is involved in a full self-splitting versus self-cohesion to persons and events in the delusive but organized reality. The surrounding social environment such as family, work setting, community and interpersonal interaction are most oppressive or stressful. In no way, the individual is able to develop a good and cohesive self-system to face an oppressive and stressful environment and life frustration. For example, the individual is not only bullied or oppressed by his/her boss and colleagues, s/he is also being engulfed and imploded by his parents and his/her spouse. In both situations, s/he needs to be engaged in a self-splitting versus self-cohesion in order to survive within these two important but oppressive contexts. In the family, his/her self-system needs to split an external part that coincides with the self-organization of his parents to preserve the inner self from being abused by them. Similarly, s/he needs to overtly be obedient and accept all related bullying from his/her bosses and colleagues. In doing so, his/her self-system also splits part of it to relate with his/her oppressive colleagues and boss so that s/he can appear as obedient, submissive and tolerating in continuation of his/her employment and stable income. In both ways, the self-splitting versus self-cohesion mechanism is the only way for the individual to maintain a stable family and a stable employment. However, in this process, her self-system is severely split and the dilemma of self-cohesion and self-splitting prevails. That means, in each oppressive environmental context, the only way s/he can survive is to involve in a self-splitting versus self-cohesion mechanism. S/he needs to adhere with the external object to serve two functions. The first function is united with the external object's self-boundary as well as the self-ingredient to strengthen the individual's weak and poor self-organization. The second function is to split the part of self-system (in terms of false self in Laing's concept of divided self in schizophrenia) that united with the oppressive others to ensure the security of the inner self. The first function is self-cohesive and the second function is self-splitting. As the split parts become more and more, the split parts unite with the oppressive others more and more, and the residual self-system decreases more and more. Finally, the self-splitting versus self-cohesion prevails in a way that fractures the self-system of the individual and severely weakens the ego functioning of the residual self-system. The residual self-system loses its power to maintain its own boundary, identity, and sense of reality. At this stage, it nurtures various types of symptoms including positive, negative, and first rank symptoms.

Stage 4: Highly Confused Self-Splitting versus Self-Cohesion to Highly Delusive and Disorganized Reality

In this stage, the prevailing self-splitting versus self-cohesion dynamic force does not only happen in every aspect of life making the individual's schizophrenic symptoms manifest fully.

This dilemma further intensifies to an extent that it turns into a highly confused manner. For example, an individual who is continuously oppressed by his/her colleagues, boss, parents and family members may finally develop a delusion that people around him/her are sent by a nasty demon to destroy his/her whole life. As his/her self-boundary is highly diffused, s/he may even presume that this nasty demon has inserted a computer chip into his/her mind. His self-splitting versus self-cohesion dynamic force turns into a highly confused manner. Everywhere s/he goes and any person s/he encounters, s/he deludes that this person is sent by the nasty demon. S/he gets a feeling that through the nasty demon, this person can read his/her mind and think in his/her brain. In doing so, s/he immediately splits her residual self-system into two subsystems; one unites with the person s/he encounters through the nasty demon. One remains as his/her self. As the process goes on, more and more parts of his/her self system is split off and projects outwards, the more and more diffused his/her self boundary becomes, and the more and more s/he is confused with himself/herself and his/her surrounding environment. Underlying this is a prevailing fear that sooner or later his/her own being or self-system will be totally occupied by anyone in the environment through the nasty demon. The highly confused self-splitting versus self-cohesion mechanism makes the individual construct a highly delusive and disorganized reality. Within which, the individual becomes highly ambivalent that s/he may fail to have a clear boundary about himself/herself, and persons as well as objects in the immediate environment. In many cases, his/her own self-identity is changed accordingly. The individual is no longer himself/herself, s/he turns into a self-grandiose identity so as to face the prevailing threat from the environment. His/her projected his/her self split parts to join with external objects leaving a prolonged and unfilled vacuum in the fragile self system, the individual needs to create a new grandiose and delusive self-identity so that s/he can survive within the prevailing paranoia developed from the interpreted threat from the environment. For a person with a persecutory delusion that a powerful demon is following him/her everywhere, s/he may finally develop a grandiose identity that s/he becomes a powerful god that can diminish any demon not only in him/her but also in other persons' mind and body. The conflict between persecutory delusion and grandiose identity further speeds the self-breaking and tearing to a degree that s/he becomes highly confused in mind, with rapid shifting from one delusion to another delusion. S/he can also hear different tracks of voices arguing with one another.

Self-Concealment versus Self Visibility

Existence and Non-existence within Oppressive Environment

As mentioned above, the self-system has three inherent forces including, splitting, destructing and concealing forces. Concealing force means that part of the self-system is being suppressed and even repressed. Within a coping and strengths based orientation, the concealing force enables the individual to protect other parts of self-system being hidden from the oppressive others. Within a dynamic and dialectic view, self-concealment versus self-visibility co-exist together. While one is trying to withdraw from the reality and from others attention, the best strategy is not to have total non-existence, which is never possible, as s/he still needs to survive in daily functioning with an apparent existence in various social and physical contexts. Thus, the best way to conceal this is to use the techniques of `wearing a mask' or `appearing to be a different person', so that the actual self can be concealed and protected from being exposed to criticism and oppression. Laing (1960) described this mechanism in terms of false self and/or unembodied self. The concealing mechanism, psychologically, can be understood as the mechanism of `dissociation' in which unpleasant and traumatic experiences are being repressed. In acute stress disorder, individuals even numb all their senses on their own body, mind and environment so that they can survive even in the most extremely adverse environment. Underlying the process of dissociation, individuals only manifest a limited amount of ego functioning in the immediate social environment. What is invisible and concealed in the highly adverse, oppressive, risky, and dangerous environment is the individual's body and mind. They become apathetic, with an absence of feelings and thinking. It is a kind of appearance of the unembodied self or even the false self by helping the individual to try all means to survive within the highly risky environment.

Projective Identification: Social Camouflage

In fact, in the animal world, while facing an unavoidable but dangerous environment, the best strategy is the use of camouflage in which the animal appears as a part of the environment. Camouflage is the best concealment mechanism, as it exists in the same color, and same shape as the objects in the environment. That means, in camouflage, concealment, and visibility work together. The best concealment is a visibility in which the enemies regard the animal as part of the environment. In the process of self-fragmentation, a similar mechanism also occurs, by means of projective identification, the individual conceals himself by being identical with the oppressive external objects. In doing so, s/he also enmeshes with the bad nature of the oppressive others. The bad nature is, in fact, according to Freud, common among human beings. That means it is also embedded within the individual's self-system. They are the components of the bad self of the individual. In being identical with the bad others, the bad self will thus increase drastically in a way that is intolerable and unacceptable to the individual, which s/he needs to project out. In other words, within the projective identification mechanism, the individual visualizes himself/herself by being identical with his/her bad others so that s/he can conceal his/her good self without being swallowed by oppressive others. However, in doing so, the more s/he identifies with the bad others, the more s/he feels threatened by others, the more withering and deteriorating the good self becomes and the more fragile and vulnerable his/her self organization is and the more s/he needs to conceal himself/herself from the threatening environment.

Mental Observers As a Way to Self-Concealment

Laing (1960) affirmed that in the process of self-fragmentation, the individual, in facing the inescapable and unavoidable oppressive environment, tends to distance himself/herself from his/her own body. S/he becomes a 'mental observer', looking at his/her body doing everything with the oppressive environment. In other words, the individual's mind and consciousness is detached or concealed, but his/her body is still visible and present.

> `the normal individual, in a situation all can see to be threatening to his being and to offer no real sense of escape, develops a schizoid state in trying to get outside it, if not physically, *at least mentally; he becomes a mental observer, who looks on, detached and impassive, at what his body is doing or what is being done to his body*. If this is so in the normal, it is at least possible to suppose that the individual whose abiding mode of being in the world is of this split nature is living in what to him, if not to us, is a world that threatens his being from all sides, and from which there is no way to exist. (Laing, 1960: 79)

The feeling of being invisible/concealed from the environment but the body is visible can get worse and worse in the prevailing projective identification. Finally, the sense of being a mental observer may come to a stage that the individual is no longer himself/herself; s/he becomes another person. That means s/he addresses himself/herself as another person. That is, a complete concealment to be another person both in identity and in consciousness. In other words, his/her body as well as his/her mind are identical to someone else or she/he becomes another in the oppressive environment. However, his/her own good and real self may be concealed.

> `She would refer to these diverse aspects as 'he' or 'she' or address them as 'you'. That is, instead of having a reflective awareness of those aspects of herself, 'she' would perceive the operation of a partial system as though it was not of 'her', but belonging outside. She would be hallucinated (Laing, 1960: 180).

Concealment and Visibility in Paranoid and Grandiose Delusion

In other words, s/he is no longer himself/herself but a person that is observing himself/herself. In a delusive paranoid state, s/he is being obsessively betrayed and followed by others. S/he is deeply afraid of being visible. S/he tries hard to hide and becomes invisible so that s/he will not be hurt by bad others who exist everywhere. In a delusive grandiose state, the delusively paranoid concealment turns into a highly visible grandiose figure, such as a mighty god, powerful heroes, and/or a supernatural being coming from outer space. In doing so, s/he has supernatural powers to penetrate others' mind and brain. S/he is able to read others' ideas and thinking. Within this grandiose delusion, the individual's real and original identity is properly concealed, what becomes visible is only the delusive grandiose and supernatural being. The concealment and visibility dilemma, in the process of self-fragmentation, turns into a delusive paranoia and delusive grandiosity dilemma. Within the paranoid state, it is the withering and weakening of the self-system with intensive fear towards prevailing bad others. The grandiose state is total concealment of the real self by dressing up a highly grandiose but delusive self to fight back the highly oppressive others.

Stages of Development of Self concealment versus self visibility dynamic force

In the process of psychotic self-fragmentation, because of the prevailing mechanism of projective identification, similar to the stages of development in the self-splitting versus self-cohesion dynamic forces, there are also various stages in the development of self-concealment versus self-visibility dynamic force. They are described in the following table.

Stage of Self concealment versus self visibility dynamic force	**Forms of Concealment and Visibility**	**Content and Process of Self concealment versus self visibility**
Temporary Self concealment versus self visibility	Reflective Concealment vs Actual Participatory Visibility	As the oppressive environment exists temporarily, the individual only uses the self-concealment versus self-visibility shortly. In facing others' critical comments and embarrassing situations, s/he cannot avoid or escape, s/he may first take a reflective distance from it and evaluate whether s/he has done something wrong or is there any means to deal with that sort of oppression. Then s/he tries to use that means to have participatory visibility in the temporarily oppressive environment. For example: in a formal meeting, a man is suddenly criticized and excluded by his colleagues. To face this situation, he needs to use humor to turn the embarrassing situation into a joke. By means of this, he can make the formal criticism and exclusion just in a form of casual teasing. In doing so, he needs to take a reflective concealment in which he tries to keep a distance from the criticism and have a quick but temporary reflection so he can desert such criticism. Instead of being totally withdrawn from the situation or respond in an angry way, he takes on the situation actively by participating in a humorous way. It is visualization in a form of humorous existence. However, if the use of humor cannot ease him out the embarrassing situation, he needs another temporary reflection by being detached from the interaction from a while, thinking that he has already been self-humiliated informally but they still push on with their criticism and exclusion. This time, he may suddenly turn into an angry visualization by arguing back and taking an active stance to fight back all these criticisms and exclusions. The reflective concealment and actual participation is only a temporary measure to deal with the embarrassing situation and critical comments in the social environment. Once such situations change, the individual can regain normal spontaneous social interaction with others. S/he does not need to be caught within this dilemma constantly.

(Continued)

Stage of Self concealment versus self visibility dynamic force	Forms of Concealment and Visibility	Content and Process of Self concealment versus self visibility
		In fact, reflective concealment, to a suitable extent, may help the individual have a good reflection about what s/he has done to others and make him/her have better self-control in interpersonal interaction.
Partial Self concealment versus self visibility	Detached Concealment vs Dissociative Participatory Visibility (mental observer and wearing mask)	In that situation, the oppressive environment is ongoing, even if the individual uses reflective concealment to deal with the oppressive situation, s/he does not find any faults, misdeeds, or inappropriate attitudes or manner that s/he needs to change, or even if s/he changes, the oppressive environment still prevails. Similarly, actual participatory visibility cannot ease the situation. Instead, the more the individual uses actual participation, the more s/he feels being oppressed and the more s/he feels angry with the oppressive others. However, there is no way s/he can express this sort of anger, for it may invite further oppression and unfair treatment. Thus, the best way to survive within this sort of constant oppressive environment is by detached concealment and dissociative participatory visibility. Detached concealment means that the individual is cognitively or emotionally detached from the oppressive environment. S/he physically exists in the environment but emotionally and mentally s/he is detached from the related interaction and activities within the oppressive environment. Dissociative participatory visibility implies that the individual is highly dissociative from external stimuli and related objects, persons and issues in the oppressive environment. S/he shows no response or seriously numbs his/her senses of anger, hate and inferiority in being humiliated, isolated, teased and criticized by oppressive others. In doing so, within Laing's (1960) terms, the individual acts like he/she is wearing a mask or being a mental observer watching what s/he and others are doing within the oppressive environment. *For example, B is spontaneously bullied and humiliated by his/her oppressive boss and supervisor.* No matter how hard s/he reflects, evaluates, and even improves himself/herself, the humiliation, oppression, and bullying are still there. However, B needs this job to support his family; he cannot quit it or find another one. To survive within all the continuous oppression, bullying and humiliation, s/he needs to engage in a detached concealment and dissociative participatory visibility. He is emotionally and mentally detached in this working environment, in particular when the boss is bullying, humiliating, and oppressing him.

Stage of Self concealment versus self visibility dynamic force	Forms of Concealment and Visibility	Content and Process of Self concealment versus self visibility
		He numbs all his senses of self, mind, environment, and growth so that he does not feel being hurt or excluded. In this mental detachment, he is still working with his colleagues and his boss. He is visual, he is participating in his work, but he acts just like a working robot with no feelings, no self-image, and no hurt or harm. He is highly detached and dissociative in his work. He continuously reminds himself that it is only a job, a source of income, and a way to get money to support his family.
Full Self concealment versus self visibility	Camouflage Concealment vs Opponent Identified Visibility	Under the prevailing oppressive and humiliating environment, the use of detached concealment and dissociative participatory visibility can only maintain a minimum survival for the individual. The individual is thus kept with a dilemma. On one hand, the more s/he uses his/her 'unembodied self' or 'mask' and acts as a robot in his/her immediate physical and social environment, the more his/her self-system suffers from deteriorating self-isolation and self-withdrawal implying that the self-system becomes weaker and weaker. That means, s/he becomes more and more vulnerable to external oppression. On the other hand, oppression and humiliation becomes more and more intense and intolerable to a degree that even robot-like participation cannot inhibit the harm and hurt from the oppressive others. The individual faces a crisis in mental and ego survival. Facing that sort of urgency, the individual engages in camouflage concealment and opponent-identified visibility. Camouflage means that the individual has to identify or pretend to be part of his/her oppressive environment. That means, s/he identifies or even internalizes the critical comment from the oppressive others in oppressing himself/herself. S/he rationalizes that s/he is bad and needs to be oppressed by others. Opponent identified visibility implies that s/he behaves like his/her oppressive others. This can exist in two different ways. The first way is that s/he models the oppressive other to oppress the other person. Another way is that s/he oppresses himself/herself by saying that s/he deserves to be humiliated by the oppressive others. The humiliating experience makes him/her feel good and it is beneficial for his/her own development. S/he may even engage in some self-punishment behaviors to please the oppressive others. In doing so, s/he can totally conceal his/her own anger, and his/her real inner self from the oppressive environment. In other words, s/he is not only a mental observer but also a controller. S/he can control himself/herself to fool the oppressive others.

(Continued)

Stage of Self concealment versus self visibility dynamic force	Forms of Concealment and Visibility	Content and Process of Self concealment versus self visibility
		In terms of projective identification, the individual's bad self is projected outside and identifies with the bad others, so that the individual's good self can be concealed and protected from the oppression. *There are two representations of the bad self (BS). The first representation is regarding oneself as bad and deserves to be punished by others (BS1). The second is a manifestation of one's deep-seated anger and seeks to take revenge and diminish others (BS2). Similarly, the good self (GS) can exist in two ways. The first one is regarding one as tolerable, endurable and surviving within prevailing oppression (GS1). The second one is regarding one is good and should not oppress other (GS2). The bad others (BO) can also exist in two ways. The first are those who substantially and overtly oppress the individual (BO1). The second are those who seem to be going to and/or planning to covertly oppress the individual (BO2).* There can be many combinations of projective identification in the camouflage concealment versus opponent identified visibility**.** The first one is BS1 + BO1 + GS1. The individual internalizes the substantial negative comment from the oppressive others (BO1) admitting that s/he deserves to be punished and oppressed by the bad others (BS1). In doing so, the individual's good-self assumes that one is tolerable, endurable, and surviving (GS1). Under this condition, oppression can thus be concealed and protected. That means, the individual appears as though s/he deserves to be punished. He tends to be visual as the opponent's form and style. The more s/he is punished, the more s/he ensures himself/herself is tolerable and endurable in the oppression. The second combination is BS2 + BO1 + GS2**.** The individual harbors an intensive anger and a strong urge to take revenge (BS2). S/he identifies with the substantial oppressive others (BO1). S/he joins with the oppressive others. S/he becomes part of the oppressive group and oppresses others (BS2 + BO1). His/her prevailing anger and feelings of hatred from being oppressed by others can be transferred and released to those s/he oppresses. In doing so, s/he successful conceals his good self (GS2) that s/he does not deserve oppression by others.

Stage of Self concealment versus self visibility dynamic force	**Forms of Concealment and Visibility**	**Content and Process of Self concealment versus self visibility**
		The third combination can be BS1 + BO2 + GS1. The individual internalizes that s/he is bad and deserves punishment (BS1). However, what s/he is afraid of and internalized does not substantially exist. Instead, the bad others are all surrounding the individual (BO2) and are all planning and conspiring together to oppress, to harm or even to kill the individual. When BS1 and BO2 are combined, that means the individual harbors a prevailing paranoia that every one surrounding him/her is conspiring to harm him/her. The paranoia is greatly intensified by thinking that s/he is bad and deserves punishment. In doing so, s/he actually conceals the thinking and believes that s/he has special tolerance to cope with the all the torture and oppression (GS1). There are many combinations in projective identification. The more intensively and frequently and durably the individual is engaged in camouflage concealment versus opponent identified visibility, the more vulnerable and sensitive he/she is to external oppression and the more weak and fragile the individual self-identity, image and boundary is. In addition, s/he may become more and more detached from himself/herself as well as the substantial reality. For example, in the case B, even he frequently engages in the detached concealment and dissociative participatory visibility, he cannot cope with the oppressive environment. In the humiliation by his boss, even if B tries to numb his senses towards such criticism and behave as if he is highly detached (detached concealment), his boss still curses that B does not have good concentration to reflect his own fault. His boss also accuses B that he does not have a good commitment to his job since he does everything like a robot (dissociative participatory visibility) without any emotional commitment. Even worse, aside from his boss, other colleagues also come in to oppress B, saying and gossiping that B does not have commitment to his job. He just wants money in his job. As B still needs this job for financial support of his family B needs to transfer his detached concealment and dissociative participatory visibility to camouflage concealment versus opponent identified visibility. In this dilemma, the mental observer can no long be effective. Instead, B needs to identify himself with the oppressive comments from his boss and colleagues. Within the projective identification mechanism, B has various ways to engage in the camouflage concealment versus opponent identified visibility.

(Continued)

Stage of Self concealment versus self visibility dynamic force	Forms of Concealment and Visibility	Content and Process of Self concealment versus self visibility
		The first way is BS1 + BO1 + GS1. In terms of camouflage concealment, he needs to internalize the negative comments from his boss (BS1). In doing so, he needs to undergo a critical process of identifying himself as bad and unacceptable. Whenever his boss and his colleagues criticize, tease, and humiliate him (BO1), he immediately criticizes, teases, and humiliates himself. The process of self-punishment is done in an intensive way, so that his oppressive boss and colleagues admit that he is self-punishing and has a deep sense of repentance. He also becomes a target of teasing and bullying. In doing so, his good self is tolerating, enduring the oppression (GS1) so it can be concealed and protected. He perceives himself as a suffering hero. The second way is BS2 + BO1 + GS2. Instead of self-punishment, he also turns himself into an oppressive other (BO2). He joins with the oppressive boss and colleagues (BO1) and oppresses other colleagues. He identified a colleague who is a newcomer in the company. Whenever his oppressive boss oppresses or blames him, he will transfer the blame and oppression to this newcomer. He also oppresses his subordinates complaining that they have done something seriously wrong that invites the blame and oppression from his boss. In doing so, he tends to conceal and protect his good-self, thinking that he is perfect and does not deserve any punishment and oppression. The third combination can be BS1 + BO2 + GS1. B admits and internalizes that he/she deserves the oppression and punishment from the oppressive boss and colleagues (BS1). However, instead of confining that oppression comes from substantial blaming and bullying, B assumes that most colleagues in the company join with the oppressive boss to oppress him. Even though he cannot hear or visualize their substantial gossiping, oppression, and exclusion, he still assumes that they are doing that (BO2). The combination of BS1 and BO2 means that B thinks his performance is not faulty with errors and thus invites others comments and criticism. Within all this camouflage, his good self (being highly tolerant, and enduring as well as having an intensive will to improve himself) is being protected (GS1).

Stage of Self concealment versus self visibility dynamic force	**Forms of Concealment and Visibility**	**Content and Process of Self concealment versus self visibility**
Confused Self concealment versus self visibility	Prevailing Paranoid Concealment vs. Grandiose Visibility	As time goes by, the individual faces tremendous and prevailing oppression. Together with this is drastic projective identification that splits the integrity and cohesion of the individual's self-system. The merging of the bad self and bad others with protection of the good self implies that there is a constant splitting of the self-system. The opponent identified visibility BS1 or BS2 in merging with BO1 or BO2, though, provides camouflage concealment on GS1 or GS2, but also have a prevailing splitting effect on the individual self-system. *The more the individual inclines toward camouflage concealment versus opponent identified, the more his/her self-system is split, with diffused self-identity and boundary.* In addition, his/her sense of reality and ego functioning to cope with stress and oppression also deteriorate. Gradually, the individual develops a confused self-concealment versus self-visibility in a form of prevailing paranoid concealment versus grandiose visibility. *Prevailing paranoid concealment means that the bad others (BO2) grow tremendously* in a way the individual gradually assumes that all people around him/her are gossiping and planning to harm him/her. It gradually becomes a paranoid community. *First, it includes persons within the individual's social circle such as work, family, and peers (BO2a).* That means the individual gradually develops the thought that related persons in his/her family or job all cooperate and conspire together to harm and oppress the individual. Even if there is no substantial evidence or experience, the individual still assumes that they are oppressing him/her. *Secondly*, as the situation gets worse, the individual even thinks that *everyone in the neighborhood, environment, or society is conspiring to harm and oppress him/her (BO2b).* Furthermore, the individual may even think that even *people far away, may use certain media such as wavelength, computer, light, and other things to control, and oppress the individual (BO2c).* Parallel with the growth of bad others (BO2), *there is growth of the bad self (BS2)*, the individual first thinks that s/he *deserves to be punished by members in his/her social circle, including work, family and peers (BS2a).* Then, the individual may go one step forward, thinking that s/he *deserves negative attention, feelings of hatred and even rejection from anyone in the immediate physical and social environment (BS2b).* Finally, the individual is fully aware and assumes s/he is bad but important enough to be *punished or chased by imaginative circles or groups of persons* (BSc).

(Continued)

Stage of Self concealment versus self visibility dynamic force	Forms of Concealment and Visibility	Content and Process of Self concealment versus self visibility
		In facing the prevailing paranoid delusions, the individual tries every means to escape from them by avoiding going outside, seeing people, hiding with all sorts of measures to avoid being hurt and being harmed by the delusive others. All these concealment measures are continuously modified according to the self-constructed nature of the oppressive others. For example, if the oppressive others are highly powerful in computer internet control; the individual may avoid using the computer or use some anti-measures in internet intrusion. If the oppressive others are present in the neighborhood or the working environment, the individual may persistently avoid going there. If the individual suddenly discovers the people around in the physical environment are planning or gossiping about him/her. S/he leaves the physical environment immediately despite any on-going activities and others' response. Grandiose visibility implies that the individual, in facing the prevailing but delusive paranoia, can no longer conceal or avoid. That means paranoid concealment is not effective or workable. *As the bad others, from BO2a to BO2c, grow tremendously, the individual actually has no way to hide, escape, or avoid it.* The paranoid prevailing bad others are, in fact, everywhere, in the immediate physical environment or the self-constructed environment. They are using every means, through substantial eye contact, or through imaginative and penetrating media such as air, internet, magic powers and many others. The prevailing bad others create intolerable and intensive fear and so the individual needs to develop defensive mechanisms. *The best defensive and protective mechanism is to develop grandiose visibility.* It implies two particular and important aspects in grandiose visibility. The first aspect is that, within the projective identification mechanism, the *bad self (BS1) grows as the bad others (BO2) grow in parallel.* On the one hand, we can regard the growth of BO2 as an increasing sense of inferiority or diminishing self-identity and competence. On the other hand, *we can regard BO2 as an increase of self-attention and specialization that the individual thinks that many people in the world*, even those who do not appear in the reality, want to harm or hurt him/her.

Stage of Self concealment versus self visibility dynamic force	Forms of Concealment and Visibility	Content and Process of Self concealment versus self visibility
		The second aspect is that as the bad others *(BO) and bad self (BS) combine powerfully. It shares the power of the good self (GS) as the possibility of encountering good others (GO)* in the actual reality is getting thinner and thinner. *Thus, the only chance to fight back the delusive but overwhelming bad others is to combine the GS and GO together in a delusive way.* That means, the individual constructs a delusively grandiose self-system in coping with the prevailing but delusive bad others. There are many combinations is doing so. As mentioned, there are two sorts of good self (*GS1: the individual is highly tolerating and enduring to external oppression; GS2: the individual is perfect and good and should not be oppressed by others*) and two sorts of bad others (BO1: the oppressive others are substantially present; BO2 the oppressive others are not substantially oppressing the individual but they plan, motivate or are inclined to do so.). Thus, there should also be two types of good others (*GO1, the supportive others are substantially present and caring towards the individual; GO2, the supportive others are not substantially supporting, but they are going, planning, or willing to support the individual.*). That means, BO2 grows in the form of BO2a, BO2b and BO2c, as GO2 grows accordingly. Firstly, *GO2a implies that the client assumes that someone within the client's social circle is planning or going to care, support and respect him/her.* In fact, the others are present but they have not done anything supportive. Secondly, the individual even thinks that *everyone in the immediate neighborhood, environment, or society is likely to help, support, appreciate, or even respect the individual (GO2b).* Thirdly, the individual may indulge in thoughts that *all related people far away, by means of different media, still care, support, respect, appreciate or even fall in love with the individual (GO2c).* That means, as the paranoid fear towards the bad others grow, the grandiose urge for good others also grows. To cope with the prevailing but delusive bad others who combine with the bad self in the form of over-whelming paranoid delusion, *the individual may also combine his delusive good others (GO2) with his good self (GS1 or GS2).* As the good self is gradually concealed and withers with the continuous projection of the bad self in matching the prevailing and delusive bad others, it becomes weaker and weaker.

(Continued)

Stage of Self concealment versus self visibility dynamic force	Forms of Concealment and Visibility	Content and Process of Self concealment versus self visibility
		Finally, the residual good self needs to use camouflage and change to delusive good others for survival. In that case, individuals identify changes to grandiose others. S/he may identify himself/herself as a powerful but delusive god. In extreme cases, the good others may become highly delusive and present everywhere (GO2c) combined with a highly delusive good self (GS2) (GO2c + GS2). In that situation, GS2 (the individual is perfect) and GS1 (the individual can tolerate hardship and torture) may finally change to a highly delusive self-identity (GSdel). It can be a combination of GO2 with GS1 and GS2 in a delusive way (GSdel = GO2 (a, b and c) + GS1+GS2). That means, the individual becomes an almighty and powerful figure in which s/he can tolerate and conquer any difficulties and hardships. In doing so, s/he can seem highly respectable to others. For example, Tom is a client with schizophrenia. He harbors a strong delusion that he is the Chief Disciple of the Buddha. The grandiose identity serves two purposes. The first purpose is that being Chief Disciple of the Buddha, he can or he has already suffered and tolerated a lot in his previous life and this life. That is why he is worthy to be the Chief Disciple of the Buddha (GO1). The second purpose is that being the Chief Disciple of the Buddha, he is perfect, almighty, and powerful and deserves others' respect and admiration (GO2). Apart from these two dimensions, the identity of the Chief Disciple of the Buddha also implies that he combines or even transforms his self image to a delusive supportive other, that is the Buddha who supports him anytime he is in trouble (GO2c). That means, the grandiose delusion of the Chief Disciple of the Buddha is a combination of these three components (GSDel = GO2c + GS1+GS2). In that sense, the grandiose delusion and identity (GSDel) can have different degrees. First, the grandiose identity has still some sense of self by the individual (GSDelA). That means the individual has almighty power and respect because of ownership of power from a common religious and powerful figure in society. In Tom's case, he is still Tom, but the Buddha gives him power to endure torture or to save others from hardship. In doing so, Tom's own self-identity does not have any changes or distortion.

Stage of Self concealment versus self visibility dynamic force	Forms of Concealment and Visibility	Content and Process of Self concealment versus self visibility
		Second, the grandiose identity has moved from a `subject' to an `object' stand (GSDelB). That means the individual becomes an 'object' in terms of a follower, a disciple, a son, a child, or a sibling of the almighty figure. That means, the individual's self-identity changes accordingly. S/he is no longer himself/herself before the grandiose identity. S/he is the child, sibling, son, or disciple of the almighty powerful figure. Finally, the grandiose identity moves one step further (GSDelC). That means, the individual simply becomes the almighty figure himself/herself. That means the individual's own self identity is totally submerged. Instead, s/he becomes the delusive and grandiose figure. S/he owns almighty power to fight back all oppressive figures in his/her environment by himself/herself. Also, with all the almighty power, the individual can also win others' respect and even worship. In Tom's case, Tom becomes the Buddha himself. He is no longer the disciple of the Buddha. He is the Buddha. In doing so, his own identity 'Tom', being the son of his father, or the worker in his company, changes accordingly. He even tells others that he is not the son of his father. Instead, his real father is the King of Heaven. That is why he is born to be the Buddha. He is also sent by the King of Heaven to detect all evils in this world. With all these mighty powers and important duties, he is able to earn the respect of all humanity. Also, in no way, is he afraid of his oppressive boss and colleagues now. With almighty power, as a Buddha, he knows that they are all evils in their previous life. They come to the world to destroy good men. That is why he is being oppressed but they do not know that he is the mighty Buddha. Now it is the time for him to disclose their evil deeds. One day, Tom dresses like a Buddha and goes to his company. He loudly proclaims to others that he is the real Buddha and comes to curse and fight with the evils, the boss and colleagues. No doubt, in the full manifestation of grandiose delusion, Tom is thus taken by the police to a nearby mental hospital with a diagnosis of schizophrenia.
Highly Confused Self concealment versus self visibility	Frequent shifting of delusive identity and paranoid delusion	In the prevailing paranoid concealment versus grandiose visibility, the individual faces the prevailing combination of bad others and bad self (From BO2a to BO2c combined with BS2a to BS2c), s/he needs to develop a grandiose delusion in terms of combination of unrealistic good others and good self (GSDel = GO2c + GS1+GS2).

(Continued)

Stage of Self concealment versus self visibility dynamic force	**Forms of Concealment and Visibility**	**Content and Process of Self concealment versus self visibility**
		That means the individual is constantly engaged in a dilemma of delusive paranoid concealment and delusive grandiose visibility BO2c + BS2c Vs GSDel (GO2c + GS1+GS2). Either the paranoid concealment or the grandiose visibility can be a stable and constant stage. Instead, *it is highly unstable and deteriorating*. The more one engages in delusive prevailing concealment the more s/he needs to use delusive grandiose visibility, and the more the individual becomes fragile in coping with stress in the environment. Finally, the individual may *absorb in a highly fluctuating shifting between prevailing delusive paranoid concealment by avoiding any delusive harm from the immediate environment and overwhelming delusive grandiose visibility*. In doing so, the individual's mental state is highly unstable, with intensive detachment from immediate reality and high absorption in delusive paranoia and grandiosity. His/her social and ego functioning also deteriorates. Apart from frequent shifting between delusive paranoid concealment and delusive grandiose visibility, individuals may even be unstable in paranoid delusion and grandiose delusion. Instead of having one stable and organized and grandiose delusion, the individual may have several. S/he may constantly shift around these delusions. For instance, if the individual has 3 delusive paranoid concealments (Pa, Pb, & Pc) and has 3 delusive grandiose visibilities (Ga, Gb, & Gc). The individual may thus shift around Pa and Ga; Pb and Gb; as well as Pc and Gc. In intensive psychotic cases, the individual may even develop dialogue between the different paranoid delusion and grandiose delusion. For example, an individual may delude that there are two tracks of voices dialoguing with one another in his/her ear/brain/abdomen. Also, s/he may delude that s/he is not only one grandiose and delusive person but a combination of two or three of these grandiose figures. In Tom's case, he is the Buddha, but with special and continuous fighting and struggling with a powerful demon, who chases him wherever he goes. That means, he is constantly shifting between delusive paranoia as well as delusive grandiosity. When he encounters the powerful demon, he is fearful and tries to avoid going to some places, doing something, or saying some words. He tried to conceal himself saying the demon is so powerful and is everywhere watching his performance.

Stage of Self concealment versus self visibility dynamic force	Forms of Concealment and Visibility	Content and Process of Self concealment versus self visibility
		To defend against this demon, he needs to use the power of a Buddha. The powerful magic of the Buddha is highly visible. He may wear a full Buddhist garment, murmuring Buddhist spells and performing Buddhist rituals. In doing so, he is able to control or diminish the power of the demon. Sometimes, he may even say the power of Buddha and the power of the demon fight with one another in his own abdomen making him have diarrhea. If they fight within his lungs and nose, he suffers from high fever and influenza. If they fight within his leg, he suffers from crippled legs. In some situations, he even speaks with two voices, one in a low tune representing the demon, and one in a high tune representing the Buddha.

Self-Destruction and Self-Preservation

The Instinct to Destruct and to Preserve

Within the dilemma of self-splitting versus self-cohesion, an individual with schizophrenia involves the self-splitting mechanism to maintain his/her pseudo-self cohesion within a highly oppressive but unavoidable environment. Within the dilemma of self-concealment versus self-visibility, the individual needs to be self-concealed so that s/hc can be invisible in front of his/her prevailing opponents. The best concealment is being visible as the opponents. In the dilemma of self-destruction and self-preservation, the individual involves a self-destruction of part of his/her own self-system to preserve the remaining self-system. It represents the individual's inherent drive to fight, to diminish, and to attack. *In normal circumstances, human beings fight, attack, and diminish others as a defense for external danger or a way to fight for one's physical or psychological survival.* That means, *the inherent destructive force is closely linked with the inherent preservation force.* Thus, the self-destructive force is also linked with the urge for self-survival and preservation. It is easy to understand that a solider commits suicide after failure in the battle. He kills himself before anyone kills him. As he kills himself, it also means no one can kill him anymore.

Similarly, the death instinct and other inherent instincts are also for the sake of survival.

> `Freud's reduction of the many instinct to Eros and Thanatos - sexual and death instinct. Freud argued that every instinct to preserve life is in itself constituted of some components of both Eros and Thanatos. Eros unites and ties together the living elements and preserves the living structures in continuous antagonism to Thanatos, which endeavors to separate these elements and structures, to kill them, to bring them back to the inorganic phase of death out of which all life developed. According to these concepts, all ego instincts are characterized by their localization; *self preservation may then be considered due to pre-established order of the contest between the sexual and death instinct in every organism*.' (Federn, 1953)

That means, both the sexual instinct and death instinct is in fact, for the sake of self-preservation. It is understandable, within an intolerable trauma or torture; the individual is always inclined to kill himself/herself so that s/he can immediately terminate the unbearable psychological and/or physical pain. It is an inherent self-defense and preservation mechanism to protect the individual from overwhelming painful external stimuli.

Defensive Self-Destruction in Fantasy

As mentioned above, as the individual with schizophrenia is spontaneously engulfed, imploded, and depersonalized, the only way to get rid of the overwhelming and unavoidable oppression is to develop a self-split false self-system in which the individual depersonalizes, implodes, and engulfs himself/herself. In doing so, his/her real self can be free from or shielded from further depersonalization, implosion, and engulfment by oppressive others. Within the false self-system and the process of self-implosion, engulfment, and depersonalization, the individual is undergoing an intensive self-destruction process. *However, within the inner real self-system, the individual is undergoing a process of self-preservation, in which s/he tries to save and maintain his/her own self-image, self-identity, and autonomy.* Nevertheless, the more oppressive the external environment is, the more vigorous the individual needs to undergo the destructive mechanism on his/her self-system. That means, the larger the false system, the smaller is the inner real self-system. As a consequence, the individual may need to *transform his self-system into a delusive system in which both the destructive and preservative mechanisms occur not only in the substantial reality but also in the fantasy.*

> 'Without an open two-way circuit between fantasy and reality, anything becomes possible in fantasy. Destructiveness in fantasy goes on without the wish to make compensatory reparation, *for the guilt that prompts towards preserving and making amends loses its urgency.* Destructiveness in fantasy can thus rage on, unchecked, until the world and the self are reduced, in fantasy, to dust and ashes. In the schizophrenic state, the world is in ruins, and the self is (apparently) dead. No amount of frantic activity seems to have the power to bring life back again. (Laing, 1960: 85)

Destruct Oneself to Destruct Other

In other words, the external oppressive reality is also destructed within the false self-system. Self-destruction like self-harm is, in fact, painful, intolerable, and even unacceptable for an individual. No one likes to cut or harm himself/herself. However, if s/he regards his/her own body as others, the self-destruction act and mechanism becomes moralized, acceptable, and tolerable. Within the projective identification mechanism, the bad self is projected outwards; it is identified and united with the bad others. As the oppressive others in the external environment is highly dominating, oppressive and powerful, the individual cannot destroy it. *However, if the bad self is united and identified with the oppressive others, if s/he destroys the bad self, s/he can convince himself/herself that s/he also destroys the bad others.* In other words, the self-destruction is moralized and justified and regarded as a means to destroy the oppressive others. As a consequence, the individual punishes, destructs and even diminishes himself/herself as 'delusive' ways to punish, destruct and diminish the oppressive others to convince himself/herself s/he is secure and protected.

Externalized and Self-Perceived Dangerous Destructiveness

The more s/he engages in it, the more the individual needs to destruct his/her own self-system. S/he needs to convince and ensure his/her own destructiveness so that s/he believes that s/he can possess the power to destruct the oppressive others. *The more s/he believes in his destructiveness, the more s/he thinks s/he is able to delusively destruct oppressive others by destructing his/her own bad self that unites with the oppressive others.* By doing so, s/he can preserve his/her own inner real self without being attacked by oppressive others.

> 'If there is anything the schizoid individual is likely to believe in, it is his own destructiveness. He is unable to believe that he can fill his own emptiness without reducing what is there to nothing. He regards his own love and that of others as being destructive as hatred. To be loved threatens his self; but his love is equally dangerous to anyone else. His isolation is not entirely of for his own self's sake. It is also out of concern for others. A schizophrenic patient would not allow anyone to touch her, not because they would do her some harm, but because she might electrocute them.' (Laing, 1960: 93).

Inherent Fear within Prevailing Destructiveness

However, in the process of destructing oppressive others, the over-whelming destructiveness may also mean, at the same time, that it can destruct the support of good others. Thus, when the self-destruction prevails by pushing the bad self into uniting with bad others and destructing both of them, the individual takes a risk that s/he can also destruct the good others consciously or unconsciously. In that case, s/he has to be very cautious about his/her own destructiveness as s/he may harbor the following fears and risks.

1. Someone within the oppressive environment, without his/her consciousness or without his/her own defense may take away his/her destructiveness by touching them or uniting with them.
2. Some good others, by touching or uniting with them, may also be destructed or hurt by their destructive power. That means s/he may diminish the good others, in a way it also means that there is no one to support or unite with their good self.
3. The externalized destructiveness may gradually become uncontrollable to a degree that it may destruct his/her residual good self also making himself/herself become a total inner vacuum and ontological emptiness.

Interestingly, these fears are a chain response of the self-destruction versus self-preservation dilemma. The individual starts with a fear that external oppressive others may finally destruct him/her both mentally and ontologically. To preserve himself/herself from this external destructiveness from oppressive others, s/he needs to defend himself/herself by creating his/her own destructiveness. At least, s/he has to convince himself/herself that s/he possesses sufficient power to destruct the destructive others to defend and preserve himself/herself. However, the more s/he believes that his/her destructiveness is highly powerful, the more s/he is afraid that such destructiveness is out of his/her control and manipulation. Thus, to avoid these overwhelming fear and risks, the individual may thus, on one hand, exhibit his/her intensive power of destructiveness proving that s/he has power to destruct any external oppressive others. On the other hand, s/he may avoid touching or uniting with others, making his/her destructiveness out of control. *That sort of dilemma may intensify to a degree that it gradually deteriorates the individual's normal contact of reality and relationship with others. S/he may become more and more self-isolated and delusive with both paranoid (avoid being stolen by destructive power) and grandiose (possessing high destructiveness) hallucinations.*

Ultimate Destruction of the Substantial Self-System and the Reality

As the destructiveness of the individual increases drastically, it may risk finally destruction of the individual's self-system and the actual reality. The destruction of the self-system means that not only is the bad self projected outward and being destructed mentally, but also the good self is also at risk for possible self destruction. The destruction of the actual reality implies that not only the bad others in the oppressive reality are mentally destructed by the individual but also the good others. *That means, both the self-system and substantial reality turn into a massive delusive world. In doing so, the individual tries to preserve his/her meaning of survival and meaning of existence in terms of delusive good-self and delusive good others.*

Delusive Self-destruction versus self-preservation in 'The Ghost of the Weed Garden'

1. Loss of sense of substantiality and autonomy

That sort of delusive existence could be illustrated by Laing's (1960) case '*The Ghost of the Weed Garden'* in which Julie was a 17-year-old female suffering from schizophrenia.

> `She said the trouble was that she was not a real person; she was trying to become a person. There was happening in her life and she was trying to find happiness. She felt unreal and there was an invisible barrier between her and others. She was empty and worthless. She was worried that she was too destructive and was beginning to think it best not to touch anything in case she caused damage. She had a great deal to say about her mother. She was smothering her, she would not let her live, and she had never wanted her. Since her mother was prompting her to have more friends, and to go out to dance, to wear pretty dresses, and so on, on the face of it these accusations seemed palpably absurd.' (Laing, 1960:179).

Julie's condition clearly showed that her prevailing destructiveness deconstructed her totality and substantiality of self-system thus she felt that she was not a real person. In doing so, she tried to preserve her delusive autonomy that she could choose her own path, own thing, and own action. That means, she destructed her actual self-identity, image, and sense of substantiality in a way both her and related reality were also diminished so that delusively she could become a real person again. She was kept in an ontological dilemma that on one hand, she felt she was not a real person. On the other hand, she was trying to become a person, an autonomous person with full vigor to search for happiness. As she fully recognized that the search for autonomy was uncertain and vague, and the sense of non-existence was highly uncomfortable and intolerable, thus she was threatened by her own prevailing destructiveness. She worried that she was too destructive and could destroy the world around her. She avoided touching anything around her. To preserve her delusive autonomy, she had already destroyed everything including her own self and her immediate environment. That was why she felt dreadfully empty and worthless. Everything including herself becomes empty ash within her destructiveness. She was facing an unresolved dilemma; either to destroy everything including herself and the immediate reality to gain her delusive autonomy or to tolerate the engulfing and pressing reality that her mother, who tended to suffocate her in every aspect of life, making her feel dead, totally passive, and inert in everyday life. Thus, she declared that 'a child had been murdered'.

> `However, the basic psychotic statement she made was that '*a child had been murdered*', She was rather vague about the details but she said she had heard of this from the voice of her brother (she had no brother). She wondered, however, if this voice may not have been her own. *The child was wearing her clothes when it was killed. The child could have been herself. She had been murdered either by herself or by her mother*, she was not sure. She purposed to tell the police about it.' (Laing, 1960: 179)

2. Destruction (murder) of the good self by the bad mother (bad other)

It was certain that the murdered child, was, in fact herself. She tried to voice her self-destruction versus self-preservation dilemma; that she was destructed by her engulfing mother ever since she was a child. However, while she was mentally admitting this murdered child was her, she could not preserve her strive for autonomy. Thus, she tried to regard this murdered child as another person unrelated or distant to her. According to Laing (1960), this destructed part of the self-system was part of the real self or the inner self. The good compliant child instead said it was her false self. It serves a callous layer to seal up the real self from external harm. However, as the real self comes out, striving for autonomy and substantiality, it was then murdered by her bad mother. *She proclaimed this murdered child was wearing her clothes while she was killed. This murdered child pretended to be her but was not actually her.* By doing so, her strive for autonomy was secured and preserved. Nevertheless, the self-destruction made the whole self-system became weak, fragile, and diffused. Julie's ability to ensure her substantial existence was also deeply threatened. That means, what she could preserve was also a delusive existence of autonomy. *She needed external validation of this murder to reconstruct her sense of substantiality.* That was why she needed to call the police or say that her delusive brother had witnessed the whole killing process. In doing so, the self-destruction versus self-preservation dilemma became prevailingly powerful to destroy both her outer good self, bad others, as well as her self-identity, self-image, self-boundary and perception of the actual substantial reality.

3. The fight for autonomy: the rebellious but real self

Julie's struggle was a long and hard one in trying to escape from her mother's overwhelming control and influence on her. Laing (1960) had interviewed various people around Julie. They all agreed in seeing her life in three basic states in which her destructiveness developed gradually.

> `Now, although each of the various people interviewed had his/her point of view on Julie's life, they all agreed in seeing her life in three basic states of phases. Namely, there was a time when
>
> a. The patient was a good, normal, healthy child, until she gradually began
> b. To be bad, to do or say things that caused great distress, and which were on the whole 'put down' to naughtiness or badness until

c. This went beyond all tolerable limits so that she could only be regarded as completely mad.

... it does supply us with the important information that the original pattern of her action was entirely in conformity with what her parents held to be good and praiseworthy. Then she was for a time `bad', that is everything her parents most did not want to see her do, or hear her say, or to believe existed in her, she came out with.' (Laing, 1960:182)

From Laing's description, it was clear that in facing her mother's high engulfment and control (her mother's destructiveness towards Julie), she was initially obedient and complying. However, that sort of engulfment and control suffocated her self-development as well as her senses of substantiality and autonomy in her self-system. That means, *Julie needed to rebel to struggle for ontological existence of the whole self-system by preserving her own good self.* On that moment, she was no long obedient and submissive. Instead, she became rebellious, that was the turning from good child (being compliant but loss of autonomy and substantiality: the false self) to the bad child (rebellious and fighting for autonomy and substantiality: the real self) in the eyes of others, in particular her mother. In no way could the rebellion turn her mother's engulfment and control into genuine and facilitating freedom. Instead, her mother might increase control or engulfment to ensure Julie would not deviate from her 'right track'.

'Both parents of Julie 'accepted the patient's false self as good and rejected every other aspect of her as bad....Not only did they reject as bad all of Julie, apart from the compliant lifeless shadow, which passed in their eyes for a real person, they completely refused to take to heart any of the reproaches that Julie had against them. Julie and her mother were at this time both desperate people. Julie in her psychosis called herself '*Mrs. Taylor. What does this mean? It means `I am tailor-made*. I was fed, clothed, and tailored. Such statements are psychotic, ...What I feel must have been the most schizophrenogenic factor of this was not simply Julie's attack on her mother, or even her mother's counter attack, but the complete absence of anyone on her world who could or would see some sense in the point of view, whether it was right or wrong..' (Laing, 1960: 192)

That means, once Julie developed her own defensive destructiveness (being a rebelliously bad child), her mother's destructiveness towards Julie increased accordingly. Facing her mother's over-whelming and prevailing destructiveness (control and engulfment); it was a really hard battle for Julie to fight for her existence.

`She was not fighting to win an argument, but to preserve her existence, in a way, Julie was not simply trying to perceive her existence, she was trying to achieve existence.... When her mother said she was bad, Julie felt this as murder. It was the negation of any autonomous point of view on her part. *Her mother was prepared to accept a compliant, false self to love this shadow, and to give it anything....But she had never recognized the real disturbing presence in the world of a daughter with her possibilities.* The existential truth in Julie's delusion was that her own true possibilities were being smothered, strangled, murdered...Julie needed to be allowed to project some of her bad self onto her mother, and to be allowed to take some goodness out of her mother, not merely to be given it at all time....She began to convert existential truth into physical facts. She becomes deluded. If she began by accusing her mother of never letting her live, in an existential sense, she ended by talking and acting more than half as though her mother had, in an legal sense, actually murdered an actual child.' (Laing, 1960:193).

The only way for Julie to preserve her own autonomy and substantiality was to be mad by assuming and proclaiming that her mother 'murdered' a child that resembled her. In doing so, Julie could be delusively be released from her mother's control and engulfment.

`We cannot at present say why this was so. But that she was capable of saying and doing such things that were almost incredible to her parents. All that emerged was totally unsuspected. They tried at first to discount it, but as the offenses grew, they strove violently to repudiate it. It was a great relief, therefore, when, instead of saying that her mother would not let her live, she said that her mother had murdered a child. Then all could be forgiven.' (Laing, 1960: 182)

With reference to Laing's (1960) description of Julie's case, the development of the self-destruction versus self-preservation dynamic force can be described by the following table:

Table. Stages of Self-Destruction versus Self-Preservation

Stages of Self - destruction versus self-preservation dynamic force	**Degree of Self - Destruction**	**Degree of Self-Preservation**	**Others' perception and response of the self-system within the self-destruction and preservation dilemma**	**Self-perception of Self-system within the self-destruction and preservation dilemma**
Stage One: No Need for Development of Self Destruction and Self Preservation	No need to develop self-destructive mechanism. Self-destruction is only limited to inherent sex and aggressive drive that is well under controlled by the individual	The environment is supportive and adaptive. The individual feels secure, safe, and certain. S/he did not need to develop any defensive self-preservation mechanism consciously or unconsciously.	Good and happy individual (As the significant others are reasonable and supportive, occasionally, the individual is perceived as a happy and obedient one)	Good and Adaptive Individual (The individual finds happiness and has good adaptation to others' needs and demands)
Stage Two: Initial Development of Self-destruction versus self-preservation Dilemma: The Development of Unembodied Self	The individual needs to develop initial self-destructiveness as s/he may internalize negative demand and command from oppressive others.	The individual needs to develop initial self-preservation mechanism as s/he has to protect him/her from negative commands by oppressive others. S/he may appear as obedient by actually rebellious in doing other things s/he likes secretly and occasionally.	Good but unhappy individual. (As his/her significant others are oppressive, the individual is perceived as good but unhappy in following others' command.)	Unhappy but compliant individual (Facing continuous oppression, the individual develops unembodied self to follow others' unreasonable demands)
Stage Three: Gradual Development of Self destruction versus self-preservation Dilemma:	The individual develop a process of self-destruction s/he tends to absorb and acts according to the demand of others' oppression and criticism.	The individual develops a continuous process of self-preservation by being cognitively, emotionally, and mentally distancing from the oppressive and critical others.	Non-compliant Individual (In facing the continuous oppression of the significant others, individual becomes highly non-compliant.	Unhappy individual loss of autonomy and substantiality (Full development of unembodied self tends to suffocate the real self.

(Continued)

Stages of Self - destruction versus self-preservation dynamic force	Degree of Self - Destruction	Degree of Self-Preservation	Others' perception and response of the self-system within the self-destruction and preservation dilemma	Self-perception of Self-system within the self-destruction and preservation dilemma
	In doing so, s/he diminishes his/her own negative feelings and response and acts like a mechanical robot in doing so.	In following others critical and oppressive other, s/he hides his/her own real feelings and responses. S/he convinces himself/herself that the oppressive and critical others, in fact, cannot actually control and manipulate him/her.	S/he appeared as compliant and obedient but with a sense of being distant, apathetic, and alienated to others).	The individual uses unembodied self to comply with others' demands and oppression, but feels sad, angry, and inferior inside.)
Stage Four: Externalization of Self-Destruction and Self-Preservation: Rebellion of the Oppressive Other to Preserve Autonomy and Substantiality	In being rebellious to oppressive others, the individual tries to destruct his/her unembodied-self so that s/he could be free from the compliance of the oppressive others as well as destructing the influence of the oppressive others. As the oppressive others are also their significant others, thus, the diminishing of the influence of the oppressive others as well as the complying unembodied self may mean *destructing individual supportive system, as well as part of his/her identify and self system. As a consequence, s/he also destructs his/her overall ability to be autonomous and independent and unique.*	In being rebellious to oppressive others, the individual tries to preserve his/her inner real self in terms of own decision-making, autonomy and independency. However, as s/he has long been complied and internalized his/her oppressive others' negative comments. *In being rebellious, s/he is also oppressing his/her bad self by projecting it out to link up with the oppressive others.* In doing so, s/he aims to preserve his/her own good self.	Bad and rebellious individual. The individual actually rebels, opposes. and turns against his/her significant others. S/he no longer appears as obedient and compliant. *His/her significant others may have two responses.* Firstly, s/he may be shocked by his/her sudden change from obedience to rebellion. On the other hand, they may think that the rebellious acts are not the individuals' own will but rather bad influence by others.	Individual tries to struggle for autonomy and substantiality in reality. In doing so, s/he tries to oppose and rebel against oppressive others. In doing so, *s/he is facing a great dilemma in self-perception.* On one hand, s/he perceives himself/herself as right and good in struggling for autonomy and substantiality. On the other hand, s/he absorbs others' criticism that s/he is bad in the struggle for autonomy.
Stage Five: Internalization of Self-Destruction and Self-Preservation: Diminishing Unembodied Self and Development of False Self	As the rebellion and the struggle for autonomy and substantiality finally fails the individual loses his/her autonomy and substantiality. S/he feels painful and hopeless in facing his/her oppressive others. *The more s/he is aware of the oppression of the reality, the more pain s/he feels.*	The distancing from reality and environment may mean that the individual tries to lessen the destructive effect of the oppressive others so that s/he can preserve his/her but concealed autonomy and substantiality.	The individual's sense of reality, rational response to external demand becomes more and more confused. In a way, his/her significant others thought that the individual is 'crazy', 'insane' or 'mad'.	The struggle of autonomy and substantiality finally fails as the significant others' become more and more oppressive and controlling.

Stages of Self - destruction versus self-preservation dynamic force	**Degree of Self - Destruction**	**Degree of Self-Preservation**	**Others' perception and response of the self-system within the self-destruction and preservation dilemma**	**Self-perception of Self-system within the self-destruction and preservation dilemma**
	Thus, the individual tries to dissociate his/her sense of reality so that the pain can be lessened. In doing so, *the diminishing un-embodied self in the rebellious stage turns into a new state of 'false self'*. It is a state of getting out of touch with reality. A mental distancing of oppressive others. It is a destruction of participatory motives and actions in related environment.	As the oppressive others can diminish the individual's rebellion overtly, the individual learns to protect the real self (the urge for autonomy and substantiality) **by** means of active appearance of the false self. It can be inappropriate and confused response to others. It can be a form of self-isolation in front of others. All these enable the oppressive others fail to control the individual.	That means, people around cannot predict, or make sense of the individual's responses.	Thus, the individual feels that s/he actually loses his/her autonomy, identity and substantiality. S/he is 'murdered' or 'diminished' by the oppressive significant others.
Stage Six: Intensive Development of Self-Destruction and Self-Preservation: Full Development of False Self	The full development of false self also means an intensive dissociation and distancing of the oppressive reality and a strong weakening of individual ego functioning. The individual becomes more and more *involved in false self related delusive reality in which normal social functioning, social interaction, social response are gradually deteriorated.*	The full development of false self implies a concealed self-preservation of the individual's fragile autonomy and substantiality. As the individual is involved in false self-related delusive reality, his/her *strive for self-autonomy and substantiality can only be attained in an unrealistic or even delusive way.* That means, his/her good self can only be preserved by transforming in a delusive way. On one hand, the individual may *become highly protective by being oversensitive to external threats* - bad others (development of paranoid delusion). On the other hand, the individual may develop a powerful and omnipotent delusive identity (development of delusively good self).	The full representation of the false self is actually perceived by others as a manifestation of insanity and madness **in** the eyes of others. The false self-projected by the individual is a part of his/her bad self in front of others.	In development of false self to replace the unembodied self, individual uses the false self to hide his/her true self. That means, *inappropriate and confused responses to external environment are actually a method to conceal his/her inner `true self"*. That is the struggle for autonomy and substantiality. The false self is an opposite and confused representation of the true and autonomous self. That means, if the inner true self is good, then the false self appears as bad. If the inner true self aspires for autonomy, the false self appears as stagnant. If the inner true self feels inferior, the false self appear as superior. In doing so, the individual uses the projected bad self, not only to protest the bad others but also to conceal and preserve the inner true self.

(Continued)

Stages of Self - destruction versus self-preservation dynamic force	**Degree of Self - Destruction**	**Degree of Self-Preservation**	**Others' perception and response of the self-system within the self-destruction and preservation dilemma**	**Self-perception of Self-system within the self-destruction and preservation dilemma**
Stage Seven: Over-whelming Development of Self-Destruction and Self-Preservation: Destruction and Splitting of the False Self and True Self	As the false self develops fully, it not only dissociates and distances the individual from the oppressive reality but also suffocates the freedom of the inner true self from the contact of reality to an extent that is intolerable and unbearable for the individual. In doing so, the individual needs to be free from the concealment of the false self to have some minimal contact of the reality. The individual consciously or unconsciously tries to diminish his/her false self by regarding it as a foreign lifeless body that should be rejected. It manifests in a form of self dialogue and self talk in which the individual represents two voices one bad figure arguing with one good figure in which the good figure tries to be free from the control of the bad figure. In other words, the destruction of the false self implies that it further splits into the inner false self and outer false self. *The outer false self may intermingle with the residual unembodied self, forming a delusive negative reality* for the individual. The inner false self may intermingle with the inner self in forming a *delusive positive reality* for the individual. In doing so, individual ego boundary becomes totally diffused with difficulties in distinguishing self and reality.	The diminishing of the false self aims at freeing the fragile inner self. The struggle for autonomy and substantiality actualizes not only in a delusive way but also in a fragmented, diversified, and unstable way. That means, the individual not only develops paranoid hallucinations and delusive omnipotent identities, s/he even shifts around these two sides or creates several omnipotent and delusive identities as well as several paranoid figures. His/her inner self, even though being eagerly preserved and delusively restored but it is gradually fragmented by the paranoid and grandiose delusions and hallucination. In preserving the individual fragile true self-system, the individual may further split it into outer true self and inner true self. The outer and inner true self may totally transform into two different omnipotent identities to fight against the delusive negative reality. As the delusive negative reality is created by the outer false self and unembodied self, it is comparatively stagnant, under controlled, and can be effectively dealt with by the omnipotent delusive identities.	Individual's mental state is highly confused, fragmented, and ambivalent. S/he is perceived by others as highly insane and very confused. For those with strong religious or superstitious beliefs, they may even regard the individual as being possessed by demons. Most of them believe that the highly confused mental state is not understandable and should be *detained and institutionalized immediately*. Many of them agree that the individual is in a state of psychiatric emergency that may contain high risk or tendency of unpredictable violence to the community.	Within that sort of splitting of inner false and outer false self as well outer true self and inner true self, the individual faces an intensive dilemma. On the one hand, the individual feels highly confused that the delusive and negative reality (outer false self in fusion with the residual unembodied self) is getting bigger and bigger. It gradually becomes uncontrollable *with rapid shifting and changes of reality, body, mind, and spirit.* On the other hand, the frequent shifting from different omnipotent figures formed by the inner false self and outer true self can make the individual highly autonomous and free to do what s/he wants in a delusive way. In doing so, the individual becomes more and more confused and diffused with fast changing and highly fluid self-identity and self-boundary.

Stages of Self - destruction versus self-preservation dynamic force	Degree of Self - Destruction	Degree of Self-Preservation	Others' perception and response of the self-system within the self-destruction and preservation dilemma	Self-perception of Self-system within the self-destruction and preservation dilemma
		In doing so, the individual's self-system becomes highly fluid and changes quickly from one figure to another figure.		

From Self-Fragmentation to Self-Integration

All the above-mentioned theories and concepts of self-fragmentation of persons with schizophrenia have strong implications for mental health recovery for persons with schizophrenia. Burnham (et al., 1969) affirmed that dividedness exists in several forms such as splitting, dissociation, segregation, segmentalization, and sejunction.

There may be various degrees in the process of self-fragmentation. It starts with a form of dissociation between mind and body, inner and outer, reality and self-consciousness. Then, it proceeds to a form of self-splitting in which the fragmentation becomes obvious and the self-system is split into two sub-systems.

They can be the unembodied self and the embodied self, as mentioned by R. D. Laing. They can also be the good and bad self, as described by Klein. The self-splitting can go further and further making the self-system finally split into different sub-systems. It can be the residual unembodied self, outer false self and inner false self, outer true self and inner true self, along Laing's line of thinking. It can also be an externalized good self, externalized bad self, inner bad and inner good self, along Klein's thinking. These two types of systems suggested by Laing and Klein can be combined, in which the false self-system can be the bad self. The outer false self can be the externalized bad self and the inner false self can be the inner bad self. The greater the degree of the fragmentation, the more confused and delusive the individual becomes, and the more diffused and alienated towards the external reality. In the process of self-fragmentation, individuals, in facing the external oppressive but unavoidable reality, may try to split off the bad-self to retain the good self with a result of ambiguity of external and internal, confusion of his/her own needs, and others' demands, as well as overlapping of his/her own self-identity and delusive and constructed identities (Frosch, 1983). There are various causes of self-fragmentation, such as lack of experiences of wholeness as well as oppressive environments in forms of implosion, engulfment, and depersonalization. Apart from external causes, there can also be internal causes such as prolonged problems in object relationships in which the individual has low self-confidence. S/he always harbors fear in disturbing others and being abandoned by others. S/he has a strong need to cling to objects but with intensive fear of being diminished by objects. All these have a negative impact on individual's ego, id, and superego. S/he may always have an auxiliary ego (incomplete or non-confident ego) that is unable to perform good social functioning; a primitive harsh superego that internalizes external unreasonable demands; and a highly disturbing and uncontrollable id with prevailing desires (Burnham et al. 1969). The situation is further complicated by the need and fear dilemma in which the individual, on one hand, seeks to cling to others, but, on the other hand, avoids being abandoned by others

(Burnham et al. 1969). Bion (1984) affirmed that self-fragmentation is due to the interaction between the problematic environment and personality. There are four types of problematic personalities, overwhelming destructive impulses, hatred of internal reality, unremitting dread of imminent annihilation, and premature formulation of object relationship. In terms of projective identification, Bion (1984) articulated that the individual projects part of his/her self (usually bad self) to the external object. Together with that is also identification of this object to preserve his/her self (usually good self). However, the more the individual engages in this, the more self-split the individual becomes. Arieti (1974) described that psychotic self-fragmentation can exist in two forms. The first form is that part of the self-system that acutely detaches from the whole. The second form is that the whole self-system that chronically separates from the part.

In all these theories and concepts, self-fragmentation tends to be a confusion and ambiguity in the following:

a. A confusion and ambiguity of reality and fantasy
b. A confusion and ambiguity of the internal and external world
c. A confusion and ambiguity of what one needs and what is actually available in the environment
d. A confusion and ambiguity of one's own self-identity
e. A confusion and ambiguity of presence of external objects

Laing (1960) further elaborated that self-fragmentation can exist in two forms, molar (personality) and molecular (thought, behavior, attitude) fragmentation (Laing, 1960). For each split partial self-system, it has its own identity center of awareness (Laing, 1960). Bion (1984), based on Klein's concept of depressive position, described that in the process of psychotic self-fragmentation, the breaking of the ego system occurs when the individual fails to use reparation in resolving conflicts in projective identification.

Putting all these together, the process of psychotic splitting can be roughly described in the following stages:

Stage 1: Dissociation (dissociation of mind and body, past and present, inner and outer, and self and others)

Stage 2: Splitting occurs when dissociation fails (good and bad self, embodied self and unembodied self, as well as true and false self)

Stage 3: Molar fragmentation of personality (breaking into more than one partial-self systems within which may or may not be conflicting to one another)

Stage 4: Molecular fragment of thoughts within each split/fractured partial-self system (confusion of thoughts, perception and interpretation within every fractured sub-self system),

Stage 5: Further fragmentation of all these divided and fractured partial self-systems (Each fractured partial self-system may have its own delusive identity, boundary and interpretation of external reality)

Stage 6: There are spontaneous and continuous conflicts and ambiguities within and between these divided and fractured partial self-systems (The individual may shift from one delusive identity to another one, has constant manifestation of running tracks of auditory hallucinations with one arguing with one another, with thought insertion and thought broadcasting.)

Stage 7: The self-fragmentation of all these partial self-systems can be continuous until reparation is impossible. (The individual is in a state of severe mental confusion and has a very poor sense of reality, which may lead to a psychiatric emergency and possible harm to oneself and another.)

Underlying this self-fragmentation process are three unresolved dilemmas and dynamic forces, self-splitting versus self-cohesion, self-concealment versus self-visibility and self-destruction versus self-preservation. Self-splitting versus self-cohesion exists in a form of pull and push forces. The individual needs to split his/her self-system to maintain a fragile or even delusive cohesion in facing the extremely oppressive social environment. It consists of a process with the following stages of development.

Stage one: Temporary self-splitting versus self-cohesion to significant others.

Stage two: Partial self-splitting versus self-cohesion to persons and events in the reality.

Stage three: Full self-splitting versus self-cohesion to persons and events in the delusive but organized reality.

Stage four: Highly confused self-splitting versus self-cohesion in the highly delusive and disorganized reality.

The second dynamic force is self-concealment versus self-visibility in which the individual tries to maintain a dilemma of existence versus non-existence within an oppressive environment. In fact, projective identification is a form of normal social camouflage in which the individual tries to identify with his/her oppressive others. The whole process of development of this dynamic force with psychotic self-fragmentation can be described by the following stages:

Stage one: Temporary self-concealment versus self-visibility (reflective concealment versus actual participatory visibility)

Stage two: Partial self-concealment versus self-visibility (detached concealment versus dissociative participatory visibility)

Stage three: Full self-concealment versus self-visibility (camouflage concealment versus opponent identified visibility)

Stage four: Confused self-concealment versus self-visibility (prevailing paranoid concealment versus grandiose visibility)

Stage five: Highly confused self-concealment versus self-visibility (frequent shifting of delusive identity and paranoid delusion)

The third dynamic force is self-splitting versus self-preservation. This dynamic force starts with the individual's inherent instinct to destruct and to preserve one's own self and others in facing danger and threat in the external environment. Individuals with schizophrenia, are involved heavily in a delusive self-destruction mechanism in which they try to destruct themselves mentally so that the oppressive others cannot destruct them. In a way, this is the only delusive way to preserve the individuals' own inner self, such as self-image, self-identity, and autonomy. This is also a way to destruct oneself to destruct others.

There are also different stages in self-preservation versus self-destruction in the development of schizophrenia.

Stage one: *No need* for development of self-destruction versus self-preservation (self destruction is only limited to inherent sex and aggressive drive, which is under control of the individual.)

Stage two: *Initial development* of self-destruction versus self-preservation (the individual may internalize negative comments from external oppressive environment)

Stage three: *Gradual development* of self-destruction versus self-preservation (the individual tends to absorb and acts according to the demand of others' oppression and criticism. But it is too painful and unbearable. Thus, s/he tries to dissociate his/her own sense of reality to lessen his/her negative feelings and inner pains.)

Stage four: Externalization of self-destruction versus self-preservation by rebellion of the oppressive others to preserve one's autonomy and substantiality. (The individual destructs his/her un-embodied self to diminish the influence of oppressive others. In doing so, s/he also diminishes his/her external parts of self-images and identities.)

Stage five: *Internalization* of self destruction versus self preservation by *diminishing unembodied self and development of false self* (the individual dissociates himself/herself from a painful reality completely by diminishing his/her un-embodied self and builds up a false self. The individual is largely withdrawn from participation of normal social interaction and daily activities.

Stage six: *Intensive development* of self-destruction versus self-preservation: *Full development of false self* (The full representation of the false self can be a full manifestation of psychotic symptoms. Other may perceive the individual is seriously insane and mad.)

Stage seven: *Overwhelming development* of self-destruction and self-preservation: Destruction and *splitting of the false self and true self* (the individual regards the false self as a foreign lifeless body that should be rejected. The residual but diminished un-embodied self and false self becomes a delusive negative reality.)

In fact, these three dynamic forces intermingle and reinforce one another in the self-fragmentation process. In facing the unavoidable oppressive environment, since the individual is weak in an object relationship, his/her harsh superego and stormy personality is unable to defend him/her from all the external oppression and humiliation. Instead, s/he tends to internalize all the oppression and humiliation. S/he also identifies with all these oppressive and humiliating but significant others. In doing so, the individual is highly painful and self-fracturing. Thus, these three dynamic forces, self-splitting versus self-cohesion, self-concealment versus self-visibility, as well as self-destruction versus self-preservation become the mechanisms for the individual to lessen his/her pain and increase his/her endurance in his/her self-fracturing process. On one hand, self-splitting, self-concealment and self-destruction enables the individual to separate, cover-up, and diminish parts of his/her self system that coincides, overlaps, internalizes and identifies with the oppressive significant others. On the other hand, self-cohesion, self-visibility and self-preservation allows the individual to protect, to glue together and to manifest his/her residual self-system that has not been influenced by the oppressive significant others.

These three dynamic forces, self-splitting versus self-cohesion, self-concealment versus self-visibility, and self-destruction versus self-preservation serve different functions in the process of self-fragmentation. The self-splitting versus self-cohesion tends to be the force in fracturing and pseudo-maintenance of the major infrastructures of the self-system. The self-concealment versus self-visibility tends to be the force in disguising and visualizing the self-image and identity. The self-destruction versus self-preservation is the force diffusing and modifying the sense of existence of the self-system. In the coming chapters, the writer will describe the impact of these three dynamic forces in positive, negative, and first rank symptoms. Strictly speaking, these three dynamic forces, within the oppressive environment, are destructive forces leading to self-fragmentation. However, within a supportive, empathic, and caring environment, these three dynamic forces may turn out to be the constructing forces leading to a full recovery of self-integration.

Implications to Mental Health Recovery

The Three Dynamic Forces as Basic Components and Natures of Self System

As mentioned above, the three dynamic forces in self-fragmentation of schizophrenia is a pull and push force in splitting, concealing and destructing the self-system in facing continuously oppressive others in terms of engulfment, implosion, and depersonalization. Within these dynamic forces, it is highly negative in terms of splitting, concealing, and destructing the self-system. Underlying these is also a strong urge to preserve, to visualize, and to integrate the self-system. In fact, these three dynamic forces represent different components and natures of the self-system that can be represented in the following:

1. Self-Splitting versus Self-Cohesion: It represents the forces in maintaining the structure of the self-system. To maintain its functioning, the self-system needs to have a constant and regular structure. When the self-system loses or breaks its basic structure, its basic function is hindered.
2. Self-Concealment versus Self Visibility: It represents the *connection and linkage* of the self-system with related issues, objects, and persons in the social environment. A healthy self-system needs to have constant, regular, and meaningful connection with related issues, objects, and persons in the actual reality. In doing so, the self-system is appropriately visualized and presented. Self-concealment is done to protect the individual from external threats by being detached from external objects, issues and persons in the actual reality. This dynamic force also represents the sense of existence and non-existence of the individual. In self-concealment, the individual tries to be non-existing with an oppressive environment. In self-visibility, the individual tries to be a high profile o visual his/her sense of existence within an accepting and supportive social environment.
3. Self-Destruction and Self-Preservation: It represents the strengths and energy of the self-system. If the energy and strengths is properly challenged and directed, the self-system preserves itself, and maintains its survival as well as further development. If

> the energy is inappropriately challenged and directed, the self-system destructs itself and faces a process of deterioration and extinction.

The three components, strengths and energy, connection and linkage, as well as structure, are basic ingredients of self-system. In mental health recovery, it is really a restoration of one's strengths and energy, connection and linkage as well as structure in a healthy and constructive self-system.

Life and Death Instincts in Dilemmas of Self-Fragmentation and Self-Integration

Life Instincts

Freud (1920/1961) affirmed that that are two types of instincts in our life. One is the life instincts (Eros). Another one is the death instinct. Life instincts actually come from our survival needs and bodily desires. It is the `Id' including sex, thirst, and hunger, and pain avoidance. Human beings need this for basic survival of oneself and the whole human species. It is also pleasure seeking, which the individual enjoys in gratifying all these bodily desires. Energy created by all these basic instincts is called 'libido'. Apart from being energized by bodily desires `id', Eros is also concerned with love and intimacy with others. It is a powerful energy guiding human behaviors. The suppression and repression of all these bodily desires, love, and intimacy may make all this energy turn inward in forms of various kinds of neurosis. Life instincts are important to support one's survival intrapersonally and interpersonally. Intrapersonally, they support us to feel alive and possess enough psychic and physical energy in daily living, and in facing challenges and difficulties. However, when our physical and social environment is continuously oppressive and abusive, energy from life instincts are suffocated and hindered.

Death Instincts

As an opposite of life instincts, Freud (1920/1961) further described that there are the death instincts 'Thanatos'. Freud, taking a pessimistic existential stance stated that 'the goal of all life is death' (Freud, 1920/1961). He observed that people with traumatic experiences always recall, re-bounce or self-induce all these experience with an unconscious death wish to end up their torture and pain in life. Freud (1920/1961) concluded that all self-destruction is sparked by energy from death instincts. When this energy turns outwards, it becomes aggression and violence towards others.

Life and Death Instincts in Psychotic Self-Fragmentation

In other words, the self-fragmentation of clients with schizophrenia is originated from the energy and power of the death instincts. That means, self-destruction, self-splitting, and self-concealment, are all energized by the death instinct. As an opposite, self-cohesion, self-visibility, and self-preservation are all energized by life instincts.

According to Freud, we all possess Eros and Thanatos. That means, the above-mentioned three dynamic forces, self-preservation versus self-destruction, self-concealment versus self-visibility, and self-splitting versus self-cohesion not only presents in clients with schizophrenia, but also present in all human beings. The difference is that for normal persons within an acceptable and caring social environment, they only manifest or are conscious of self-preservation, self-visibility and self-cohesion within an actual reality. His/her Eros with smooth development and manifestation of his/her libido activates his/her daily life and social interaction. His/her self-destruction, self-concealment, and self-splitting are hidden or concealed within unconscious level. His/her death instinct does not manifest. However, once the immediate reality and social environment becomes highly oppressive or even abusive, the opposite happens. That means, self-concealment, self-destruction, and self-splitting become overt and are fully activated and developed by the death instincts. At the same time, self-preservation, self-cohesion, and self-visibility can only be suppressed or it turns to an unconscious or subconscious level. By doing so, various forms of mental and emotional problems may evolve gradually. To survive, the individual may try every means to avoid the death instinct manifestation and try to turn the life instinct alive again. This serves as an internal driving force for the individual to avoid the oppressive environment and search for a positive and nurturing social environment.

For clients with schizophrenia, they are continuously and spontaneously engulfed, victimized, depersonalized, and imploded by the oppressive environment. Prolonged suppression of libido and Eros are intolerable for them. The only way they can handle it is to distort their perception of the oppressive reality or simply detach from it by engaging in self-destruction, self-splitting, and self-concealment. As mentioned above, in doing so, they destruct, split, and conceal oppressive others by destructing, splitting, and concealing themselves. All these are highly painful. To keep them alive mentally, they can only numb all these painful feelings on one hand, or become involved in delusions and hallucinations on the other hand. Their delusions and hallucinations become their delusive reality in which they can actualize their self-preservation, self-cohesion, and self-visibility.

Mental Health Recovery from Psychotic Self-Fragmentation Dilemma

All these have strong implications to mental health recovery for persons with schizophrenia. That means, recovery of clients with schizophrenia should be a holistic recovery from psychotic self-fragmentation dilemma. It should be a holistic recovery in the following aspect:

1. Recovery by activating life instincts within a supportive actual reality
2. Recovery by proper channeling of energy in death instincts
3. Recovery by restoring the energy, structure and connection of the self-system
4. A multi-dimensional recovery

Recovery by Activating Life Instincts within a Supportive Actual Reality

Firstly, for a holistic recovery, the life and death instinct should be properly exercised. That means, self-preservation, self-cohesion, and self-visibility should be properly manifested with a supportive and caring social environment. That means, life instincts can be nurtured and actualized. Death instincts in terms of self-splitting, self-concealment, and self-destruction are gradually submerged. In doing so, the three dynamic forces in life, self-preservation versus self-destruction, self-cohesion versus self-splitting, as well as self-visibility versus self-concealment, are properly articulated and normalized. Secondly, the life instinct should be gradually and naturally developed. For any intervention and interacting that is controlling and coercive, it actually re-activates clients' death instinct and reinforces clients' urges for self-concealment, self-destruction, and self-splitting, with a result reinforcing manifestation of negative symptoms. Thirdly, in activating life instincts, clients with schizophrenia may be facilitated to join in some pleasurable activities and enjoyment in a morally and socially acceptable way, such as:

1. Going out for meals and enjoying good food with supportive caregivers, workers, and/or other clients in services. In doing so, their life instinct is certainly sparked and intensified by desires and satisfaction of enjoying favorite foods with friends and peers.
2. Facilitate clients to have normal and moral courtship, love, and sex with supportive and caring spouses. In doing so, their life instincts are certainly sparked and intensified by gratifying the desires for sex, love, and intimacy.
3. Encourage clients to engage in interesting games, exercises, and interactions with others. By doing so, their life instincts are initiated and intensified by enjoying and involving interacting and interesting activities with others.
4. Facilitate supportive others to recognize, to appreciate and to share positive feelings with clients with schizophrenia. By doing so, their life instincts are sparked and intensified by mutual sharing, mutual acceptance, and mutual support with one and others.

Once, clients' life instincts are sparked and intensified within a caring and supportive reality, their self-preservation, self-cohesion and self-visibility are powerfully activated. All these self-integrations can be actualized within a reality context. Clients with schizophrenia no longer need to stay in their delusive and hallucinated inner world for pseudo self-preservation, cohesion, and visibility. That means, once their life instincts are activated, their positive symptoms in terms of hallucinations and delusions alleviate accordingly. In the same way, they become more activated, and motivated in participating in daily activities and interaction with supportive others. By doing so, their negative symptoms can also be enlightened. All these may be shown by the self-narration of a client with schizophrenia, Tom. Related parties' consensus was sought in their stories for academic purposes. For the sake of confidentiality, personal information, and personal identity were properly disguised. What was bracketed was the writer's elaboration. In this case, the writer was the professional consultant of the concerned psychiatric rehabilitation service agency:

> Tom: I had suffered from schizophrenia for several years. When I was small, my mother was very controlling and manipulating. My father never appeared as he engaged in an extra-marital relationship with another woman. I grew up within my mother's anxious control. I never had my own choice. In fact, I felt highly suffocated under my mother's control.
>
> Gradually, I learned to detach from her anxious blaming and enmeshment. Physically, I was listening to my mother's comments but mentally I was detached from her. Gradually, I used this form of self-detachment to face my teacher's and my classmates bullying and oppression. They always bullied me as weak, inert, and girlish. In fact, I split myself into two parts, one part facing the cruel reality, and another part as my own autonomous self (*self- splitting versus self-cohesion dynamic forc*e). I could never let my own autonomous self out, because whenever I tried to say anything against

my controlling mother, abusive teacher, and bullying classmates, they would impose even greater control, abuse, and bullying on me. It was much better to conceal my own self inwards *(self-concealment versus self-visibility dynamic force)*.

With that sort of concealment, I was free inside, but cut off from outside. This was an interesting game. I played this well when I was only twelve. While I was inert, dull, or appearing as silly and submissive outside, I could imagine my own fantasy inside (self-destruction versus self-preservation). At first, I imagined all my dreams came true. I became a strong man with mighty power to fight against my bullying classmates and teacher. Sometimes, I imagined that I came from a wealthy family and my father was a very rich businessman. As I had a lot of money to spend, many girls chased me around but they could never get me.

As my mother, teacher, and classmates became more and more controlling, oppressive, and bullying; my time engaging in imagination and fantasy increased. It really disturbed my daily functioning; I could no longer concentrate on my studies, interact with others, or eat properly. Instead, the delusive inner world absorbed me (self-destruction versus self-preservation dynamic force). One day, when I walked on the street, a beggar came and followed me closely. Even though I had tried my best to avoid him, he still followed me. I ran and ran and finally I crossed the road but was knocked down by a running class.

When I woke up in the hospital, the entire world changed. I heard a voice from the heaven saying that I was originally an almighty God in my previous life. There were many jealous evil spirits around trying to steal my godly power away. All these made me felt highly ambivalent. On one hand, I was happy about my power and godly identity in my previous life. On the other hand, I was afraid of all kinds of evils spirits around. The voice said that my controlling mother, oppressive teacher, and bullying classmates were actually sent by evil spirits to steal my godly power away. I was in a panic state. No sooner, I was sent into a mental hospital. The psychiatrist there affirmed that I had suffered from schizophrenia for quite a number of years already. I had to receive a heavy dosage of anti-psychotic medication. It really made me feel dull, inert, and dizzy. At first, I refused to take that medicine. They imposed injections on me. After the medical injection, the whole world was slowing down. My inner world autonomy also slowed down. I was inert and emotionless. I did not have an interest in the outside world. I simply sat still and my mind was blank (negative psychotic symptoms and effects of institutionalization and heavy dosage of anti-psychotic medication).

I stayed in the mental hospital for two years. I refused to return home. At that time, I was already 21 years old and I had already finished my secondary school education but with a very poor public examination. The medical social worker referred me to a psychiatric half way house. In there, there was a kind and empathic social worker, Jack. He empathically listened to my own stories. At that moment, I thought I was hopeless. As a patient with schizophrenia, I did not have any future. All I could do is to sit still in the half way house staring at the television for the whole day. I was inert, withdrawn, and passive, having no interest to engage in household cleaning or other activates. Occasionally, some residents approached me but I had no interest in engaging with them. I just felt that I was just a dead man (the loss of life instincts).

While I assumed that my whole life should be frozen by inertness and withdrawal, my social worker Jack, still held on. To stir me up, together with some other residents, he always invited me to have afternoon tea. At first, I refused them. After several invitations, I joined them. We enjoyed afternoon tea at a Chinese restaurant. Dim sum there was really good. They did have some good sharing of their life experiences. They invited me to share my life experiences too. I felt quite inert and tired. For me, life was just meaninglessness and in vain. I felt I had nothing to share.

Among them, there was a beautiful young woman, Jane. She also joined in the afternoon tea. Indeed, she was young and pretty. She said she also had schizophrenia and

> was on the road to recovery. She worked as a waitress in a Chinese restaurant nearby. She was kind and empathic. Other residents also said she was a pretty lady, and encouraged me to start dating her. It was really a big challenge. If I was a normal young and energetic guy, I would certainly started my dating immediately. But now, I was a useless schizophrenic patient. How could she be interested in me? In my mind, I really aspired that she could be my girlfriend. A few days later, she approached me in the halfway house saying that there was a vacancy of a waiter in her Chinese restaurant. She asked whether I was interested in it. Of course, I was interested in it. This should be a golden chance for me. From that time onwards, I tried to convince myself that I had to recover from my schizophrenia. I could recover as well as Jane.

Tom's self-narration clearly showed his psychotic self-fragmentation was strongly influenced by three dynamic forces, self-splitting versus self-cohesion, self-destruction versus self-preservation, and self-concealment versus self-visibility. As his psychotic symptoms prevailed, Tom's life instincts declined accordingly. Instead, his dead instincts increased drastically. He became inert, withdrawn, and passive in most aspects in life. The empathic social worker, Jack, with the help of other residents, tried every means to spark Tom's life instincts. Going out for meals, enjoying food with other supportive residents, and dating with a beautiful young lady in the halfway house all served as effective means to initiate and intensify Tom's life instinct. Once his life instincts were generated, Tom's urge and will to recover were consolidated.

Recovery by Proper channeling of Energy in Death Instincts

Apart from generating and intensifying life instincts, facing the three dynamic forces, it is crucial that related professionals should also help clients with schizophrenia properly channel death instincts. For clients with schizophrenia, because of prolonged oppression by their engulfing, imploding and depersonalizing significant others, their life instincts are deactivated but their death instincts are highly activated. However, their aggression cannot turn outwards in fighting against their oppressive but attached oppressive others. Instead, they direct the anger towards themselves in forms of self-splitting, self-concealment, and self-destruction. In severe cases, all these death instincts driven forces are symbolized in forms of intense paranoid, grandiose, or catatonic delusions and hallucinations, as well as severe inertness, detachment, and withdrawal in negative symptoms. Thus, for a holistic recovery, it is necessary for related professionals to channel clients' negative emotions, such as feelings of inferiority, fear, anger, loneliness, worthlessness, helplessness and/or emptiness behind highly symbolized positive symptoms (paranoid, grandiose, or catatonic delusions and hallucinations), as well as negative symptoms (blunt affect, ahedonia, alogia and avolition). By doing so, the destructive energy from death instincts can be properly released and ventilated together with negative emotions and urges. Related interventions in this aspect can be listed in the following:

1. Related professionals should have patience and interest in observing, listening and understanding details, contents, and related contexts of clients' manifestation of their positive and negative symptoms
2. Related professionals should have a full recognition of related meanings, emotions, functions and purposes behind clients' positive symptoms and negative symptoms

3. Related professionals should help clients to recognize, ventilate and express all these negative emotions, functions, and purposes behind their positive symptoms and negative symptoms within a highly supportive, caring and accepting social environment. In doing so, their energy from their death instincts can be properly released.

After a good release and ventilation of destructive energy from death instincts, the self-splitting, self-destruction, and self-concealment can be properly alleviated. Together with the gradual growth and intensification of life instincts with a supportive, caring and accepting social environment, the dilemma of self-fragmentation and self-integration can be gradually normalized.

All these could be illustrated in Tom's case. The emphatic social worker, Jack tried to release Tom's internalized death instincts energy. The following was Jack's verbatim recording in a counseling session with Tom. At that moment, Tom had already started a constant courtship with Jane, the beautiful young lady living in the same half way house as Tom. He also worked as a waiter in the same Chinese restaurant as Jane. As Tom's life instincts were fully sparked and intensified, he was no longer inert, withdrawn and passive. With good psychic energy, he was able to elaborate his anger towards his controlling mother, abusive teacher, and bullying classmates as well as other bad people in his life.

Tom and Jack were sitting in the interview room in the psychiatric halfway. Before that, they had just finished the dinner.

Jack: How is your work?

Tom: Fine, I learned how to be a waiter in a large and busy Chinese restaurant.

Jack: Jane must help you a lot.

Tom: Yes, indeed, she is a good waitress. She taught me many things I don't know.

Jack: You are dating her.

Tom: Yes, I loved her and she seemed to have interest in me. I am lucky to have such a beautiful young lady as my girl friend.

Jack: So you are so proud of her. How is she comparing with your mother and your former girl friend (Jack had to lighten Tom's life instincts before he could channel his hidden energy in his death instincts?)

Tom: Frankly speaking, Jane is my first girl friend. Of course, she is much better than my mother. My mother was so controlling, she simply regarded me as her toy to manipulate and control. In front of her, I was never a complete person.

Tom began to elaborate his anger towards his mother.

Jack: So, you hated her…..

Tom: It was really hard to say. She brought me up. Ever since my father was involved in an extra-marital relationship, my mother was the only one I relied on. But she did not care about my feelings.

Jack: So you felt really suffocated and uncomfortable in front of her. Didn't you?

Tom: I simply felt that she grasped my throat and I could not breathe properly in front of her.

Jack: So, you think your whole life was being ruined by her.

Tom: Not so, apart from her, there were my abusive teachers and my bullying classmates. They were all bastards.

Jack: It was really good that you could air out your deep hatred feeling towards your mother, your teachers and your classmates. How do you feel now?

Tom: Thanks a lot. I have never been so comfortable in my life. No one really liked to listen to me. They simply said I was insane. When all these hatred feeling stored up in your mind, it simply eats up your soul.

Jack: So be relaxed.

Interestingly, after Tom could fully ventilate his deep hatred feelings towards his oppressive others, his delusions, and hallucinations were much alleviated. Despite working very hard in the Chinese restaurant, he was happy and contented. It was clear that after self-directed but concealed anger once released, Tom felt enlightened and much more energetic than before.

Recovery by Restoring the Energy, Structure and Connection of the Self-System

As mentioned above, the three dynamic forces imply three different aspects and components of the self-system. Self-preservation versus self-destruction implies strengths and energy of the self-system. Self-splitting versus self-cohesion implies structure of the self-system. Self-visibility versus self-concealment implies connection and linkage of the self-system.

These three dynamic forces properly fracture the structure, disturb the connection and linkage, as well as misuse clients' psychic energy in their self-system. In the acute psychotic state, the structure is split. Related psychic energy is misused in forms of highly disturbed delusions, hallucinations and odd and bizarre behaviors; the connection of reality is distorted. In chronic psychosis, the structure of the self-system becomes highly diffused. Their psychic energy in the self-system is exhausted. Their connection of reality is highly detached. All these make negative symptoms prevail.

In other words, *holistic recovery should imply proper connection with persons, issues, and objects within supportive and caring reality.* At the same time, clients' ego strengths should be nurtured and their structure in their self-system should be properly structured.

Intervention Strategies to Improve the Structure Self System

In actual clinical practice, structure of the self-system can be restored by the following:

1. Structural physical and social environment with constant and regular presence of secure and supportive objects, persons, and issues.
2. Scheduled and structured normalized daily life including a regular daily schedule, regular activities and secure interaction with others.
3. Structured programs and services and stable and caring workers and staff

The structured life, programs and service should be designed to resolve the self-splitting versus self-cohesion dynamic force for clients with schizophrenia. To help the client with schizophrenia to regain his/her self-cohesion in actual reality, rather than within delusive reality, all these structured life programs and services should be provided regularly and continuously. By doing so, related clients with schizophrenia can gradually formulate their normal patterns and structure in life, normal patterns and structure in self-perception, and normal patterns and structure in social function. With the structured and continuous support from their significant others; including related professionals and caregivers, they are able to restore a cohesive self-system in actual reality. All these could be illustrated in Tom's case. Below was the narration of the social worker, Jack, in describing how he provided structured life, programs, and services in helping Tom to develop a cohesive self-system within a supportive reality.

> Jack: under the supervision of our professional consultant, I tried to provide a structured life, and programs for Tom. Indeed, it was very important for his mental health recovery. Under his mother's tight control, in his whole life, deep down in Tom's mind, he was quite rebellious. He wrongly assumed that living a confused life was a manifestation of autonomy. He wanted to stay up very late at night and wake up at any time he wanted. If he did not have enough sleep, his mental health got worse.
>
> Also, having been bullied by his classmates for quite a number of years, he became quite sensitive to others' comments and rejection. He was easily irritated by others. Sometimes, his responses were a bit exaggerated. I understood that sometimes, his residual paranoia and/or grandiose delusions and hallucinations disturbed him deeply. Apart from that, he also harbored a sense of intense insecurity. Despite this, he had a stable job as a waiter and started dating Jane; he still felt that his job and his courtship were very vulnerable. All these made him oversensitive in dealing with his relationship with Jane.
>
> To resolve this, I tried to encourage and facilitate Tom to have a structured life schedule. I woke him up every day at seven o'clock and accompanied him to have morning joking. At first, he refused. After a few days practice, he began to enjoy it. Regular vigorous exercise improved his health and his sleeping conditions were much improved. Later, I invited Jane to join in the morning joking. They joked for half an hour, enjoyed breakfast together in the half way house, and took a bath before they went to work. This daily structure improved their health and mental health as well as stabilized their courtship. Gradually, a few residents joined in the morning joking. They became a stable mutual support group and had more regular gatherings, such as going out for dinner, and casual chatting in the half way house.
>
> I grouped them together and formed a structured self-help and social group. They had a group meeting every Wednesday evening. One of them was selected as the group leader, Tom was elected as the duty group leader, and Jane was the secretary. Giving Tom a clear sense of responsibility was very good to structure his response with others. He began to follow rules and regulations as well as advising others to following the house rules. He demonstrated respect to authority figures. His unconscious rebellion and anger were greatly resolved.
>
> Tom's recovery benefitted a lot from this structured life schedule, stable and patterned social interaction, and formal responsibility and roles. It seemed that his inner dynamic force of self-splitting and self-cohesion was greatly alleviated. Tom began to have a strong sense of security and confidence in daily interaction. His mental health and physical health were more stable than before.

Intervention Strategies to Develop the Strengths and Energy of the Self System

Strength and energy of the self-system can be developed by appreciating and manifesting clients' strengths, potentials, and talents. Energy can be regained by good food, good exercise, and good rest. In fact, there are many *energy sources* in our inner psychic forces.

They are:

1. Psychic energy from our will power
2. Moral energy from our superego or social norms
3. Self-actualization energy from actualizing our aspirations and self identity/
4. Emotional energy in manifestation of our mood and ventilation of our positive and negative mood.
5. Physical energy in health and body conditions
6. Desire energy (Eros) in gratifying our desires.

All these energies should be properly activated, making clients with schizophrenia gradually regain positive energy in daily life, in interacting with others, in fulfilling their responsibility and asserting their own right within a supportive and caring environment. Clinically, there are many ways to develop the strengths and energy of the self-system, in particular the self-actualization energy.

1. Identify, recognize, and develop client's talents, strengths, capacity and ability.
2. Regularize client's manifestations of his/her talents, strengths, capacity and ability
3. Openly appreciate client's manifestations of his/her talents, strengths, capacity and ability
4. Facilitate clients to internalize manifestations as his/her unique self-identity and position.
5. Encourage clients to take up responsibility and develop his career according to his/her talents, strengths, capacity, and ability.
6. Apart from developing client's actualization energy, client's other sources of energy can also developed by the following:
   a. Develop one's will power by fulfilling one's life aspiration and searching a for a good meaning of life
   b. Develop one's moral energy by taking up moral responsibility and actualizing one's morality in the society and social circle
   c. Develop one's physical energy by proper and regular physical exercises
   d. Develop one's emotional energy by sharing positive feelings and emotions.
   e. Manifest clients' Eros and life instinct

Below was the narration of the social worker, Jack showing that how he developed Tom's strengths and energy in the self-system in mental health recovery.

> Jack: the structured life, programs and services really help Tom. He became mentally and emotionally stable. With that, upon the advice of our professional consultant, we began to develop Tom's strengths and energy. I thought that it was crucial for his mental health recovery. All along, Tom was inferior and had a weak self-identity. That was why he was so sensitive to others' comments, rejection, and isolation. That was also why he harbored a grandiose delusion that he possessed godly power and could control others. In the same way, he harbored a paranoid delusion with voices saying that he was timid, bad, and untrustworthy. Another voice even said he was entirely rubbish in the world.
>
> We tried to use various means to develop Tom's strength and energy. In fact, after being elected as the deputy leader of the self-help group, Tom became vary moral, righteous, and caring. He always advised other group members to do morning exercise, to

sleep early and to maintain good physical health (Tom's moral energy was properly developed).

Apart from that, we also recognized that Tom had special talents. He actually had special talents in cooking and appreciating Chinese dishes. In the Chinese restaurant where he was working, he tried to memorize various favorable dishes on the menu. Occasionally, he went to the kitchen and observed how the chef there cooked these favorable dishes. To encourage him to manifest his talents, we arranged one dinner being prepared by Tom with his favorable dishes. He prepared several main dishes that were really enjoyable by all residents in the half way house. Tom's talents and strengths were thoroughly recognized and appreciated by others. Tom was very happy about that. He said, in his childhood, his mother had no interest in cooking, she always urged him to prepare the meals. That was why he was so skillful in this area.

(It was clear that Tom's talents was properly recognized and appreciated by all residents in the half way house. All these were able to develop his self-image and self-identity.)

After that, I had a short chat with Tom, apart from appreciating his talent, I encouraged him to receive formal training in this aspect. With the support from his girlfriend, Jane, he had enrolled a part time certificate course in cooking in Vocational Training Institute (By doing so, we could formalize and pattern Tom's talents and ability). At first, Tom was a bit reluctant in doing so, saying that he was not qualified and not ready to receive formal training.

Later, Jane frankly said that she loved Tom and wanted him to be a qualified and experienced cook so that they could earn enough money to get married and build up their own family. (In doing so, Tom's life instincts were highly enlightened. At the same time, his meaning of life, to have a happy marriage and family, was constructed. His will power increased accordingly). With that encouragement, Tom tried all his best to study in this course. In the daytime, he worked as a part time waiter in the Chinese restaurant. In the evening, he studied hard in this course.

Intervention Strategies in Improving Connection and Linkage of Reality of the Self System

In resolving clients' dynamic force of self-concealment and self-visibility, it is crucial that clients are encouraged to restore linkage and connection of objects, persons, and issues in the actual but supportive reality. In actual clinical practice, this can be attained by the following intervention strategies:

1. Build up a supportive social environment for clients with schizophrenia. If clients' significant others are oppressive and abusive, related professionals should construct a caring and supportive social environment within the service contexts.
2. Encourage clients to connect and interact with supportive others gradually to build their trust and sense of security in interacting with others in the reality.
3. Facilitate mutual and spontaneous interaction among clients and supportive others.
4. Regularize all these constructive interactions as a constant daily pattern.
5. Encourage clients to develop proper social interaction with persons in various social circles.

All these can be shown in Tom's case. Below was the narration of the social worker, Jack, showing how important social connection and linkage was in mental healthy recovery.

Jack: Thanks for our professional consultant's advice, according to his suggested intervention strategies; Tom was on the road of recovery. He studied very hard in the cooking certificate course. He was one the brilliant students in the course. His performance was very good. After two years' of hard work, he graduated with an excellent result. No sooner, he was employed by a hotel as a trainee in cooking.

This indeed, was a great improvement for Tom.

When he first came to our half way house, Tom was a bit shameful in relating to others. In addition to that, because of his active negative symptoms due to prolonged institutionalization, he was inert, passive, and withdrawn. He also harbored active positive symptoms that many people around were trying to steal his godly power. All these hindered his connection and linkage with others. That means, his dynamic force self-concealment versus self-visibility prevailed. In his life, he was accustomed to concealing himself in front of his controlling mother, oppressive teacher, and bullying classmates. The more he concealed himself within paranoid and grandiose delusions and hallucinations, the more he could prevent the harm of oppressive others but the more he fractured his self-system.

Thus, for his mental health recovery, it was crucial to establish constructive and meaningful connections, and linkage with supportive others within a caring reality. That was why I tried my best to build up a supportive and caring social environment for Tom. As his mother was highly controlling, we constructed a supportive peer system for him in the half way house. However, I could not do this in a formal way, as Tom was quite sensitive to others' rejection. Thus, I had to do this in an informal way. I and other residents invited him for tea. In addition, I encouraged him to have morning exercise with me. The most important was that all these activities should be regularized as daily activities so that Tom could relate and interact with others in a normal, gradual and natural way.

Apart from that, two more linkage and connection with others were crucial to resolve his self-concealment and self-visibility. The first one was to restore Tom's urge and trust on intimate relationships. The second one was to rebuild Tom's normal social interaction with others in various social contexts. The first one was attained by facilitating the courtship of Jane and Tom. The second one was gradually achieved by supporting Tom to be a waiter in a large Chinese restaurant.

Certainly, all these were great challenges for Tom, in particular when he felt inferior and insecure. In fact, in the first two months as a waiter in the Chinese restaurant, he sought my advice every day. I patiently helped Tom to resolve any difficulties in his job. Sometimes, with the help from Jane, I did role-play with him so that he could learn how to relate to different types of customers appropriately. Regarding his intimate relationship with Jane, I performed courtship counseling with them, helping them to communicate with one another smoothly. Jane also had some unpleasant past experiences in courtship. I had to help her to express and shared these with Tom.

When Tom properly learned how to relate to others in various social contexts within a non-threatening reality, his dynamic force of self-concealment and self-visibility was resolved and normalized. Furthermore, when Tom had already established his career as a good cook, we encouraged him to use his expertise to serve the community and society as being a volunteer instructor of cooking classes for clients with mental problems, single mothers, deprived family and juvenile delinquents. All these community contributions greatly enhanced Tom's competence and his sense of identity as well his sense of agency and influence towards others.

A Multi-dimensional Articulation of Recovery

In Tom's case, it was clear that his mental health recovery not only limited to his self-system. Instead, it gradually spread to other aspects of Tom's life. Firstly, after Tom started dating, Jane, and enrolled the cooking course, his meaning of life was no longer empty and meaningless. Instead, he had a clear and specific life goal, to be a good and professional cook and save money to marry Jane, and have a family. This was certainly a highly valuable and constructive life goal for a man. Within this specific life goal, his psychic and self-actualization energy prevailed. Following this, his emotions, his cognitive and social functioning improved accordingly. On one hand, it created tremendous strengths for Tom. On the other hand, it also meant stress and pressure in study, in work and in courtship. Fortunately, the social worker, Jack provided spontaneous support and caring to Tom and Jane. Within Jack's intervention, he did not limit himself to casework and counseling. Instead, he also organized group work (self-help groups with Jack, Jane and other residents in the half way house), programs, casual but regular interaction and activities (morning exercise and afternoon tea), career development (encourage Tom to manifest his cooking talents, enroll in cooking course, and facilitate Tom to study hard in this course), and courtship counseling (helping Jane and Tom to communicate fluently with one another) for Tom as well as for Jane. All these showed that Jack provided recovery-based interventions within intrapersonal, interpersonal, organizational, community and societal levels. Multi-dimensional intervention strategies implied a multi-dimensional recovery. In fact, all intervention strategies should follow or comply with ten recovery principles mandated in 2004 by the US Department of Health & Human Service. They are: '

1. Self Direction
2. Individualized & Person Centered
3. Empowerment
4. Holistic
5. Non-Linear
6. Strengths Based Orientation
7. Peer Support
8. Respect
9. Responsibility
10. Hope

(US Department of Health & Human Services, 2004)

Indeed, Tom's recovery is *self-directed* and *person-centered.* Jack facilitated Tom to choose his own life long partner, Jane, and his life long career. He *empowered* Tom to be assertive in starting to date Jane, to share his difficulties and frustrations in the past. Tom's recovery was *holistic* including career development, courtship, accommodation, physical exercise, and peer relationship. Tom's *strengths* and talents in cooking were fully developed. He learned and trained to take up *responsibility* in his work, in his courtship, and serving the community and society. Tom's recovery was a *non-linear path.* There were ups and downs. Tom's faced his downs when he felt insecure and inferior in taking his job and his dating. He needed Jack's counseling, Jane's encouragement, and other residents' support in getting through all these hindrances. Certainly, Tom's talents and his endeavor in cooking earned others' *respect* and nurtured his *hope* in building his own career, marriage, and courtship in life.

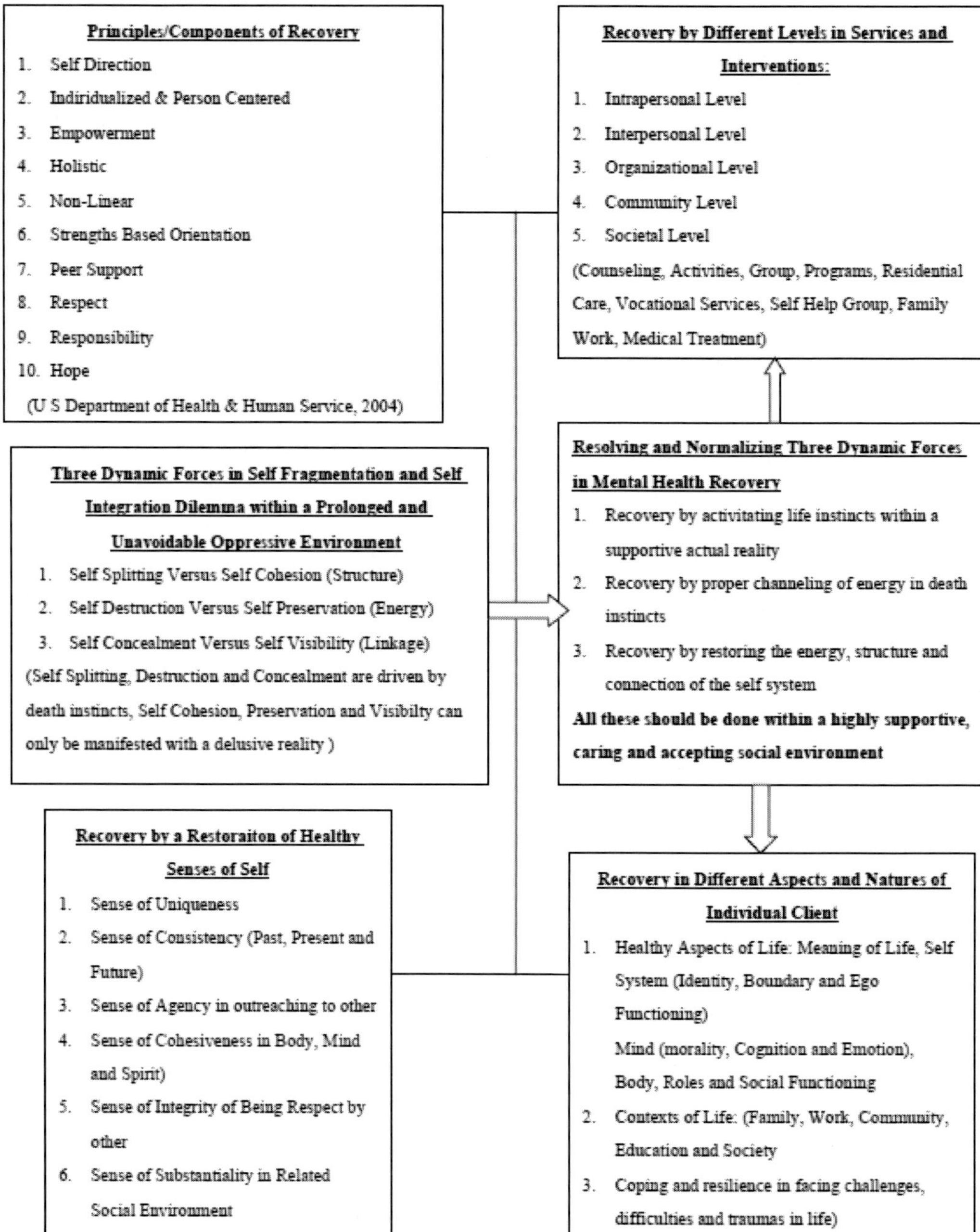

Figure. A Multi-Dimensional Articulation of Mental Health Recovery.

By means of all these multi-dimensional perspective and interventions, Tom's senses of self were gradually improved. His *sense of uniqueness* certainly was gradually attained as his cooking talents were recognized and developed. He became more and more identified as a professional cook. In doing so, his aspiration of being a good cook was his aspiration in the past, present, and the future. That means he could develop his *sense of consistency* continuously. The whole recovery process also enabled him to reach out to others. Instead of staying within his psychotic positive and/or negative symptoms, Tom was able relate to other residents, his girlfriends, and customers in the Chinese restaurant. He was able to convince and demonstrate that he was a capable cook, a helpful person, and an expertise in cooking. In doing all these, his *sense of agency* could be achieved. Furthermore, since he could live up to his own aspirations, he could do what he wanted to do, and as he could manifest his own talents in helping others, in initiating his courtship, and get married to Jane, and prepare for his life long career as a professional cook, he was highly coherent in his word and deeds, mind, body and spirit (*sense of cohesiveness*). He became a man with integrity that could earn others' respect fully (*sense of integrity*). From that time onwards, his life was no longer a vacuum; rather, it was a substantial attainment of life achievement of career, family, position, and respect in various social contexts *(sense of substantiality)*.

This multi-dimensional and holistic process of recovery can be summarized in the following figure.

Conclusion

As a conclusion, this chapter is a comprehensive discussion about the various theoretical underpinnings of the self-fragmentation and self-integration dilemma in clients with schizophrenia. Among various perspectives in psychosocial interpretation of schizophrenia, Frosch (1983), Laing (1960), Arieti's (1974), Burnham (et al., 1969) and Bion (1984) all contributed to the richness and details in psychotic self-fragmentation.

Frosch's (1983) showed that fragmentation of the self-system, or perception of others, mainly serves two functions, splitting the self-system into good and bad parts, as well splitting perception of others into good and bad parts. Following this splitting is a delusive diminishing of the bad part of the self, and the bad part of perceptions of others to preserve the self-system and to make the external environment a non-threatening one.

Laing's (1960) affirmed that because of unavoidable engulfment, implosion, and depersonalization, individuals with schizophrenia undergo a process of self-fragmentation. The self-system splits into the unembodied self and the inner self. Later, as the sense of ontological insecurity prevails, the inner self further splits into the true self and the false self. Finally, the true self can further split into an inner true self and an outer false self. Apart from this primary and secondary splitting, there is also the molar and molecular splitting. Molar splitting is a splitting of personality, self-identity and structure. Molecular splitting is a confusion of behaviors, attitudes, cognition, and emotions in each split part.

Arieti (1974) affirmed that for people with schizophrenia, in their pathological developmental process, their perception of the whole is gradually affected and weakened. As the environmental process is highly oppressive, the individual tries to detach their attention from the whole (abusive and oppressive others) to those parts that feel better and more secure. As the psychotic symptoms become more and more severe, the individual is more and more detached from the actual reality. His/her perception of the whole deteriorates more and more and his/her perception and attention on the delusive parts become stronger and stronger. In the very chronic state, the individual is inert, passive, and withdrawn and highly institutionalized. His/her perceptions on the environment may become inert and fixated. His/her perceptions on details of parts may decrease accordingly as his/her psychic energy in concentration and attention on parts deteriorates accordingly.

Burnham (et al., 1969) provided another important aspect in describing the fragmentation process in schizophrenia. Burnham (et al., 1969) affirmed that the individual cannot separate himself from the oppressive others. Instead, s/he needs the oppressive others to construct his own self-system. In that sense, he internalizes the negative comments from the oppressive other/s that is highly painful and intolerable. In other words, s/he enters into a need and fear dilemma. It is the need and fear dilemma that speeds up the process of psychotic self-fragmentation. The individual only has a fragile internal structure and lacks power to differentiate oneself from others in feeling, thinking, decision and perception. S/he harbors a strong need to depend on external objects as well as a prevailing fear of separation of external objects. The individual is sensitive, vulnerable, and breakable to others' domination, enslavement, or engulfment. His/her self-boundary and structure can be easily fractured and dissolved by all these external domination, enslavement, and engulfment.

The process of self-splitting from projective identification to fragmentation, described by Bion (1984), can be summarized into five stages. In the first stage, the individual faces an oppressive external environment as well as a weak personality. Bion (1984) tends to focus on the weak personality. In the second stage, the oppressive environment tends to intensify the weak personality of the individual. In stage three, the individual frequently involves projective identification. S/he tends to expel the bad part of the ego outside and merges with the external object. In stage four, the individual enters into a state of psychotic projective identification. The prevailing oppressive environment makes the individual unable to transform his paranoid schizoid position back to the depressive position. Instead, more and more expelled ego particles merge with related external objects. Finally, both the individual's ego and the external object are also split. That means, the individual's psychotic self-fragmentation goes on. Together with these are three unresolved dilemmas in the process of self-fragmentation. The first is the dilemma of dissociation and re-association. The second dilemma is the manifestation and disguise or visibility and concealment. The third one is the dilemmas of approach and avoidance.

Based on all these theoretical underpinnings, the writer attempts to construct three dynamic forces within the self-fragmentation and self-integration. They are the self-splitting versus self-cohesion force, self-concealment versus self-visibility force, as well as the self-destruction versus self-preservation forces. Various stages of these three dynamic forces are fully described. In fact, self-cohesion, self-visibility, and self-preservation forces are originated from one's inherent life instincts. Self-splitting, self-concealment and self-destruction come from one's death instincts. In psychotic fragmentation, individual's life instincts are being suppressed and deprived within a highly oppressive environment. Instead, the life instincts can only manifest within a delusive reality. As an opposite, one's death instincts prevail in which the individual tries to destruct, to split and to conceal himself/herself to destruct, conceal, and split the oppressive others. Based on these, mental health recovery should be initiated by sparking one's life instincts within a supportive and caring reality. Following this should be a full ventilation of one's negative emotions within one' death instincts. Then a full recovery should be founded with a full elaboration of the structure, energy, and connection of supportive others within actual reality. A multi-dimensional recovery can thus be gradually attained in various aspects of life by means of different types of intervention in various levels.

References

Arieti, S. (1974). Interpretation of Schizophrenia (2nd edition): *Completely Revised and Expanded,* London: Crosby Lockwood Staples.

Bemporad, J. R. (1967). Perceptual disorder in schizophrenia, *American Journal of Psychiatry,* 123:971-975.

Bion, W. R. (1984). Second Thought: Selected Paper on Psycho-Analysis, New York: Jason Aronson.

Burnham, D. L., Gladstone, A. I. & Gibson, R. W. (1969) *Schizophrenia and the Need-Fear Dilemma,* New York: International University Press.

Federn, P (1953). Ego Psychology and the Psychoses, London: Imago Publishing Company.

Freud, S. (1920/1961). *Beyond the Pleasure Principle (The Standard Edition). Trans. J. Strachey.* New York: Liveright Publishing Corporation.

Freud, A. (1967). *The Ego and the Mechanisms of Defense,* New York: International Universities Press.

Frosch, J. (1983). The Psychotic Process, New York: International University Press.

Klein, M. (1935). A Contribution to the psychogenesis of manic-depressive states', *International Journal of Psychoanalysis,* XVI: 145-174.

Kohut, H. (1985). *The Analysis of Self: A Systematic Approach to the Psychoanalysis Treatment of Narcissistic Personality Disorder,* New York: International University Press.

Laing R. D. (1960). *The Divided Self,* London: Tavistock Publication.

McWilliams, N. (1994). *Psychoanalytic Diagnosis: Understanding Personality Structure in the Clinical Process,* New York: Guildford Press.

Segal, H. (1973). *Introduction to the Work of Melanie Klein.* Hogarth; reprinted Karnac, 1988.

United States Department of Health and Health Sciences (2004). *National Consensus Statement on Mental Health Recovery,* Washington, DC: United States Department of Health and Health Sciences.

Index

A

B

D

E

I

J

K

L

M

N

O

P

Q

R

S

T

U

V

W

Y